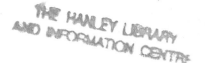
CRACKING THE
MRCS Viva

CRACKING THE
MRCS Viva
A revision guide

Iain Au-Yong MA (Cantab) BMBCh(Oxon) MRCS(Ed)
Specialist Registrar, Department of Radiology, Queens Medical Centre and
Nottingham City Hospital, Nottingham, UK

Simon Howarth MA (Cantab) BMBCh MRCS(Eng) MRCS(Glas)
Honorary Specialist Registrar, Department of Neurosurgery, Cambridge University
Hospitals NHS Foundation Trust and Clinical Research Associate in Neuroimaging,
Department of Radiology, Cambridge University, Cambridge, UK

Tjun Tang MA (Cantab) MB BChir MRCS(Glas)
Specialist Registrar in General Surgery, Eastern Deanery; currently Research
Registrar in Neuroimaging, Departments of Radiology and Vascular Surgery,
Cambridge University Hospitals NHS Foundation Trust, and Cambridge University,
Cambridge, UK

Robert Sayers MD FRCS
Reader in Surgery, Department of Surgery, Vascular Surgery Group,
Leicester Royal Infirmary, Leicester, UK

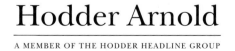

Hodder Arnold
A MEMBER OF THE HODDER HEADLINE GROUP

First published in Great Britain in 2007 by
Hodder Arnold, an imprint of Hodder Education and a member of the Hodder Headline Group,
338 Euston Road, London NW1 3BH

http://www.hoddereducation.com

Distributed in the United States of America by
Oxford University Press Inc.,
198 Madison Avenue, New York, NY10016
Oxford is a registered trademark of Oxford University Press

British Library Cataloguing in Publication Data
A catalogue record for this book is available from the British Library

Library of Congress Cataloging-in-Publication Data
A catalog record for this book is available from the Library of Congress

ISBN-10 0 340 906464
ISBN-13 978 0 340 906460

1 2 3 4 5 6 7 8 9 10

Commissioning Editor: Sarah Burrows
Project Editor: Francesca Naish
Production Controller: Joanna Walker
Cover Design: Nichola Smith
Indexer: Lawrence Errington

Typeset in 10/13, Berling Roman by Charon Tec Ltd (A Macmillan Company), Chennai, India
www.charontec.com
Printed and bound in Malta by Gutenberg Press

What do you think about this book? Or any other Hodder Arnold title?
Please visit our website: www.hoddereducation.com

To Amy, for her endless patience and support.
IAY

To my Grandfather who guided me so well and whom I will miss so much.
SPSH

To Mummy and Papa for their love and tireless support over the years.
TT

To Patty
RS

Contents

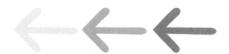

PART 4: APPLIED SURGICAL PATHOLOGY

PART 5: PRINCIPLES OF SURGERY

CONTENTS

Foreword

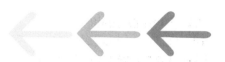

This book is aptly entitled 'Cracking the MRCS Viva'.

Most of us have been involved over the years in both taking exams and acting as examiners and understand the problems that are faced by the examinee: what to learn, what to say and most importantly what not to say. There is no book on the market that can take the MRCS viva for you, however the authors of this volume have done their best to do just that; they are all experienced at both taking exams and being examiners and are therefore well qualified to set out the potential pitfalls that may exist in viva situations. The book is divided into sections, beginning with an introduction, which details useful tips on how to take a viva and sets out the ways in which the candidate would do well. For example, do not lie and never get angry seem obvious bits of advice but are terribly important. The sections that follow on applied surgical anatomy, operative surgery, applied surgical pathology, principles of surgery, applied surgical physiology and critical care are all set out in a similar fashion and are extremely useful. I have always thought that passing a viva in any examination depends upon a number of factors, which include presentation (knowing what to say and what not to say), knowledge, composure, empathy with the examiners, and some luck. This volume will educate you on how to do all of these things and do them well. If you read this book and take note of the advice given then the percentage influence of luck will be reduced considerably and the pass rate for the exam undoubtedly increased. With the increased complexity of examinations and the importance placed on the viva voce element of them, this book is a must for all potential MRCS candidates because it not only tells you how to behave in a viva but also gives you a very comprehensive list of possible viva questions related to each topic and then goes through the responses that are required in some detail.

Sir Peter Bell
Emeritus Professor of Surgery
University of Leicester
Leicester
UK

Preface

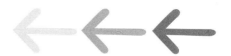

The viva section of the MRCS exam is a difficult hurdle that many surgical trainees find troublesome. There have hitherto been very few educational resources available to aid the trainee in preparing for this exam, and a lack of understanding of viva technique and what is expected of the candidate has hindered many candidates' efforts in the past.

Cracking the MRCS Viva provides a selection of common viva topics, all of which have featured in the three collegiate exams. The authors consist of a team of registrars who have all recently passed the MRCS exam at London, Edinburgh and Glasgow, as well as a senior examiner for the current intercollegiate exam.

This book incorporates a novel layout, suggesting an exhaustive list of possible questions related to each topic and a comprehensive accompanying text designed to equip the candidate with a full knowledge of each topic. This is in contrast to the style of many existing books that answer specific questions, which might not be asked in the same manner in the actual exam.

There is also a novel and thorough system of cross-referencing throughout the entire book so that all of the topics are cross-referenced to each other to enable ease of use and to enable pairs or small groups of candidates to practise real-time viva technique with each other.

The text is interspersed with boxes of example viva questions containing high-yield facts on the topic, and key learning points are highlighted throughout.

The book incorporates an exhaustive list of simple to reproduce line diagrams for the exam, as well as a list of important definitions that often constitute the opening question of the viva, and are important to get exactly right to avoid the inevitable examiners' traps. We also present a list of commonly requested equations, and a system for tackling all sorts of questions.

This book is not a comprehensive textbook, although each viva topic is considered in some detail.

The authors sincerely hope that their logical approach to viva technique helps you through what is no doubt a stressful experience, and arms you with the tools to do well.

IAY
SPSH
TT
RS

Acknowledgements

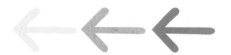

Thanks to Mr James R Seaward, MA(Cantab), MRCS(Eng), Registrar, Plastic Surgery, Royal Devon and Exeter Hospital for his major contribution to the writing of this manuscript.

We thank Sarah Burrows, Georgina Bentliff, Naomi Wilkinson and Francesca Naish of Hodder Arnold Publishing, and would also like to acknowledge our families and friends, without whose support this book would never have been published.

Abbreviations

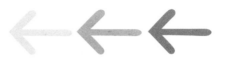

1,25-DHCC	1,25-dihydroxycholecalciferol
5FU	5-fluorouracil
5-HIAA	5-hydroxyindoleacetic acid
β-hCG	β-human chorionic gonadotrophin
A&E	accident and emergency department
AAA	abdominal aortic aneurysm
ABG	arterial blood gas
ACEI	angiotensin-converting enzyme inhibitor
ACS	abdominal compartment syndrome
ACTH	adrenocorticotrophic hormone
ADH	antidiuretic hormone
AF	atrial fibrillation
AFP	α-fetoprotein
AIDS	acquired immune deficiency syndrome
AP	abdominoperineal
APER	abdominoperineal excision of rectum
APTT	activated partial thromboplastin time
ARDS	acute respiratory disease syndrome
ARF	acute renal failure
ASA	American Society of Anesthesiologists
ASIS	anterior superior iliac spine
AST	aspartate transaminase
ATLS	advanced trauma life support
ATN	acute tubular necrosis
AV	arteriovenous
BD	twice daily
BERT	bag for the endoscopic retrieval of tissue
BMI	body mass index
BNF	*British National Formulary*
BPH	benign prostatic hyperplasia
BP	blood pressure
BXO	balanitis xerotica obliterans
CABG	coronary artery bypass grafting
CAPD	continuous ambulatory peritoneal dialysis
CC	craniocaudal
CCA	common carotid artery
CCK	cholecystokinin

CDK	cyclin-dependent kinase
CEA	carotid endarterectomy or carcinoembryonic antigen
CI	confidence interval
CIN	cervical intraepithelial neoplasia
CME	continuing medical education
CMV	cytomegalovirus
CNS	central nervous system
CO	cardiac output
COPD	chronic obstructive pulmonary disease
CPAP	continuous positive airway pressure
CPK	creatine phosphokinase
CRF	chronic renal failure
CPP	cerebral perfusion pressure
CRH	corticotrophin-releasing hormone
CRP	C-reactive protein
CSF	cerebrospinal fluid
CT	computed tomography
CVA	cerebrovascular accident
CVP	central venous pressure
CVVH	continuous venovenous haemofiltration
DCIS	ductal carcinoma *in situ*
DHS	dynamic hip screw
DIC	disseminated intravascular coagulation
DIEP	deep inferior epigastric perforator
DJ	duodenojejunal
DPG	2,3-diphosphoglycerate
DRE	digital rectal examination
DSA	digital subtraction angiography
DVT	deep vein thrombosis
ECA	external carotid artery
ECF	extracellular fluid
ECG	electrocardiogram
EGF	epidermal growth factor
ELND	elective lymph node dissection
EPSP	excitatory postsynaptic potential
ERCP	endoscopic retrograde cholangiopancreatography
ESR	erythrocyte sedimentation rate
ET	endotracheal
EUA	examination under anaesthetic
EVD	external ventricular drain
FAP	familial adenomatous polyposis coli
FBC	full blood count

FEV_1	forced expiratory volume in 1 s
FGF	fibroblast growth factor
FFP	fresh frozen plasma
FNAC	fine-needle aspiration cytology
FOB	faecal occult blood
FRC	functional residual capacity
FSH	follicle-stimulating hormone
GABA	γ-aminobutyric acid
GCS	Glasgow Coma Score
GI	gastrointestinal
GH	growth hormone
GIP	gastric inhibitory peptide
GIT	gastrointestinal tract
GMC	General Medical Council
GnRH	gonadotrophin-releasing hormone
GOJ	gastro-oesophageal junction
GORD	gastro-oesophageal reflux disease
GTN	glyceryl trinitrate
HDL	high-density lipoprotein
HDU	high dependency unit
HEPA	high efficiency particulate air
HIV	human immunodeficiency virus
HNPCC	hereditary non-polyposis colorectal carcinoma
HPV	human papillomavirus
HR	heart rate
HTLV-1	human T-cell leukaemia virus 1
IAP	intra-abdominal pressure
ICA	internal carotid artery
ICAM	intercellular adhesion molecule
ICF	intracellular fluid
ICP	intracranial pressure
IGAP	inferior gluteal artery perforator
IL	interleukin
IHD	ischaemic heart disease
IMHS	intramedullary hip screw
INR	international normalized ratio
IPPV	intermittent positive-pressure ventilation
ITU	intensive therapy unit
IV	intravenous
IVC	inferior vena cava
JVP	jugular venous pulse
LCIS	lobular carcinoma *in situ*

LDL	low-density lipoprotein
LFT	liver function test
LH	luteinizing hormone
LDH	lactate dehydrogenase
LIF	left iliac fossa
LMM	lentigo maligna melanoma
LMW	low molecular weight
LOS	lower oesophageal sphincter
LSV	long saphenous vein
LVEDV	left ventricular end-diastolic volume
MDT	multidisciplinary team
MEN	multiple endocrine neoplasia
MI	myocardial infarction
MMPs	matrix metalloproteinases
MODS	multiple organ dysfunction syndrome
MRI	magnetic resonance imaging
MRSA	methicillin-resistant *S. aureus*
MSSA	methicillin-sensitive *S. aureus*
NJT	nasojejunal tube
NGT	nasogastric tube
NHL	non-Hodgkin's lymphoma
NICE	National Institute for Health and Clinical Excellence
NIPPV	non-invasive positive-pressure ventilation
NM	nodular melanoma
NMJ	neuromuscular junction
NNT	numbers needed to treat
NPC	nasopharyngeal cancer
NPI	Nottingham prognostic index
NSAID	non-steroidal anti-inflammatory drug
OGD	oesophagogastroduodenoscopy
OPSI	overwhelming post-splenectomy infection
OPSS	overwhelming post-splenectomy sepsis
ORIF	open reduction and internal fixation
PA	pulmonary artery
PAF	platelet-activating factor
PAFC	pulmonary artery flotation catheter
PAN	polyarteritis nodosa
PAOP	pulmonary artery occlusion pressure
PAWP	pulmonary artery wedge pressure
PCA	patient-controlled analgesia
PCT	proximal convoluted tubule
P_{CO_2}	partial pressure of carbon dioxide

PCWB	pulmonary capillary wedge pressure
PDGF	platelet-derived growth factor
PDS	polydioxanone sulphate
PE	pulmonary embolus
PEEP	positive end-expiratory pressure
PEG	percutaneous endoscopic gastrostomy
PEJ	percutaneous endoscopic jejunostomy
PIP	peak inspiratory pressure
Po_2	partial pressure of oxygen
PP	pancreatic polypeptide
PPI	proton pump inhibitor
PR	per rectum
PSA	prostate-specific antigen
PTFE	polytetrafluoroethylene
PTH	parathyroid hormone
PVS	persistent vegetative state
RAP	right atrial pressure
RCT	randomized controlled trial
RIF	right iliac fossa
RLN	recurrent laryngeal nerve
RSD	reflex sympathetic dystrophy
SFJ	saphenofemoral junction
SGAP	superior gluteal artery perforator
SIADH	syndrome of inappropriate ADH secretion
SIMV	simultaneous intermittent mechanical ventilation
SIRS	systemic inflammatory response syndrome
SLE	systemic lupus erythematosus
SLNB	sentinel lymph node biopsy
SSM	superficial spreading melanoma
SV	stroke volume
SVR	systemic vascular resistance
T_3	triiodothyronine
T_4	thyroxine
TAP	transperitoneal
TB	tuberculosis
TCD	transcranial Doppler
TDS or t.d.s.	three times daily
TEP	total extraperitoneal
Tg	thyroglobulin
TGF-β	transforming growth factor β
TIA	transient ischaemic attack
TIPSS	transjugular intrahepatic portosystemic stent shunt

TNF	tumour necrosis factor
tPA	tissue plasminogen activator
TPN	total parenteral nutrition
TPR	total peripheral resistance
TRH	thyroid-releasing hormone
TRAM	transverse rectus abdominis myocutaneous
TRUS	transrectal ultrasonography
TSH	thyroid-stimulating hormone
TV	tidal volume
UC	ulcerative colitis
U+Es	urea and electrolytes
UICC	Union Internationale Contre Le Cancer
UTI	urinary tract infection
UV	ultraviolet
VC	vital capacity
VIP	vasoactive intestinal polypeptide
VLDL	very-low-density lipoprotein
V/Q	ventilation/perfusion
VT	ventricular tachycardia
VUJ	vesicoureteric junction
WCC	white cell count
WHO	World Health Organization
WLE	wide local excision

INTRODUCTION

1 Examination technique and useful tips

WHEN DESCRIBING A CONDITION

Consider using the following headings:

Disease:
Definition:
Incidence: Common/Uncommon/Rare
Age:
Sex: M:F
Geography:
Aetiology and risk factors:
Pathogenesis:
Pathology: Macroscopic
Microscopic
Spread: e.g. tumour: haematogenous/lymphatic/local/transcoelomic
Where commonly?
Transmission route for infections
Presentation: Symptoms
Signs
Investigations:
Treatment:
Prognosis: 5- and 10-year survival rates depending on stage of disease

---

↑ Mnemonic to remember

'In A Surgeon's Gown Even Physicians May Make Some Incredibly Tentative Progress!'

In	I	Incidence
A	A	Age
Surgeon's	S	Sex
Gown	G	Geography
Even	(A)e	Aetiology and risk factors
Physicians	P	Pathogenesis/Presentation (symptoms/signs)
May	M	Macroscopic (pathology)
Make	M	Microscopic (pathology)
Some	S	Spread
Incredibly	I	Investigations
Tentative	T	Treatment
Progress!	P	Prognosis

When working out **causes** to a condition use the **surgical sieve**.

⬆ **Mnemonic to remember**

'INVITED MD'

I	Infection
N	Neoplasia
V	Vascular
I	Inflammatory/Idiopathic
T	Traumatic
E	Endocrine
D	Degenerative
M	Metabolic
D	Drugs

Candidates are encouraged to start off by giving a **definition** if appropriate.

Example: What is Crohn's disease?

'Crohn's disease is an inflammatory bowel disease of unknown aetiology, that can affect any part of the bowel from the mouth to anus, and which is associated with a full thickness inflammation of the bowel wall.'

First impressions are **vital** in these vivas because there is a **limited amount** of time to judge the candidate and most candidates are much alike. If you start well, the examiner will pass you and you can then try to earn extra marks.

Try to **keep talking** to **minimize** the **number of questions** asked by the examiners. By getting into the habit of doing this, you can steer the viva the way that you want and try to pre-empt questions from the examiners!

Start broad and *become more specific* during your answer. Give **examples** along the way to illustrate the principle or show your breadth of knowledge.

Example 1: 'What can you tell me about the complications of gallstones?'

Answer: Many gallstones are **asymptomatic**

Complications can be divided into those:

- **Within the gallbladder**: common examples include:
  - biliary colic (chat briefly)
  - cholecystitis (ditto)
  - mucocele
  - empyema

- **Within the biliary tree**:
  - ○ obstructive jaundice
  - ○ ascending cholangitis
  - ○ pancreatitis
- **Outside the gallbladder**:
  - ○ gallstone ileus.

Rare but **interesting** complications include, for example, gallstone ileus or carcinoma of the gallbladder.

Example 2: see 'Functions of the liver', Chapter 96, page 384

Try to be a good undergraduate rather than a year 5 or 6 specialist registrar!

Pyramid principle
Stick to the **basics** first and work up! Try to be **methodical** as well as **logical** while progressing through your answer. Examples:

1. Mention **bedside** and **blood tests** *before* **CT/MRI!**
2. When asked how to make a diagnosis always say '**history, examination and investigation**'.
3. If the examiner is asking about a **surgical emergency** tell them that this is so and start with '**airway, breathing and circulation**' to show that you appreciate the gravity of the problem and that you need to intervene promptly. Often you need to mention that you would **resuscitate** the patient before surgery in the operative surgery viva before detailing surgery.
4. When talking about **tumours** say *benign, malignant, primary and secondary*.
5. Try to **avoid** the '**medical student syndrome**' and mentioning **rare causes** before the more common ones. This greatly irritates the examiner! Try to put important causes, such as cancers, high on the list too.
6. When talking about **complications**, discuss under the headings of **immediate, early and late**' and/or '**general versus specific**'.
7. With regards to **operative surgery** try using the headings '**preoperative, intraoperative and postoperative factors**'.
8. In the **operative surgery** section don't forget **preoperative preparation** and **consent**.

If you get stuck try to use the **mnemonic** mentioned on page 3 if asked about a particular condition or tumour, or the **surgical sieve** if you get stuck for causes of a condition. For the **surgical sieve**, use the mnemonic '**INVITED MD**' (infective, neoplastic, vascular, inflammatory, etc.). The **surgical sieve** is for looking for **causes** of something and the **surgeon's gown** is for describing a **condition**.

If you truly don't know the answer, say so! What may happen is that the examiner may suggest a line of reasoning to help you deduce the answer. If it is something very common and obvious, say 'of course!' and everyone will know that you have just forgotten in the stress of the exam. If it is something obscure, with any luck the examiner will spend the next 2 minutes telling you about it!

Do not lie to the examiners! If they find out they will most probably fail you for **poor integrity** or passing you off as **unsafe** and **not knowing your limitations**! Try to avoid waffling because this does not go down well and gives the impression that you do not know the answer and have not listened carefully to the question!

Several of the authors have said in their vivas: 'Sir, I do not know the answer to your question but using first principles I would deduce this … from this. etc.'

Never get angry or disagree with the examiner even if you know that you are right!

Look mainly at the examiner who is asking you the question but keep a regular eye on the *other* examiner who may give you surprising **non-verbal help** or **encouragement**.

Don't forget to have a **sense of humour** – remember that your pair of examiners will be completely bored, having examined numerous candidates before you.

Remember the '**KISS**' principle – *'Keep It Simple Stupid!'*

And **avoid** the '**KICK**' principle – *'Keep It Complicated and Knotty!'*

2 Diagrams and equations that you should be able to draw and write quickly for the examination

TIPS

- These will be mainly for **physiology** and **critical care vivas**.
- Do not start drawing a graph if you are unable to label the **axes** and unable to express the units that they are in. A graph without axes and units is meaningless!
- Bring a **blank piece of paper** and **pen** with you into the exam. It looks impressive if you can bring it out and start drawing to explain an answer! Shows thought and organization!

DIAGRAMS

Physiology and critical care

Nerves and muscles
- Schematic diagram of a myelinated axon
- Action potential (cardiac and peripheral nervous)
- Sarcomere
- Neuromuscular junction.

Cardiovascular system
- Frank–Starling curve of the heart
- Cardiac cycle:
  - jugular venous pulse (JVP): describe the 'c' wave, 'a' wave, 'v' wave, 'x descent'
  - arterial pressure waveform
  - heart sounds
- Swan–Ganz catheter wedge trace
- Draw the compartments of the heart and what the pressures are within the jugular vein, right atrium, right ventricle, pulmonary artery, left atrium, left ventricle and aorta at rest
- Oxygen-dissociation curve: causes for a right and left shift; Bohr shift
- Myoglobin curve
- Fetal haemoglobin curve
- Cardiac action potential: explain on your diagram where the different ions efflux and influx

- Starling's law of flux: oedema
  - need to know the oncotic, osmotic, capillary and hydrostatic pressures
  - the pressure differences between the arterial and venous ends of a capillary

Respiratory system
- Static spirometry trace: label vital capacity (VC), tidal volume (TV), functional residual capacity (FRC)
- Flow–volume loops for restrictive and obstructive airway disease:
  - compliance curve in a stiff lung
  - pressure–compliance curve in a mechanically ventilated patient
- $\dot{V}A/\dot{Q}$ profile in a standing patient
- Dead space versus a shunt
- PO_2 – chemoreceptor firing
  - graph showing $\dot{V}A$ versus PO_2 (mmHg or kPa)
  - graph showing $\dot{V}A$ versus PCO_2 (mmHg or kPa).

Kidney
- Nephron (from glomerulus to collecting duct):
  - what is absorbed where
  - permeability of the different parts
- Concentration of sodium within the loop of Henle
- Describe the thin and thick portions of the loop of Henle
- The countercurrent exchange mechanism
- Functions of the glomerulus and Bowman's capsule:
  - proximal convoluted tubule or PCT
  - distal convoluted tubule
  - collecting duct
- Volumes of the various body fluid compartments.

Endocrinology
- Feedback loops: calcium metabolism flowchart.

Pathology and principles of surgery

- Audit and the feedback loop
- Cell cycle
- Anal fistulae.

Anatomy and operative surgery

- Surgical incisions
- Schematics of the different colonic resections along with blood supply
- Whipple's procedure: the different anastomoses.

EQUATIONS

- Cardiac output:

$$CO = SV \times HR$$
$$BP = SV \times TPR$$

- Fick's principle (for measurement of cardiac output)
- Blood flow
- Vascular resistance (Poiseuille–Hagen formula)
- Wall tension (Laplace's law)
- Parkland's formula or at least one formula for fluid replacement in burns
- Creatinine clearance (Cockcroft–Gault) equation
- Henderson–Hasselbalch equation
- Oxygen delivery and consumption equation.

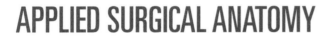

APPLIED SURGICAL ANATOMY

3 Abdominal aorta

Possible viva questions related to this topic

→ What are the branches of the abdominal aorta?
→ In what order do they come off?
→ At what level does the aorta bifurcate?

Related topics		
Topic	**Chapter**	**Pages**
Kidney	9	26
Aneurysms	46	165

LANDMARKS AND RELATIONS

The abdominal aorta **starts** at level **T12** as it traverses the diaphragm. It passes downwards in the **midline** in the retroperitoneum.

• Anterior relations: left renal vein, pancreas, lesser sac
• Posterior relations: anterior longitudinal ligament and vertebral bodies
• Right: cisterna chyli, thoracic duct, azygos vein
• Left: duodenojejunal (DJ) flexure.

It **ends** at **L4**, where it **bifurcates** into the **common iliac arteries**.

BRANCHES

PAIRED BRANCHES (CRANIAL → CAUDAL)	LEVEL	SUPPLYING
Inferior phrenic artery (inferior)	T12	Adrenal gland and diaphragm
Adrenal artery	T12	Adrenal gland
Renal artery	L2	Kidneys, adrenal glands, ureter
Gonadal artery	L2–3	Gonads, ureters
Lumbar arteries (four pairs)		Segmental supply of lumbar musculature
Iliac arteries (terminal branches)	L4	Legs, pelvic viscera
Coeliac trunk	T12	Foregut (oesophagus to second part of the duodenum) plus liver, spleen and pancreas
Superior mesenteric artery	L1	Midgut (duodenum to two-thirds along transverse colon)
Inferior mesenteric artery	L3	Hindgut (transverse colon to rectum)
Median sacral artery	L4	Sacrum

4 Anal canal

Possible viva questions related to this topic

→ What is the anatomy of the anal canal?
→ What is the embryology of the anal canal?
→ What are the differences between the anal canal above and the anal canal below the dentate line?
→ How is faecal continence maintained?
→ What is the sequence of events in defecation?

Related topics

Topic	Chapter	Page
Anorectal surgery 3: injection sclerotherapy and haemorrhoidectomy	25	73

EMBRYOLOGY

The gut starts off as an endoderm tube. The ectoderm invaginates and meets the endoderm to form the anal canal. Hence, the **distal half** of the anal canal is **ectoderm** (proctodeum) derived and the **proximal half** is **endoderm** derived. This is important in understanding the differences in characteristics of the two parts.

RELATIONS

- Posteriorly: anococcygeal body and coccyx
- Laterally: ischiorectal fossa
- Anterior: perineal body (both), penis (male), vagina (female).

STRUCTURE

The structure differs above and below the **dentate line**, which forms the embryological dividing line between ectoderm and endoderm.

This is a common MRCS question.

ABOVE	BELOW
Lined by **columnar epithelium**	Lined by **squamous epithelium**
Autonomic sensory **nerve supply**. Hence injections above the line are not painful and this is the target in haemorrhoidectomy	Somatically innervated inferior rectal nerve
Sensitive to **stretch**	Sensitive to **pain/touch/temperature**
Hindgut arterial supply – **superior rectal artery** from **inferior mesenteric artery**	Arterial supply is **inferior rectal artery** from **internal pudendal artery**
Venous drainage into inferior mesenteric vein (portal)[a]	Venous drainage into internal pudendal vein (systemic)
Lymphatic drainage follows the arterial supply (**superior rectal** and **inferior mesenteric** nodes)	Lymphatic drainage into **internal pudendal** and **internal iliac nodes**
Anal columns are present	No anal columns

[a]Note that this is a site of a **portosystemic anastomosis** (see Portal vein and portosystemic anastomoses, Chapter 14). In portal hypertension varicosities can form here, resulting in rectal varices.

SPHINCTERS

The **external sphincter** is under voluntary control. It is divided into **three parts**: subcutaneous, superficial and deep.

The **puborectalis** sling around the anal canal/lower rectum blends with this. This sling causes the distal rectum to join the rectum at an acute angle. This mechanism also helps to maintain continence.

The **internal sphincter** is under autonomic control. It forms an external muscle coat at the upper end of the anal canal.

DEFECATION

Faeces arrive at the rectum from emptying of the distal large bowel, giving rise to the urge to defecate. The intra-abdominal pressure rises with increase in diaphragmatic and abdominal muscle pressures. Anal sphincters now voluntarily relax and the faeces are evacuated.

5 Biliary tree and gallbladder

Possible viva questions related to this topic

→ What is the anatomy of the biliary tree?
→ What is a portal triad?
→ What is the anatomy of the porta hepatis?
→ What is Calot's triangle?
→ What is Pringle's manoeuvre?

Related topics		
Topic	**Chapter**	**Page**
Portal vein and portosystemic anastomoses	14	39
Liver	10	28
Laparoscopic cholecystectomy and laparoscopy	34	112

DUCTS WITHIN THE SYSTEM

The biliary system is divided into intrahepatic and extrahepatic systems.

The biliary tree starts as bile canaliculi, which divide into bile ductules and small interlobular tributaries of the bile ducts. These join each other to form larger ducts.

The right hepatic duct drains the right lobe of the liver and the left hepatic duct drains the left lobe. These two ducts leave the liver at the porta hepatis to become extrahepatic. They amalgamate to form the common hepatic duct. Distal to this it accepts the **cystic duct**, and at this point it is called the **common bile duct**.

The common bile duct travels with the hepatic artery to its left and the portal vein behind it in the **free edge of the lesser omentum** at the porta hepatis. At its most distal aspect it accepts the **pancreatic duct**. The common bile duct terminates at the **sphincter of Oddi/ampulla of Vater**. This structure is identified as a papilla in the second part of the duodenum and is cannulated at endoscopic retrograde cholangiopancreatography (ERCP).

The sphincter of Oddi opens into the **medial aspect** of the **second part** of the **duodenum**.

RELATIONS OF THE COMMON BILE DUCT

• It is **8 cm** in length.

- It has a **6 mm** upper limit of normal diameter, but gets 1mm larger every 10 years after the age of 60. It is also larger post-cholecystectomy.
- It travels in the free edge of the lesser omentum, in the porta hepatis, with and to the right of the **common hepatic artery**; both of these structures are in front of the **portal vein** (Fig. 5.1).

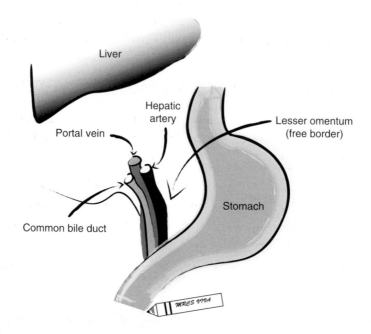

Figure 5.1

↑ **Example viva question**

What is Pringle's manoeuvre?

Pringle's manoeuvre involves placing a clamp over the **free edge of the lesser omentum** and occluding the vessels described above.

It is a useful, **temporary** measure for **controlling heavy bleeding** from the liver, e.g. in trauma, by occluding the liver's blood supply, because it can be done quickly.

The common bile duct is divided into **three parts**:

1. First part: anterior to the opening of the **lesser sac.**
2. Second part: posterior to the **first part of the duodenum.**
3. Third part: **posterior surface** of the **head of the pancreas.**

↑ **Example viva question**

What is Calot's triangle?

It is a triangle formed by the **liver, common hepatic duct** and **cystic duct**.

The **cystic artery** runs within it. It is important in identification of this structure at dissection in a laparoscopic cholecystectomy (see 'Laparoscopic cholecystectomy and laparoscopy', Chapter 34, page 112).

HISTOLOGICAL LAYOUT OF BILIARY SYSTEM

The liver is divided into functional units, or **lobules**. At the **periphery** of each of these are triads of tubes – **bile ductule**, terminal **hepatic artery branch** and terminal **portal vein tributary**. These are the **portal triads**.

Each lobule has a central terminal hepatic **venule**.

Blood flows from the portal triad (portal vein and hepatic artery) and in the **sinusoids** to the **central venule** (from the periphery of the lobule to the centre). These venules then transport blood to the **hepatic vein**.

Bile flows through the canaliculi in the opposite direction to the portal triads peripherally.

GALLBLADDER

- Pear-shaped viscus
- Lined with **columnar epithelium**
- Contains some smooth muscle in the wall
- Can hold 50 mL bile
- Consists of **fundus, body** and **neck**
- Lies in the gallbladder fossa attached to ventral surface of the right lobe of the liver
- Neck is continuous with the cystic duct. There can be a small diverticulum at this point, called **Hartmann's pouch**. Stones can impact here.

Arterial supply

Cystic artery.

Venous drainage

Via small veins into the substance of the liver.

Lymphatic drainage

To cystic node in Calot's triangle (see box above).

6 Blood supply to the heart

Possible viva questions related to this topic

→ What is the arterial supply to the heart?
→ What is the origin of the coronary arteries?

Related topics		
Topic	Chapter	Page
Blood pressure control	87	358
Starling's law of the heart and cardiovascular equations	102	403

RIGHT CORONARY ARTERY

This arises from the **right (anterior) aortic sinus** and runs between the pulmonary trunk and the right auricle.

It gives off a **marginal branch** at the junction of the posterior interventricular groove and atrioventricular sulcus, and continues as the **posterior interventricular** artery.

The posterior interventricular artery continues in the **interventricular groove** and anastomoses with the anterior interventricular artery. The **marginal branch** descends over the front of the ventricle.

It supplies the right ventricle, sinoatrial node (60 per cent) and atrioventricular node, and part of the left ventricle.

LEFT CORONARY ARTERY

This arises from the left (posterior) aortic sinus, and divides into the **circumflex** and **anterior interventricular (left anterior descending)** artery on reaching the atrioventricular groove.

The **circumflex** travels in the **atrioventricular sulcus** to anastomose with the right coronary artery.

The **anterior interventricular (left anterior descending)** travels in the interventricular groove to anastomose with the posterior interventricular artery.

The left coronary is larger than the right and supplies the left ventricle. The anastomoses are poor and in acute occlusion these arteries are functional end-arteries.

VENOUS DRAINAGE

All veins except for the anterior cardiac veins drain into the **coronary sinus**, which opens into the posterior wall of the right atrium. The main tributaries are the **great, middle** and **small cardiac veins**.

The **great cardiac vein** travels with the **anterior interventricular artery** and drains into the left (proximal aspect of) **coronary sinus**.

The **middle cardiac vein** travels with the **posterior interventricular artery** and also drains into the **coronary sinus**.

The **small cardiac vein** also drains into the coronary sinus proximally. The **right marginal vein** travels along the inferior surface of the heart and drains into the **small cardiac vein**.

The **anterior cardiac veins** run across the surface of the right ventricle and drain directly into the right atrium.

7 The diaphragm

Possible viva questions related to this topic

→ What openings of the diaphragm do you know? What goes through these openings?

→ What are the origins and insertions of the diaphragm? What are its functions?

→ What is the innervation of the diaphragm?

→ How does the diaphragm develop?

Related topics

Topic	Chapter	Page
Phrenic and vagus nerves	13	36

↑ Key learning points

- Consists of **peripheral muscular** part and inserts via central tendon, which fuses with the pericardium
- Bi-domed, reaching the **fifth rib** at its highest extent
- Two **crura** – sites of origin of the diaphragm:
  - right crus originates in the **first three lumbar vertebrae**
  - left crus arises from the first **two lumbar vertebrae**
- The right crus acts as a sling around the oesophagus and prevents reflux
- Medial and lateral arcuate ligaments are lateral to the crura and contribute to the origin of the diaphragm
- Supplied by the **phrenic nerve** ('C3, 4, 5 keeps the diaphragm alive')

DEVELOPMENT

Develops from the **septum transversum, pleuroperitoneal membranes, paraxial mesoderm** of the abdominal wall and **oesophageal mesenchyme,** all of which contribute to it.

The **septum transversum,** which initially forms an embryonic partition between the thorax and abdomen between embryonic weeks 5 and 7, eventually becomes the **central tendon.**

The **crura** of the **diaphragm** are derived from **foregut mesenchyme.**

DIAPHRAGMATIC HERNIAS

These occur through persisting pleuroperitoneal communications (where the above contributions fail to fuse).

A **Morgagni hernia** occurs anteriorly, through the foramen of Morgagni, pushing into the anterior mediastinum.

A **Bochdalek hernia** herniates through the foramen of Bochdalek, posteriorly.

These can be diagnosed by computed tomography (CT).

Openings		
Level	Main structure passing through	Other structures
T8	Inferior vena cava	Right phrenic nerve
T10	Oesophagus	Vagus (rhymes)
T12	Abdominal aorta	Thoracic duct, azygos vein

↑ **Key learning points**

Some aide-memoires for the vertebral levels

Vena cava has 8 letters and oesophagus has 10; abdomen aorta has 12.

Or CEA for the order (cava, oesophagus, aorta)

The **subcostal nerve** is transmitted under the **lateral arcuate ligament**.

The **sympathetic chain** passes behind the **medial arcuate ligament**.

The **left phrenic nerve** pierces the muscular portion of the diaphragm.

The **greater, lesser** and **least splanchnic nerves** pierce the crura of the diaphragm.

FUNCTIONS

- Main muscle of **respiration**
- Aids **venous return** to the heart (intermittent increased intra-abdominal pressure on respiration)
- **Straining** – defecation and micturition
- **Support** to the **vertebral column**.

8 The femoral triangle

Possible viva questions related to this topic

→ What are the boundaries of the femoral triangle?
→ What are the contents of the femoral triangle and their relations?
→ What are the contents of the femoral canal and what are its borders?
→ What are/draw me the borders of the femoral triangle(?)
→ Why is it important to know the relations of the femoral canal?

Related topics		
Topic	**Chapter**	**Page**
Femoral hernia repair	32	102
Femoral and brachial embolectomy	31	98
Long saphenous varicose vein surgery	35	117

BOUNDARIES

- Superiorly: inguinal ligament
- Medially: medial border of adductor longus
- Laterally: medial border of sartorius
- Roof: fascia lata
- Floor (medial to lateral): adductor longus, adductor brevis, pectineus, iliopsoas.

CONTENTS

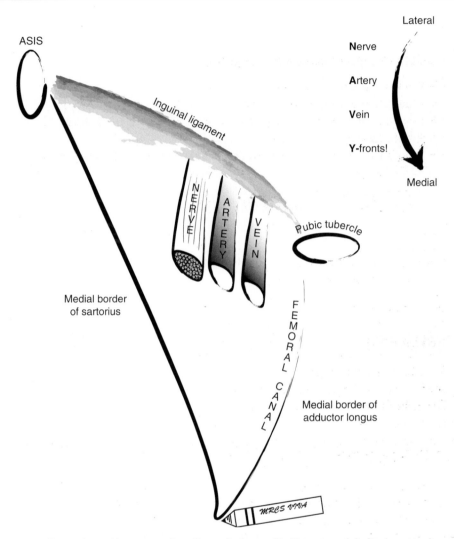

Figure 8.1   Femoral canal is a space that **allows the femoral vein to expand during increased venous return**, and contains **only fat and a lymph node** (Cloquet's) draining the clitoris/penis. (see Femoral hernia repair; Chapter 32, page 102) **Anatomy mnemonic**: NAVY (lateral to medial: **n**erve, **a**rtery, **v**ein, '**Y** fronts').

NOTE that the **nerve** is **not included** within the femoral sheath. The canal, vein and artery are, however. (The femoral branch of the genitofemoral nerve runs in the sheath and pierces it anteriorly to supply skin overlaying the triangle.)

9 Kidney

OVERVIEW OF STRUCTURE

- Retroperitoneal organs, **right lower than left** on account of the liver; 12 × 6 × 3 cm. The left **hilum** lies just above the **transpyloric plane (L1)** which passes though the **superior pole of the right kidney**.
- Enclosed in fibrous capsule and embedded in renal fat, which is itself bounded by **Gerota's fascia**. This is attached to the renal pelvis but there is an **inferior opening**, through which pus can track in renal disease.
- Divided into outer **cortex** and inner **medulla**. Cortex contains nephrons and the medullary tissue contains collecting ducts and loops of Henle.
- **Cortical pyramids** lead into the **papillae,** which lead to **calyces** that drain into the **renal pelvis**; this, in turn, leads to the **ureter.** Pyramids are separated by **columns of Bertin.**
- **Hilum** of the kidney medially transmits **vein, artery (× 2), ureter, artery (VAUA)** – this is the order from anterior to posterior.

RELATIONS

- Posteriorly: diaphragm, quadratus lumborum muscle, psoas (medially); subcostal, iliohypogastric and ilioinguinal nerves, eleventh and twelfth ribs
- Anteriorly: liver, second part of duodenum and hepatic flexure (right), spleen, stomach, pancreas and splenic flexure (left).
- Superiorly: suprarenal glands, pleural reflection (also posterior to upper poles).

BLOOD SUPPLY AND LYMPHATIC DRAINAGE

Renal arteries bilaterally, branches of aorta, renal veins drain into the inferior vena cava (IVC).

↑ **Example viva question**

What is the clinical significance of a left varicocele?

The **left testicular vein** drains into the **left renal vein** (the right directly into the IVC). A renal cell carcinoma can invade the renal vein and this will lead to obstruction of the gonadal vein. The first presenting sign of this may be a varicocele (these tumours may be silent) and these patients should undergo renal ultrasonography.

Lymphatics follow the renal arteries to **para-aortic** lymph nodes.

NERVE SUPPLY

Autonomics from the renal sympathetic plexus are distributed via the renal vessels. They mediate **pain** and **vasomotor tone**.

DEVELOPMENT AND ANOMALIES

The definitive kidney, or metanephros, is induced by the primitive ureteric bud (from the mesonephric duct) to form from the sacral **intermediate mesoderm**. This happens at day 32.

The ureteric bud itself is induced to branch by the metanephros. These branches become the calyces.

The metanephros ascends from the sacral area to the lumbar region. Failure to ascend results in a **pelvic kidney**. The kidneys may fuse during ascent and get 'caught' under the inferior mesenteric artery and this leads to a **horseshoe kidney**.

10 Liver

Possible viva questions related to this topic

→ What is the anatomy of the liver?
→ What do you know about liver segments?
→ How is the liver divided functionally and anatomically? Why does this division differ?
→ Describe the development of the liver.
→ What surface markings are useful in preparing for a liver biopsy?

Related topics		
Topic	Chapter	Page
Portal vein and portosystemic anastomoses	14	39
Biliary tree and gallbladder	5	17
Systemic response to surgery	123	514

DEVELOPMENT OF THE LIVER

The liver develops embryologically as a ventral **endoderm** bud off the gut tube.

The gut tube has a **dorsal** and a **ventral** mesentery, which attach to the posterior and anterior abdominal walls, respectively.

The liver forms within the **ventral mesentery**. The attachment of the ventral mesentery to the anterior abdominal wall becomes the **falciform ligament** and the **lesser omentum** attaches the liver to the gut tube (stomach). The free edge of the lesser omentum is the point up to which the ventral mesentery involutes embryologically.

As the liver forms within the **ventral mesentery**, in adulthood, it is almost completely covered in peritoneum, with the exception of the **bare area** of the liver.

BLOOD SUPPLY

See also 'Portal vein and portosystemic anastomoses', Chapter 14, page 39.

The liver has a **dual** blood supply:

1. **Portal system**, which carries 70% of the blood to the liver. This carries the products of digestion from the gut to the liver for metabolism.

↑ **Key learning points**

- The liver is the largest gland in the body
- It lies in the right upper quadrant of the abdomen
- It is divided into **two lobes**, right and left at the level of the falciform ligament. The **caudate** and **quadrate** lobes are included on the **left** side
- This is an anatomical division. The **functional** divide between left and right is different and follows the **blood supply**. The dividing line between the right and left lobes of liver functionally corresponds to a line drawn down the middle of the gallbladder bed, which corresponds to the divide between **right** and **left hepatic artery/portal vein territories**
- The liver is divided further (by clinicians and radiologists) into eight segments. The caudate lobe is segment 1 and 2, 3 and 4 are in the left lobe (anatomical), and 5, 6, 7 and 8 in the right lobe
- The **portal vein** and **hepatic veins** are used for division
- The **gallbladder** is attached to the undersurface of the right lobe of the liver
- Bile produced by liver hepatocytes drains into the biliary system

See 'Biliary tree and gallbladder', Chapter 5, page 17 for description of histological arrangement of lobules and biliary anatomy.

---

2. **Hepatic artery**, which carries 30% and brings oxygenated blood to the liver.

Drainage is via the hepatic veins, which drain into the IVC.

Note that embryologically, venous blood bypasses the liver via the **ductus venosus**.

RELATIONS OF THE LIVER

- Superior: diaphragm
- Inferior: duodenum, stomach, gallbladder, hepatic flexure
- Posterior: right kidney and adrenal, retroperitoneum, oesophagus, aorta, IVC.

Surface markings

Upper border level is with the sixth rib in the midclavicular line. At the upper border of the liver, the percussion note changes from dull to resonant.

The normal liver span is less than 12.5 cm.

Mesenteric attachments and ligaments of the liver

- Falciform ligament: two-layered fold of peritoneum from umbilicus to superior surface of liver, longitudinally.

- Coronary ligament: superiorly, the falciform ligament splits into its two layers; the **right** becomes the **coronary ligament**.
- Left/right triangular: formed from the **left** layer of falciform ligament.
- Ligament: most extreme part of the coronary ligament is the right triangular ligament.
- Lesser omentum: attached to **lesser curve of the stomach** and **porta hepatis** and represents the ventral mesentery. Carries the portal vein, hepatic artery and bile duct in its free edge.
- Ligamentum teres: obliterated **umbilical vein**. Joins left branch of portal vein in porta hepatis (see 'Portal vein and portosystemic anastomoses', Chapter 14, page 39).
- Ligamentum venosum: obliterated **ductus venosus**. Joins left branch of portal vein to be attached to the superior vena cava.

LYMPHATICS

Liver produces one-third of body lymph.

The lymphatics pass through the **porta hepatis** nodes and thence to the **coeliac nodes**.

NERVE SUPPLY

Coeliac plexus (sympathetic and parasympathetic).

FUNCTIONS

See 'Functions of the liver', Chapter 96, page 384.

11 Median nerve

Possible viva questions related to this topic

→ What is the course of the median nerve?
→ What does the median nerve supply in the hand?
→ How would you test the function of this nerve clinically?
→ What are the consequences of dividing the median nerve at the level of the carpal tunnel? Any differences in doing so in the arm?

COURSE

- Originates from C5, C6, C7, C8, T1 nerve roots
- Formed from the medial and lateral cords of the brachial plexus in the axilla
- Crosses in front of the brachial artery in the upper arm, having started medial to it
- Enters the antecubital fossa and passes over coracobrachialis and brachialis.

> ↑ **Key learning point**
>
> The **median nerve** is **medial** to the brachial artery in the cubital fossa.

- Leaves the antecubital fossa by passing between two heads of **pronator teres.**
- Travels in the forearm between **flexor digitorum superficialis** and **profundus.**
- Gives off **anterior interosseus** nerve in the forearm. This runs in the forearm on the interosseus membrane.
- Gives off **palmar cutaneous branch** just proximal to the wrist. This branch enters the hand superficial to the flexor retinaculum.
- Enters the carpal tunnel where it divides into terminal branches, which supply the hand.

MOTOR SUPPLY

- **Flexors of the forearm**: pronator teres, flexor carpi radialis, palmaris longus, flexor digitorum superficialis.
- **Anterior interosseus nerve** supplies flexor pollicis longus and half of flexor digitorum profundus (the other half supplied by ulnar nerve).

Intrinsic hand muscles

> ↑ **Example viva question**
>
> *What is the nerve supply of the intrinsic muscles of the hand?*
>
> Mnemonic: the ulnar nerve supplies all except '**LOAF**'
>
> Lumbricals (lateral two)
> Opponens pollicis
> Abductor pollicis brevis
> Flexor pollicis brevis

Sensory supply

The nerve supplies the **lateral three and a half fingers** and **lateral two-thirds** of the **palm of the hand**.

The **palmar cutaneous branch** supplies the lateral palmar skin. It is spared by division of the median nerve at the carpal tunnel.

If the median nerve is divided in the upper arm, this is not spared and the whole median nerve territory becomes insensate.

CLINICAL TESTS

> ↑ **Example viva question**
>
> ***What are the differences between dividing the median nerve at the elbow and wrist?***
>
> *Wrist*
> Cuts at the **wrist** or **carpal tunnel syndrome** are the most common lesions to cause loss of nerve function at the wrist. This produces loss of motor function of the small muscles of the hand as described above and sensory loss.
>
> ### Signs of loss at the wrist
> **Sensory loss** at lateral two-thirds of the hand and lateral three and a half fingers (see notes above about superficial palmar branch).
>
> **Abductor pollicis brevis** is the only muscle that will test pure median nerve function (point patient's thumb to ceiling with palm upwards and test resisted abduction of the thumb – try to push the thumb down and lateral from its base)
>
> Look for thenar wasting in the hand (long-standing injury).
>
> ### Signs specific to carpal tunnel syndrome
> ***Tinel's test***: tap the carpal tunnel and the patient will experience an electric shock sensation in the sensory distribution of the nerve.
>
> ***Phalen's test***: forced flexion of the wrist produces the same symptoms. The time to reproduce the symptoms is proportional to the severity of compression, although **nerve conduction studies** are an adjunct to clinical examination.
>
> *Elbow*
> The **long flexors** (medial half of flexor digitorum profundus, flexor pollicis longus) are lost in addition to the **pronators** (pronator teres) in lesions at the elbow. Lesions may be produced by **sharp trauma** or occasionally **supracondylar fractures of the humerus.**
>
> ### Additional clinical signs of loss at the elbow
> All of the above PLUS:
>
> Hand held **supinated**, loss of pronation.
>
> **Loss of flexion** of **distal phalanx of thumb (flexor pollicis longus).**
>
> Ask the patient to make a fist and the index and middle fingers will remain straight (loss of **flexor digitorum profundus**).
>
> In prolonged lesions loss of muscle bulk in the flexor compartment of the forearm.

12 Pancreas

Possible viva questions related to this topic

→ Tell me about the anatomy of the pancreas?
→ What are the relations of the pancreas?
→ What are the blood supply and lymphatic drainage of the pancreas?
→ Tell me about the development of the pancreas and any abnormalities
   that may arise as a result of developmental errors?
→ What is the accessory duct of Santorini and how is it derived?

OVERVIEW OF STRUCTURE

- **Exocrine** and **endocrine** gland
- **Retroperitoneal** organ, crosses **transpyloric** plane (Chapter 19, page 51)
- Divided into **head**, **body** and **tail**
- Head lies within concavity of duodenum and **pancreatic duct** drains into **second part**
- Tail lies in the **lienorenal ligament** and contacts the **hilum of the spleen**. It can be damaged in a splenectomy, leading to fistula formation.

RELATIONS

- Posteriorly (right to left): common bile duct, portal vein, splenic vein, IVC, aorta, superior mesenteric artery origin, left psoas muscle, left kidney and adrenal, hilum of spleen.
- Anteriorly: transverse colon, transverse mesocolon, lesser sac, stomach.

BLOOD SUPPLY AND LYMPHATIC DRAINAGE

- **Splenic** artery and **superior** and **inferior pancreaticoduodenal arteries**

- Corresponding veins drain into portal system
- Lymphatics follow the arteries to coeliac and superior mesenteric nodes.

NERVE SUPPLY

Sympathetic and branches of the vagus.

DEVELOPMENT AND ANOMALIES

The pancreas forms by the fusion of dorsal and ventral pancreatic buds. Both arise from the gut tube on day 26 at the level of the duodenum.

The ventral pancreatic bud migrates posteriorly around the duodenum and fuses with the dorsal bud; it becomes the **uncinate process**.

Occasionally, there are two ventral buds and if these migrate in opposite directions (anteriorly and posteriorly), this results in an **annular pancreas**.

The duct systems of the two buds becoming interconnected when the buds fuse. The ventral pancreatic duct usually becomes the main pancreatic duct and the dorsal duct involutes. If the dorsal duct persists, it is called the **accessory duct of Santorini** and it empties into the duodenum at a duodenal papilla.

13 Phrenic and vagus nerves

Related topics		
Topic	**Chapter**	**Page**
The diaphragm	7	22

PHRENIC NERVE

Provides motor and sensory supply to the **diaphragm.**

Course

RIGHT	LEFT
Arises from anterior rami of **C3–5** between **scalenus medius** and **anterior**	

> ↑ **MRCS viva**
> Mnemonic: C3, 4, 5 keeps the diaphragm alive

RIGHT	LEFT
Runs on **scalenus anterior** in the neck	
Enters the thorax via the thoracic inlet, **posterior to the subclavian vein**	
Travels anterior to the vagus	
Travels lateral to the right brachiocephalic vein and SVC	Crosses anterior to the aortic arch (compare vagus)
On surface of fibrous pericardium	**Anterior** to **left pulmonary artery**
Overlying right atrium, then IVC	**Lateral** to **left ventricle** within fibrous pericardium
Travels in **front of the root of the lung**	
Pierces diaphragm	Passes into abdominal cavity via **caval orifice**

Key learning point

Mnemonic: phrenic front

 Example viva question

What would be the effect of a spinal cord transection at C6 on respiration?

The phrenic nerves, given off already at the level of C3–5 would be intact and the patient's **diaphragm would not be paralysed**. However, the intercostals below would not be spared, leading to some difficulties with ventilation despite sparing of the diaphragm itself. Chronically, immobility and weakness of the chest wall could lead to lower respiratory tract infections.

VAGUS NERVE

- Tenth cranial nerve (X)
- **Visceral sensory** and **motor autonomic supply** to most abdominal organs
- Also has motor branches to laryngeal muscles (superior and recurrent laryngeal nerves).

Course

RIGHT	LEFT
Fibres originate from medulla	
Exit the cranium via the **jugular foramen**, forming two ganglia here	
Passes down the neck in the **carotid sheath** (posteriorly) adjacent to oesophagus	
Gives off **superior, internal and external laryngeal branches** in the neck	
Passes into thoracic cavity via thoracic inlet behind the lung	
Recurrent laryngeal nerve given off at root of neck and hooks behind **subclavian artery**	Recurrent laryngeal nerve given off at level of **arch of aorta** and hooks behind it at level of **ligamentum arteriosum**
Travels **behind** the **root of the lung** (see above)	
Travels **behind** oesophagus	Travels **in front** of oesophagus
Travel into abdomen via oesophageal opening (T10) and forms oesophageal plexus	

↑ **Example viva question**

What is the consequence of bilateral recurrent laryngeal nerve division?

This is a **surgical emergency**, because it would lead to adduction of both the true vocal cords and hence **acute airway obstruction**. Surgical cricothyroidotomy and tracheostomy are indicated. This is a rare complication of **thyroidectomy** (see 'Thyroidectomy', Chapter 41, page 144).

14 Portal vein and portosystemic anastomoses

Possible viva questions related to this topic

→ What is a portal system?
→ How is the portal vein formed?
→ What is the course of the hepatic portal vein?
→ Where are the portosystemic anastomoses?
→ What are the clinical effects of portal hypertension on the portosystemic anastomoses?

Related topics		
Topic	**Chapter**	**Page**
Biliary tree and gallbladder	5	17
Liver	10	28
Pituitary	100	397

Example viva question

What is a portal circulation? Where in the body would you find one?

• Two sets of capillaries in series
• Seen in hepatic **portal system** described here, and in the **pituitary**
• The pituitary portal system starts as capillaries in the hypothalamus, and ends as capillaries in the anterior pituitary gland. It carries releasing hormones from the hypothalamus to the pituitary (see 'Pituitary', Chapter 100, page 397).

HEPATIC PORTAL SYSTEM

This system begins as portal capillaries in the organs drained (gut organs) and ends as capillaries within the liver.

Portal vein – anatomy and relations

• Formed behind the **pancreatic neck** by union of the **superior mesenteric** and **splenic veins** at the level of **L2**, right of the midline
• Length **5 cm**

- Runs **posterior** to the **first part of the duodenum**
- Runs in the **free edge of the lesser omentum** into the **porta hepatis**, with and **posterior** to the **bile duct** and **hepatic artery**.

Portosystemic anastomoses

These are areas where the **portal capillaries** are in continuation with **systemic capillaries**. Blood does not usually flow from portal to systemic; it flows preferentially to the **liver**.

In **portal hypertension**, blood can flow from portal to systemic and these anastomoses become dilated, with clinical consequences:

Sites of anastomosis			
Site	**Portal vessel**	**Systemic vessel**	**Clinical consequence**
Lower third of oesophagus	Left gastric vein	Azygos veins	Oesophageal varices
Anal canal	Superior rectal vein	Middle/inferior rectal veins	Rectal varices
Umbilicus	Paraumbilical veins	Superficial anterior abdominal wall veins	Caput medusae
Retroperitoneal	Colic and splenic veins	Lumbar veins	Retroperitoneal bleeding
Bare area of liver	Hepatic veins	Phrenic veins	

15 Radial nerve

Possible viva questions related to this topic

→ What is the course of the radial nerve?
→ What is the effect of dividing the radial nerve?
→ What coexisting injuries would you be worried about if a patient suffers a spiral fracture of the humerus?

Related topics		
Topic	**Chapter**	**Page**
Median nerve	11	31
Ulnar nerve	21	55

COURSE

- C_5–T_1 nerve roots
- Arises from the **posterior cord** of the **brachial plexus**
- **Posterior cutaneous nerve of the forearm** is given off in the axilla
- Passes between the long and medial heads of **triceps**
- Passes adjacent to and in contact with the humerus in the **spiral groove**, posteriorly, accompanied by the **profunda vessels**
- Pierces the **anconeus** muscle, supplying it
- Continues into antecubital fossa between **brachialis** and **brachioradialis** muscles. It supplies the elbow joint
- Divides into **deep** and **superficial** branches in antecubital fossa
- The superficial radial nerve is **sensory** and supplies the hand
- The deep part is motor and continues into the forearm where it supplies the extensors of the forearm.

MOTOR SUPPLY

Radial nerve

Triceps, brachialis (small part), brachioradialis.

Deep radial nerve

Extensors of the forearm: extensor digitorum, extensor digiti minimi, extensor carpi ulnaris, abductor pollicis longus, extensor pollicis longus, extensor pollicis brevis, extensor indicis.

SENSORY SUPPLY

- Radial one and a half fingers dorsally
- Supplied by the **superficial branch** of the radial nerve
- Skin on the back of the posterior aspect of the forearm supplied by the **posterior cutaneous nerve of the forearm**.

CLINICAL ASSESSMENT

↑ **Example viva question**

What coexisting injuries would you be worried about if a patient suffers a spiral fracture of the humerus?

The examiner is asking what the effects of division of the radial nerve are at the level of the **spiral groove**.

Function of the **superficial** and **deep branches** of the radial nerve in the forearm is lost. This leads to loss of sensation and muscle power. If the radial nerve is divided the patient will suffer a **wrist drop**. This is caused by paralysis of the extensors of the forearm, leading to unopposed action of the flexors.

Loss of grip strength **occurs because** synergy of **flexors** and **extensors** is required for gripping and the paralysis results in loss of this.

Paraesthesiae should be tested for over the **first dorsal interosseus**.

16 Salivary glands

Possible viva questions related to this topic

→ What is the anatomy of the parotid and submandibular glands? Show me their surface anatomy on this skull.

→ What structures are at risk in surgery of these glands?

Related topics		
Topic	**Chapter**	**Page**
Triangles of the neck	20	53

PAROTID GLAND

Anatomy

- **Paired** glands
- **Largest** of the salivary glands
- **Serous** gland
- **Wedge** shaped
- Surrounded by **connective tissue capsule (investing layer of deep cervical fascia)**
- Divided into **superficial** and **deep** lobes by the five divisions of the **facial nerve**
- Overlies the **angle of the mandible**
- Superior margin extends behind the **temporomandibular (TM) joint**
- Anterior margin superficial to **masseter** muscle
- Deep part of gland between **medial pterygoid** and **ramus of mandible**
- **Parotid duct** from facial process of gland (anterior aspect) over **masseter**. Pierces **buccinator** muscle; course is submucosal until it opens into a papilla opposite the **upper second molar tooth**.

Contents – lateral to medial

- **Facial nerve** and branches
- **Retromandibular vein**
- **External carotid artery**
- **Parotid lymph nodes.**

These structures are at risk at surgery. At superficial parotidectomy the **facial nerve** is preserved and the plane that it forms between the superficial and deep parts of the gland is dissected.

Blood supply

External carotid artery.

Lymphatic drainage

Parotid and deep cervical nodes.

SUBMANDIBULAR GLANDS

Anatomy

- **Paired** glands
- Mixture of **serous** and **mucinous** acini
- **Connective tissue** capsule, derived from the **investing layer** of **deep cervical fascia**
- Consists of a **superficial** and **deep** part, in continuity with each other around the posterior border of **mylohyoid**, which divides the two parts
- **Superficial** part lies within the **digastric triangle (anterior triangle)** (see 'Triangles of the neck', Chapter 20, page 53).

Relations

- Lateral: medial aspect of mandible, and below this, **facial nerve** (cervical) and **facial vein**
- Medial: hyoglossus and styloglossus
- Anteriorly: anterior belly of digastric
- Posteriorly: stylohyoid, posterior belly of digastric, **lingual** and **hypoglossal** nerves
- Superiorly: **lingual nerve**
- Inferiorly: **hypoglossal nerve**.

Submandibular duct (Wharton's duct) emerges from the **anterior aspect** of the gland, and travels lateral to the tongue in the submucosa; it is crossed twice by the **lingual** nerve and opens into a papilla just **lateral to the frenulum** of the tongue.

Blood supply

Facial and **lingual** arteries.

Lymphatic drainage

Submandibular, deep cervical nodes.

The marginal **mandibular branch of the facial nerve** is at risk in submandibular surgery, so the **incision is made low**. The angle of the mouth will droop if the nerve is divided at surgery.

SUBLINGUAL GLANDS

Anatomy

- Smallest of the three glands
- Paired glands
- **Serous** and **mucinous** acini, predominantly the latter
- Situated submucosally, beneath the floor of the mouth near the midline.

Relations

- Anterior: opposite gland
- Posterior: deep submandibular gland
- Medial: genioglossus, lingual nerve
- Lateral: mandible
- Inferior: mylohyoid muscle.

Several ducts open into the floor of the mouth, adjacent to the submandibular duct opening.

17 Stomach

STOMACH

Roughly **J shaped**. It consists of:
• Fundus
• Cardia
• Body
• Antrum
• Pylorus.

Relations

Anteriorly
• Abdominal wall
• Left costal margin
• Diaphragm
• Left lobe of the liver.

Posteriorly
• **Lesser sac** – this **separates** the stomach from the pancreas
• Transverse mesocolon
• Left colic flexure
• Upper pole of the left kidney

• Left suprarenal gland
• Spleen and splenic artery.

Superiorly
• Left dome of the diaphragm.

The **lesser omentum** is attached along the **lesser curvature** of the stomach, the **greater omentum** along the **greater curvature**. These omenta contain the **vascular** and **lymphatic supply** of the stomach.

↑ **Example viva question**

What is the blood supply of the stomach?

• Left gastric artery – coeliac axis
• Right gastric artery – hepatic artery
• Right gastroepiploic artery – from the gastroduodenal branch of the
  hepatic artery
• Left gastroepiploic artery – from the splenic artery
• Short gastric arteries – from the splenic artery.

Both sets of arteries anastomose with each other on their respective gastric
curvatures and then anastomose with the supply of the other curve.

During **oesophagectomy**, the **short gastrics**, **left gastroepiploic** and **left gastric arteries** are divided to mobilize the upper part of the stomach, so that it can be pulled up to form the neo-oesophagus. The stomach then derives its blood supply solely from the right gastric and gastroepiploic arteries and their anastomoses.

Venous drainage

Corresponding veins drain into the **portal system**.

Lymphatic drainage

This accompanies its blood vessels. Stomach can be divided into **three drainage zones**:

• **Area I**: superior two-thirds drains along left and right gastric vessels to **aortic nodes**.
• **Area II**: right two-thirds of the inferior third of the stomach drains along the
  right gastroepiploic vessels to the subpyloric nodes and then to the aortic nodes.
• **Area III**: left third of the greater curvature drains along the short gastric arteries
  and splenic vessels lying in the gastrosplenic and lienorenal ligaments, then via
  the suprapancreatic nodes to the aortic group.

Clinical implication

Extensive lymphatic drainage and technical difficulty of complete removal make stomach cancer surgery difficult, with poor results. Involvement of the nodes around the splenic vessels can be dealt with by removal of the spleen and the ligaments, body and tail of the pancreas; gastroepiploic lymph nodes are removed by excising the greater omentum, but appreciate the difficulty of removing the lymph nodes around the aorta and head of the pancreas!

Gastric innervation

The anterior and posterior vagi control **motility** and **secretion**.

They enter the abdomen through the **oesophageal hiatus**.

The **anterior vagus** lies close to the stomach wall. It supplies **cardia and lesser curve,** and runs together with the **left gastric artery**. At this level, it is referred to the **anterior nerve of Latarget**. It gives branches to the anterior stomach and a large hepatic branch to the pyloric antrum.

The **posterior vagal trunk** runs down the **back** of the lesser omentum behind the anterior trunk as the **posterior nerve of Latarget**. It supplies anterior and posterior aspects of the body of the stomach. The bulk of the nerve forms the coeliac branch.

Truncal vagotomy was previously an operation for **complicated peptic ulcer disease**.

Truncal vagotomy of **both trunks** at the lower oesophagus **reduces gastric secretion** and **paralyses the pyloric antrum**. Therefore it must be coupled with a **drainage procedure** such as a **pyloroplasty** or **gastrojejunostomy** to avoid **gastric stasis**.

- **Highly selective vagotomy** divides the individual nerves as they supply the acid-producing body and antrum, leaving the pylorus intact.
- **Posterior truncal vagotomy** leaves anterior pyloric nerves intact. It is coupled with an anterior seromyotomy.

Vagotomy is a historical procedure, and these days it is very rarely performed.

18 Thyroid gland and parathyroid glands

Possible viva questions related to this topic

→ What is the anatomy of the thyroid gland?
→ Describe the nerve supply of the thyroid gland.
→ What layers of the neck need to be divided at thyroidectomy?
→ What is the blood supply of the thyroid gland?
→ What are the positions of the parathyroids? Which are more constant?
→ What colour is a normal parathyroid?
→ How might a parathyroid be identified at surgery?
→ Plus questions related to thyroidectomy topic.

Related topics		
Topic	**Chapter**	**Page**
Thyroidectomy	41	144
Triangles of the neck	20	53
Phrenic and vagus nerves	13	36
Thyroid cancer	62	244

THYROID GLAND

Anatomy

- Has two lobes (**right** and **left**)
- Connected by a narrow central **isthmus**
- **Pyramidal lobe** sometimes presents projecting up from the isthmus
- Surrounded by sheath derived from **pretracheal** layer of **deep cervical fascia**
- Found in the **anterior triangle** of the neck
- Consists of follicular tissue (produces thyroxine or T_4 and triiodothyronine or T_3) and medullary C-cells (produce calcitonin).

Relations

- Posterolateral: **carotid sheath** (common carotid artery, internal jugular vein, vagus nerve)
- Anterolateral: strap muscles

- Medially: **larynx, trachea, oesophagus, recurrent laryngeal nerve.** Branch of vagus nerve (in the groove between trachea and oesophagus) – see 'Phrenic and vagus nerves', Chapter 13, page 36.

Blood supply

Important for the surgeon to know; commonly asked in vivas.

- Two arteries (superior, inferior)
- Three veins (superior, middle, inferior)
- **Superior thyroid artery**, branch of the **external carotid artery**
- **Inferior thyroid artery**, branch of the **thyrocervical trunk**, from the **subclavian artery**
- **Superior and middle thyroid veins** drain into the **internal jugular vein**
- **Inferior thyroid vein** drains into the **left brachiocephalic vein**.

See 'Thyroidectomy', Chapter 41, page 144.

Lymphatic drainage

Deep cervical nodes.

Development

Embryologically, the thyroid gland descends embryologically from the **foramen cecum**, which lies at the divide between the anterior two-thirds and the posterior third of the tongue, guided by the thyroglossal duct, to its final position anterior to the trachea.

The duct hooks behind the hyoid bone, which is important to remember in surgery of **thyroglossal cysts** (remnants of the duct) because this part must be excised, with the central part of the hyoid bone (Sistrunk's operation).

PARATHYROID GLANDS

- **Four** in number
- Secrete **parathyroid hormone (PTH)** and mediate calcium homoeostasis (see 'Calcium homoeostasis', Chapter 88, page 362)
- **Ochre** in colour; can be stained by administration of **methylene blue**, which stains them blue
- Two superior glands lie at the posterior border at the level of the mid-thyroid
- **Two inferior glands** are much **more variable in position**, at the inferior thyroid; they can lie in the thyrothymic ligament or even the superior mediastinum
- Supplied by the **superior** and **inferior** thyroid arteries.

19 The transpyloric plane of Addison

Possible viva questions related to this topic

→ What is the transpyloric plane?
→ At what level is the transpyloric plane found?
→ What are the surface markings for the transpyloric plane?
→ What structures are found in this plane?
→ What are the surface markings of the gallbladder?
→ What is the subcostal plane?
→ At what level does the abdominal aorta bifurcate?
→ What is the interrelationship of the common iliac artery, vein and distal ureter?
→ What dermatome surrounds the umbilicus?

SURFACE MARKING OF THE GALLBLADDER

Level of the ninth costal cartilage in the midclavicular line.

THE SUBCOSTAL PLANE

This passes across the lower margins of the thoracic cage formed by the **tenth costal cartilage** on each side.

It is also at the level of the third lumbar vertebra and at the level of the origin of the **inferior mesenteric artery**.

↑ **Example viva question**

What is the transpyloric plane?

The **transpyloric plane** of **Addison** is a plane **perpendicular** to a line connecting the **jugular notch** and the **pubic symphysis**; it passes through the **body of L1 vertebra**.

It is approximately halfway between the **xiphisternum** and **umbilicus**

Surface anatomy: a hand's breadth below the **xiphoid process**

Structures found at this level: **12!**

Important structures are found at this level, which is why it is frequently asked about!

- Fundus of gallbladder (see 'Biliary tree and gallbladder', Chapter 5, page 17)
- Lower border of L1 vertebra
- Spinal cord ends
- Pylorus of stomach (see 'Stomach', Chapter 17, page 46)
- Neck of pancreas (see 'Pancreas', Chapter 12, page 34)
- Attachment of the transverse mesocolon
- Superior mesenteric artery branching off the aorta
- Portal vein formed from the superior mesenteric vein and splenic vein (see 'Portal vein and portosystemic anastomoses', Chapter 14, page 39)
- Hilum of spleen
- Hilum of both kidneys and their vascular pedicles (see 'Kidney', Chapter 9, page 26)
- Duodenojejunal (DJ) junction

TOPICS RELATED TO THE MAIN THEME

The **abdominal aorta** bifurcates at the level of the **umbilicus** or the **fourth lumbar vertebra** slightly to the left of the midline (see 'Abdominal aorta', Chapter 3, page 13).

The **umbilicus** is at the level of the **L4** vertebra and its **dermatome** is **T10**.

The **common iliac artery** lies slightly **anterior** to the **corresponding vein**. The **distal ureter** travels **anterior** to both these structures (see 'Ureter', Chapter 22, page 58).

20 Triangles of the neck

Possible viva questions related to this topic

→ What are the triangles of the neck?
→ What are the borders of the triangles of the neck?
→ What are the contents of the triangles?
→ What is the surface anatomy of the anterior and posterior triangles of the neck?
→ What structures could be damaged in a stabbing injury to the neck?

Related topics		
Topic	Chapter	Page
Thyroidectomy	41	144
Carotid endarterectomy	27	81
Tracheostomy	42	148
Salivary glands	16	43

TRIANGLES

- Posterior triangle
- Anterior triangle.

They are subdivided into: submental, digastric, carotid and muscular.

POSTERIOR TRIANGLE

Borders

- Anterior: posterior border of **sternocleidomastoid**
- Posterior: anterior border of **trapezius**
- Inferior: **clavicle**.

Contents

- Muscles (floor of triangle): splenius capitis, levator scapulae, scalenus medius (scalenus anterior), (serratus anterior)
- Nerves: branches of **cervical plexus**, spinal **accessory nerve** (travels from one-third of the way down posterior border of sternocleidomastoid to trapezius); **trunks** of **brachial plexus**
- Other: lymph nodes (occipital/supraclavicular), **subclavian artery**. Transverse cervical and suprascapular vessels.

> ↑ **Key learning point**
>
> Mnemonic: **the trunks are in the triangle** – to remind you which part of the brachial plexus is here.

ANTERIOR TRIANGLE

Borders of anterior triangle

- Midline
- Posterior border of sternocleidomastoid
- Ramus of mandible.

Subtriangles

- Carotid triangle: sternocleidomastoid, posterior belly of digastric, superior belly of omohyoid. *Key contents*: **common and external carotid artery**.
- Digastric triangle: mandible, anterior and posterior bellies of digastric. *Key contents*: **submandibular gland** (see 'Salivary glands', Chapter 16, page 43).
- Submental triangle: anterior bellies of digastric, body of hyoid. *Key contents*: **anterior jugular veins.**
- Muscular triangle: sternocleidomastoid, superior belly of omohyoid, midline. *Key contents*: **larynx** and **trachea**, **thyroid gland** and **parathyroid glands** (see 'Thyroid gland and parathyroid glands', Chapter 18, page 49).

Contents

- Muscle: suprahyoid muscles (digastric, stylohyoid, mylohyoid, geniohyoid)
- Strap muscles (thyrohyoid, sternothyroid, sternohyoid)
- Nerves: recurrent and external laryngeal nerves (from vagus nerve)
- **Vagus nerve** (in carotid sheath – see 'Phrenic and vagus nerves', Chapter 13, page 36), ansa cervicalis, hypoglossal nerve
- Vessels: **common carotid artery** and bifurcation, branches of external; internal jugular vein
- Other: **thyroid gland, parathyroid glands, submandibular gland, trachea** and **oesophagus.**

> ↑ **Example viva question**
>
> *What structures could be damaged in a stabbing injury to the neck?*
>
> This question requires the candidate to divide the neck into triangles, as above, and then to go through each region methodically in terms of structures (structures, muscles, nerves, arteries).
>
> Mention the most important structures first.

21 Ulnar nerve

Possible viva questions related to this topic

→ What is the course of the ulnar nerve?
→ What does the ulnar nerve supply in the hand?
→ How would you test the function of this nerve clinically?
→ What is the ulnar paradox?
→ What do the lumbricals do and how many are there?
→ What do the interossei do and how many are there?
→ How can you distinguish ulnar nerve injuries from other nerve injuries by examining the hand?

COURSE

- Originates from **C7, C8, T1** nerve roots
- Formed from **medial cord** of the brachial plexus in the axilla
- Runs **between axillary artery** and **vein** in the upper arm
- Lies on **coracobrachialis** in the arm, medial to the **brachial artery**
- Passes behind the **medial epicondyle** of the humerus
- Passes between the two heads of **flexor carpi ulnaris**, supplying it
- In the forearm it lies between **flexor digitorum profundus** and **flexor carpi ulnaris**
- Passes superficial to the **carpal tunnel**
- Divides into terminal branches at the **pisiform** bone.

MOTOR SUPPLY

Forearm

Ulnar half of flexor digitorum profundus, flexor carpi ulnaris.

Intrinsic hand muscles

Supplies all intrinsic muscles of the hand with four exceptions: 'LOAF' supplied by median nerve – two lateral lumbricals, opponens pollicis, abductor pollicis brevis and flexor pollicis brevis.

↑ Example viva question

What is the ulnar paradox?

Division of the ulnar nerve at the **wrist** produces severely clawed ulnar fingers as the **lumbricals** and **interossei** are lost. **Flexor digitorum profundus** is **intact**, producing further flexion. In lesions at the elbow (a more 'serious' lesion, because more nerve is lost), flexor **digitorum profundus** is now paralysed. Paradoxically, the claw hand is not as bad, because the extra flexion of the ulnar two fingers that this muscle provides is lost.

↑ Example viva question

What do the lumbricals do and how many are there?

There are **four** lumbrical muscles, the lateral two supplied by the **median nerve** (see 'Median nerve', Chapter 11, page 31) and the medial two by the **ulnar nerve**.

They originate from the **flexor digitorum profundus** tendons and insert into the corresponding **extensor expansion**.

They **flex the metacarpophalangeal** joints and **extend the interphalangeal** joints. They are responsible, in conjunction with the interossei, for coordinating **fine movements** of the fingers such as writing or playing a musical instrument.

↑ Example viva question

What do the interossei do and how many are there?

There are **four palmar** and **four dorsal** interossei.

They are supplied by the **ulnar nerve**.

Origin: metacarpal base.

Insertion: proximal phalanx base

The **palmar interossei adduct** the fingers and the **dorsal interossei abduct.**

Mnemonic: palmar adduct (PAD), dorsal abduct (DAB)

SENSORY SUPPLY

The nerve supplies the **medial one and a half fingers** and **medial third of the palm of the hand**.

CLINICAL TESTS

Wasting of the small muscles of the hand (particularly hypothenar eminence) in longstanding lesions.

Test the **interossei** by asking the patient to grip a piece of paper between middle and ring fingers, and try to remove the paper. Compare with the other side.

Froment's sign: if a patient is asked to grip a piece of paper between the thumb and lateral aspect of forefinger, he or she will flex as the thumb adductor is lost.

Test the **sensory distribution**.

22 Ureter

Possible viva questions related to this topic

→ What is the course of the ureter?
→ What is the blood supply of the ureter?
→ What are the relations of the ureter and what structures cross it?
→ Trace the ureter's course on a KUB abdominal film.
→ Where might stones be held up?

Related topics		
Topic	**Chapter**	**Page**
Kidney	9	26

KEY FACTS

- Length 25 cm
- Lined by **transitional epithelium** (hence possible site of transitional cell carcinoma)
- Blood supply superiorly by **ureteric branch of renal artery** and inferiorly by **superior vesical** and **gonadal artery**; middle part supplied by **aorta, gonadal** and **iliac** vessels
- Lymph drainage with the arteries, eventually to para-aortic nodes (superior part) and iliac nodes (inferior part)
- Autonomic nerve supply, pain fibres accompany sympathetics.

COURSE AND RELATIONS

RIGHT URETER	LEFT URETER

Retroperitoneal

Descends on psoas major (adjacent to tip of vertebral transverse processes on KUB film)

Passes over the **genitofemoral nerve** and the **gonadal vessels** pass over it

Third part of duodenum anterior	Lateral to the inferior mesenteric vessels
Right colic, ileocolic and root of mesentery anterior	Left colic vessels anterior

Point of narrowing at **pelviureteric junction**, where it crosses the brim of the pelvis

Runs over **external iliac artery** and vein

Vas deferens in the male crosses over it

'Water under the bridge'

Turns medially at the level of the ischial spine (key landmark on KUB film) and enters the bladder inferolaterally

Second point of narrowing at point of entry to bladder – **vesicoureteric junction** or VUJ.

The two points of narrowing are the most common site of impaction of ureteric stones

---

↑ **Example viva question**

Tell me the course of the ureter on this KUB film.

It passes down level with the tips of the **transverse processes** of the lumbar vertebrae, commencing at the medial aspect of the kidney (outline seen on KUB).

It turns medially at the level of the **ischial spine**. Point out the sites of narrowing described above.

OPERATIVE SURGERY

23 Anorectal surgery 1: anal fissure and lateral sphincterotomy

Possible viva questions related to this topic

→ Examiner may show you a picture of an anal fissure and ask 'what is the diagnosis?'
→ In what positions are these normally found?
→ What are the most common causes of severe anal pain?
→ What is the differential diagnosis for anal fissure, especially if atypical in location?
→ What is a sentinel pile?
→ How do you best diagnose an anal fissure?
→ How would you manage a patient with this problem?
→ What are the non-surgical treatment options for this condition? Does it work?
→ How do you perform a lateral sphincterotomy and what are the main complications?

Related topics		
Topic	**Chapter**	**Page**
Anal canal	4	15
Fistula *in ano* and pilonidal sinus	24	67
Injection sclerotherapy and haemorrhoidectomy	25	73

↑ Example viva question

What is an anal fissure?

An **anal fissure** is a **longitudinal tear** in the **mucosa** and **skin** of the **lower third of the anal canal**.

ANAL FISSURE

- **Common**: seen in **young adults** – males > females
- Peak incidence **20–30 years of age**

- **Constipation** is thought to be the **primary cause** but there is actually **no evidence for this**. The constipation could be the result of the fissure. Underlying **pathophysiology** is **local trauma** → internal and external anal sphincter dysfunction → **ischaemia**
- Anal fissures are the **most common anal abnormalities in Crohn's disease**
- Most are **posterior** in the midline (**90 per cent**)
- **Anterior** (**10 per cent**) fissure more common in **women**, especially after **childbirth** (vaginal delivery).

DIFFERENTIAL DIAGNOSIS OF SEVERE ANAL PAIN/ANAL FISSURE

- Acute fissure *in ano*
- Perianal haematoma
- Strangulated internal haemorrhoids
- Perianal and ischiorectal abscess
- Inflammatory bowel disease (IBD)
- Colorectal malignancy
- Proctalgia fugax (painful rectum).

SYMPTOMS AND SIGNS

Anal pain during or immediately after **defecation** as a result of **sphincter spasm**. This can **persist** for up to an hour.

- **Bright red bleeding per rectum** – normally on the toilet paper on wiping
- **Pruritus ani**
- **Watery discharge** from anus
- **Constipation**
- There might be a **history** suggestive of **cyclic fissuring** and **healing**
- On **examination**, the fissure is usually **concealed** by **anal spasm**. Patient is in too much pain even to let in a finger. However, you can sometimes **see** the **white circular fibres** of the **internal sphincter** muscle at the **base** of the **fissure**. On inspection you may see a **small anal skin tag** at the superficial end of the fissure (=sentinel tag). This suggests that the **fissure** is **chronic**.

The best way of **diagnosing** an anal fissure is by the **history** and **visual inspection** – **not** by digital examination or proctoscopy!

CONSERVATIVE TREATMENT

- **Conservative treatment is successful** in up to **50 per cent** of cases. Principle of management is to **reduce internal anal sphincter spasm: local anaesthetic gel** (good analgesia), **GTN ointment cream** (0.2 per cent TDS) for at least **4/52**.

- **GTN ointment** thought to exert a **local vasodilator effect** and **allow healing**.
- Patient advised to keep **adequately hydrated**, retain a **high-fibre diet** (also thought to reduce the risk of recurrence) and be prescribed **laxatives** to keep stool soft. Review in outpatients. Remember to advise using a glove for application, otherwise it will get absorbed – warn patient of potential for **headaches**. (If these occur, patient should be advised to discontinue use.)
- Can then try **diltiazem cream** (2 per cent BD) but some surgeons use this as a first line option.
- **Other options:** **botulinum toxin** injection.

Key learning point

You should know the doses of the creams available:

GTN ointment cream (0.2 per cent TDS)
Diltiazem cream (2 per cent BD)

OPERATIVE SURGERY

Anal stretch

This is **controversial** – some think it causes uncontrolled disruption of the internal anal sphincter and that reproducibility from one patient to the next is poor. High rates of **faecal incontinence** have been reported.

Lateral sphincterotomy

- **Indication:** failed medical therapy (usually two courses of GTN 6/52 prescribed before consideration)
- Usually leads to **healing** in **95 per cent cases after 4 weeks**
- Performed under a **general anaesthetic**
- Patient is placed in the **lithotomy position**
- **Per rectum examination, rigid sigmoidoscopy** and **proctoscopy** performed to confirm the **diagnosis** and rule out **synchronous pathology**
- Examine with **Eisenhammer's** or **Park's retractor**
- **Internal sphincter muscle** identified usually after developing a **submucosal plane** with **local anaesthetic**
- Insert scissors into the **intersphincteric space** and **enlarge**
- **Internal muscle fibres** are cut usually to **dentate line** away and **lateral** to the fissure

- **Fissurotomy** may be an added option
- Need to warn patient of risks of **faecal** and **flatus incontinence** and **treatment failure**.

↑ **Example viva question**

What are the complications of a lateral sphincterotomy?

Treatment failure (5 per cent)
Faecal incontinence (permanent in 5 per cent)

---

24 Anorectal surgery 2: fistula *in ano* and pilonidal sinus

Possible viva questions related to this topic

→ What is the difference between a fistula and a sinus?
→ How do you classify fistula *in ano*?
→ How would you excise a superficial fistula *in ano*?
→ What does Goodsall's law state?
→ What are the features of a complex fistula?
→ What imaging modalities can help in defining complex fistulae?
→ How does a pilonidal sinus develop and where else can it occur?
→ How do these patients normally present?
→ What are the surgical options?
→ What is the Karydakis procedure?

Key learning points

Definitions

A **fistula** is an **abnormal communication** between **two epithelial-lined surfaces**.

Example: with a **fistula *in ano*** a communication exists between the **perianal skin** and either the **anal canal** or the **rectum**

A **sinus** is a **blind-ending tract** communicating with an **epithelial surface**. This may be **normal** (e.g. carotid sinus) *or* **abnormal** (e.g. **pilonidal sinus**).

FISTULA *IN ANO*

Causes

Most fistulae start as an **abscess** as a result of:
- Crohn's disease
- Trauma
- Diabetes mellitus
- Infection: tuberculosis (TB) and HIV
- Carcinoma.

Classification (Fig. 24.1)

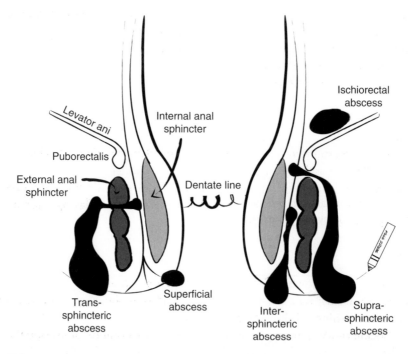

Figure 24.1

- Superficial
- Intersphincteric
- Trans-sphincteric
  - low
  - high
- Suprasphincteric.

> ↑ **Key learning point**
>
> ### Goodsall's law
>
> This law states that, if an **external opening** lies **anterior** to an imaginary **transverse line** with the patient in the lithotomy position, **bisecting the anal opening**, its **tract** will **pass directly** into the **anal canal**, whereas, if the **opening** lies **posterior** to this line, the **tract** will **curve** in a **horseshoe manner** towards the internal opening by entering the **anal canal** in the midline **posteriorly**.

Aims of management

- **Define anatomy** – identification of the internal opening is the most important determinant of successful treatment of fistula *in ano*.
- **Effective drainage** of **sepsis** (abscess and tracts)
- **Eradication** of **source** of **sepsis**
- **Preservation** of **sphincter function**
- Wound care.

Generally
- **Superficial, intersphincteric** and **low trans-sphincteric fistulae** (lie *below* puborectalis) can be **laid open** and **packed**
- **Suprasphincteric** and **high trans-sphincteric fistulae** pass *above* the **puborectalis** and should be **treated** by a **seton suture** because immediate **laying open** has a **high risk** of faecal incontinence.

Procedure

- **General anaesthetic**; patient placed in **lithotomy position**.
- **Examination under anaesthetic (EUA)** and **rigid sigmoidoscopy** used to inspect for internal openings of the fistula
- Pass a **Lockhart–Mummery probe** gently into the **external fistulous opening** and note **direction** and **depth** in which the probe goes. Remember Goodsall's law when assessing the direction of the tract.

Superficial fistula
- If the **probe** passes **superficially** the **tract** is **excised** either with a **knife** or by **diathermy**. The fistula is excised by *directly cutting down* on to the *probe* and *if necessary* dividing the **superficial fibres** of the **internal sphincter**.
- **Excise** any **overhanging skin** on *either side* of the fistula to encourage **healing** by granulation.
- **Curette granulation tissue**.

- Always send excised tissue for **histology** (look for cause).
- Apply an **alginate dressing** to raw area to **aid haemostasis**.

Deep fistula

- If the **tract** is **deep** it is likely to be complex and will require **specialist colorectal help**. If **no help is available** to deal with a **high fistula**, insert a **nylon seton** to **aid drainage** and **allow reassessment** at a later date.
- **Endoanal ultrasonography** and **magnetic resonance imaging** (MRI) can be helpful in **defining tracts** when they are obscure or form part of a complex fistula.
- If anything more than a simple low fistula is present, the **trainee** should seek expert assistance:
  - A **trans-sphincteric tract** passes across the external sphincter to the ischiorectal fossa. The **internal opening** is often at the **level** of the **anal valves**
  - *Identify* **internal opening** with the **proctoscope**
  - **Probe** the **external opening**
  - **Open** the **anal canal epithelium** to the **level** of the **internal opening**
  - If the **tract** is **below** or at the line of the **anal valves**, *divide* the **muscle**. If it is above, *insert a **seton***.

Setons

- A **seton** is a **thread** or **suture** that is *passed along* the **fistula tract**.
- **Loose seton** – *tied loosely* it acts as an **effective drain** and **allows healing** to occur (*50 per cent cases*).
- **Tight cutting seton** – tied tightly it will slowly cut through the enclosed tissue. The seton can be subsequently **tightened every 2 weeks** under local anaesthetic to cut slowly through the enclosed sphincter muscle. This allows **fibrosis** to take place behind, thus **maintaining sphincter integrity**.

Features of a complex fistula

- **Recurrent episodes** post-surgery
- **Multiple** external openings
- **Induration** felt **above puborectalis** muscle
- **Probe** from external opening **passes upwards** instead of to the anus
- Associated more with **Crohn's disease** (Crohn's perianal fistula).

PILONIDAL SINUS

Aetiology

There are **two schools** of thought:

- Congenital: a nest of hairs become enclosed as the skin closes over it. This does not explain why the hairs found at the bottom of a pilonidal abscess are demonstrably 'scalp-type' hairs. Hence this is not the current view.

- **Acquired**: chronic trauma allows a hair tip to penetrate the skin and the rolling motion of the buttocks causes the hairs to burrow in. A deep natal cleft, hairy area and occupations involving prolonged sitting also predispose to this condition.

Also found in the finger webs of people in certain occupations: **hairdressers** and **sheepshearers**. May be also seen in the **umbilicus, axilla** and **perianal** areas.

Presentation

- Asymptomatic
- Acute pilonidal abscess
- Chronic discharging sinus.

Management

Conservative
If the patient has **midline pit disease** and **minimal symptoms**, he or she can be managed conservatively with **good personal hygiene** and **regular removal of hairs**.

Surgical
Indication
Persistent or **recurrent** pilonidal sinus.

Options
- **Lay open wound and packing**: completely excising pits and lateral tracks with an elliptical excision. Wound should then be packed with a seaweed dressing.
- **Primary closure**: patient should be warned of wound breakdown and dehiscence, because midline wounds are difficult to heal. Never attempt to perform primary closure on purulent tissue.
- The **Karydakis procedure** is one of several types of operation for pilonidal disease with the **intent of primary closure**. An **advancement flap** is created so that the wound is brought away from the midline without being under tension so that healing is improved. The **natal cleft** is also **rendered shallow**.

Preoperatively
- A phosphate enema is given to prevent early postoperative defecation. **Intravenous antibiotics** (include anaerobic cover) are given at induction.
- The patient is placed **prone** on the table under **general anaesthetic** with the **buttocks strapped apart**. The **natal cleft** area is **shaved**, prepared and draped, and any areas of infection are covered.
- An **asymmetrical** (D-shaped) **ellipse** is marked on the skin to encompass both the **midline pits** and the **lateral sinus** (wider part of the ellipse). Skin is incised using **diathermy** according to the marked pattern and deepened to the **pre-sacral fascia**. The block of tissue is excised.

- The restraining tapes are removed. Skin flaps are created so that both edges can be approximated, achieving meticulous haemostasis with diathermy.
- Closure is with interrupted 1/0 Vicryl to fat and interrupted 1/0 nylon to skin. A mini-vac is placed and secured beforehand to help close down the dead space.

Postoperatively
- Drain reviewed and normally taken out at **24 hours**
- **Oral antibiotics** are given for **5 days**.

The patient is warned to **lie on his or her side**. **No sitting** for at **least 5 days** to prevent excess tension on midline wound.

25 Anorectal surgery 3: injection sclerotherapy and haemorrhoidectomy

Possible viva questions related to this topic

→ What are haemorrhoids and what are their normal functions?
→ What are the common causes of pathological haemorrhoids?
→ How do you perform injection sclerotherapy for haemorrhoids?
→ What are the indications for performing a haemorrhoidectomy?
→ How do you perform a Milligan–Morgan open haemorrhoidectomy?
→ How do you distinguish the internal sphincter from the external sphincter?
→ What are the potential complications?
→ How would you treat thrombosed strangulated haemorrhoids?
→ What are you palpating for during a per rectal examination?

Related topics

Topic	Chapter	Page
Colorectal cancer	54	200
Anal fissure and lateral sphincterotomy	23	63
Fistula *in ano* and pilonidal sinus	24	67

HAEMORRHOIDS

↑ Example viva question

What are haemorrhoids?

Haemorrhoids (piles) are **engorged vascular cushions** found within the **submucosa** of the **anal canal**. They consist of a **sacculated venous plexus** with a **rich arterial supply supported by a fibromuscular connective tissue**. They normally contribute to:

• anal continence
• protection of the sphincter mechanism during defecation.

They are found at **constant positions** within the **anal canal** (3, 7 and 11 o'clock positions).

Common causes of pathological haemorrhoids

- **Constipation** (thought to produce **shearing forces** that lead to **fragmentation of** the supporting **fibromuscular matrix**)
- **Prolonged straining** (thought to lead to **engorgement** of the **anal cushions**)
- **Pregnancy**
- **Internal sphincter dysfunction.**

Management

- Appropriate **dietary** and **defecatory** advice to prevent straining and constipation
- **Asymptomatic**: conservative
- **Symptomatic**: **injection sclerotherapy** or **banding** for **primary** and **small secondary** haemorrhoids.

↑ **Example viva question**

How do you inject haemorrhoids?

Injection sclerotherapy: outpatient setting
Warn the patient that the procedure may be **painful**, that he or she may notice **significant blood loss** after the procedure for about **48 hours** and that **repeat injections** may be required.

Ask about **nut allergy**.

Left lateral position.

Position proctoscope within anal canal.

Visualize the groups of haemorrhoids and inject with **5 per cent phenol in almond oil** into the **bases**. Do not inject too close to the **dentate line** because this can cause severe pain. Start with the **lowest haemorrhoid** first so that any bleeding **does not obstruct** the **view**.

Watch till the superficial tissues **blanch** and **swell**. This is an indication that the injection is in the **correct plane**.

Review in **outpatients** in **6 weeks**.

HAEMORRHOIDECTOMY

Indication

Prolapsing **third-degree** haemorrhoids.

Milligan–Morgan technique advocated and can be performed as a **day-case proced-ure**, although **stapled anopexy** can also be performed now with good results.

Open versus **closed** technique.

Preparation

- A preoperative **phosphate enema** should be given to allow an adequate examination under anaesthetic to be performed.
- Patient is placed in the **lithotomy** or **jack-knife** position, slightly **head down**.
- Perform a **per rectum examination** (see below) and **rigid sigmoidoscopy**, and visualize the **anal canal** and **rectum** with a **proctoscope**. Confirm the **position** of the **group** of **haemorrhoids** by introducing a dry gauze swab into the anal canal and gently withdrawing it.
- Insert an **Eisenhammer's retractor** and assess which haemorrhoids need excision.
- Inject **local anaesthetic** into each **skin bridge** and **external component** of each haemorrhoid to be excised. Apply **Spencer–Wells forceps** to the perianal skin outside the mucocutaneous junction at the **3, 7 and 11 o'clock positions**, opposite the primary pile groups. Retract on these forceps to bring the haemorrhoidal masses into view and reapply the forceps.
- Start with the most **inferior haemorrhoid (7 o'clock group)** because this prevents blood clouding the operative field. Put the internal sphincter under tension by inserting an index finger into the rectum while holding the forceps in the palm of the hand.
- Mark out amount of haemorrhoid to be excised by scoring with the cutting diathermy. This should bear a **V- or U-shaped incision** in the skin close to the haemorrhoid.
- Excise the external component with coagulation diathermy.
- Extend dissection from the anal canal, separating the haemorrhoid from the white fibres of the internal sphincter, with a combination of **blunt** (regular sweeping motion pushing the subcutaneous tissue towards the anal canal, using a piece of gauze) and **sharp dissection**. The **external fibres** look **red**.
- Some surgeons **transfix** the **vascular pedicle** with a **1/0 Vicryl suture**, although this is **not** the **authors' practice**, because this has been attributed to causing **postoperative pain**. If meticulous haemostasis is achieved gradually, the pedicle can be transected without transfixion.
- Repeat the same procedure for the remaining haemorrhoidal groups, leaving **distinct skin bridges** to **avoid anal stenosis**.
- If performing a closed technique, close skin bridges with 0 Vicryl.
- Achieve **meticulous haemostasis** because bleeding is the most common reason for taking a patient back to theatre postoperatively.
- Insert **metronidazole** 500 mg and **diclofenac suppositories** along with a **soft petroleum jelly gauze** or **seaweed dressing** into the anal canal. This is

partially to keep the mucocutaneous bridges flat against the internal sphincter.
- The patient will naturally pass this gauze in 24 hours.
- Use blue gauze or perineal pad.
- Use a firm T bandage.

Postoperative advice

- Good oral analgesia (worse pain is the first bowel motion usually on day 7)
- Stool softeners
- 5/7 oral metronidazole
- Regular baths.

↑ **Key learning point**

Principles

'If it looks like a dahlia it's sure to be a failure. If it looks like a clover your worries are over!'

Don't be too radical with your excisions; you can always come back and repeat the operation. You cannot undo any damage to the internal or external sphincters!

Thrombosed strangulated haemorrhoids, which may present as an emergency, may be treated **conservatively** (analgesia, bed rest, elevated legs and ice packs) or by **immediate haemorrhoidectomy**. One of the concerns performing a haemorrhoidectomy on strangulated piles is **sepsis**.

Complications

- **Pain ++**
- **Acute retention of urine** (caused by postoperative pain)
- **Reactionary haemorrhage** (within 24 hours of surgery)
- **Secondary bleeding** is often the result of **infection**, which occurs on days 7 or 8 postoperatively
- **Constipation** and **faecal impaction** (resulting from pain)
- **Faecal incontinence** (damage to the sphincter mechanism)
- **Perianal fistula formation**
- **Recurrence** of the haemorrhoids
- **Anal stenosis.**

↑ **Example viva question**

What are you palpating during a per rectum (PR) examination?

In **males**:

- **Anterior**: prostate gland, rectovesical pouch, vas deferens, seminal vesicles, and bimanual palpation of the bladder
- **Posterior**: sacrum, coccyx, sympathetics and splanchnic vessels
- **Laterally**: ischial spines, obturator internus and Alcock's canal

In **females**:

- **Anterior**: pouch of Douglas, uterus and vagina (posterior fornix)
- **Posterior**: sacrum and coccyx
- **Laterally**: ischial spines

Also examine for (can be bimanually):

- **Rectal masses**, e.g. rectal carcinoma (lower rectum)
- **Acutely**: pelvic appendix (mass)
- Blood, stool (superiorly)

26 Burr holes and lumbar puncture

Possible viva questions related to this topic

→ How is a burr hole fashioned?
→ For what might a burr hole be used?
→ What are the complications of performing a burr hole?
→ At what level should a lumbar puncture be performed?
→ What are the principles of lumbar puncture?
→ What is a normal opening pressure?
→ What structures are traversed by the spinal needle during lumbar puncture (from skin to deep)?

↑ **Example viva question**

What might a burr hole be used for?

Burr holes are used for procedures that require limited intracranial access:

- Immediate relief of an **acute extradural haematoma** or acute subdural haematoma as a **holding measure** before performing a formal craniotomy procedure
- Treatment of chronic subdural haematoma
- Placement of a **ventriculostomy catheter** (external ventricular drain or **EVD**)
- Placement of an **intraparenchymal pressure monitor** ('bolt')
- Access for some **stereotactic neurosurgery**, including brain biopsy for tumour pathology
- Burr holes can be used to allow insertion of a craniotome for the formation of a free bone flap in more extensive neurological operations.

POSITIONING A BURR HOLE

Principles of burr hole placement are **away** from **major venous sinuses** and air sinuses and not overlying eloquent brain. The following are common sites for placement:

- **Frontal** (usually 1–2 cm in front of coronal suture in the midpupillary line to avoid the primary motor cortex)

- **Parietal** – overlying the parietal eminence
- **Occipital**
- **Temporal** (commonly used in the case of an acute extradural haematoma).

Technique

A classic technique for the fashioning a burr hole is described below, but this is rapidly being replaced with either a relatively wide twist–drill technique or the use of a mechanical perforator (Midas Rex or similar):

- Position patient on horseshoe head cushion
- Check side on computed tomography (CT), which must be displayed in theatre
- Shave scalp and prepare it with alcohol solution
- Prepare skin and drape having **marked midline** and **incision**. Drape as if for a **craniotomy**. Plan incision so that **trauma flap** could be raised if necessary
- Incision down to bone approximately 4 cm in length
- Use **periosteal elevator** to scrape back periosteum
- Insert small self-retaining **retractor** – this should stop all skin edge and galeal bleeding
- Use the **perforator** attached to a **Hudson brace** to perforate the outer table of the skull. Continue using the instrument until the inner table has just been perforated and a small amount of shiny dura can be seen. A conical hole should be the result (in the case of an extradural, at this stage dark clot and altered blood should be expressed)
- Swap the perforator for the **burr** and **widen the hole** to its base without damaging the underlying dura
- If subdural access is needed, score the dura with a no. 15 blade and pick up with a dural hook. Cut onto the dural hook to fashion a cruciate opening of the dura
- Use **monopolar diathermy** to coagulate dural leaves
- **Closure**: 2/0 Vicryl to galea and clips or 3/0 nylon to skin.

Complications

- Extradural bleeding
- 'Plunging' and damage of underlying structures
- Infection: ventriculitis, subdural empyema
- Venous sinus damage and possible air embolism
- Cerebrospinal fluid (CSF) leak possible if dura opened.

LUMBAR PUNCTURE

Lumbar puncture should be performed **below** the **level** at which the **spinal cord ends** (L1 in an adult, but lower in a child as a result of differential growth).

It allows the sampling of CSF and the measurement of the CSF pressure.

Indications

CSF sampling
- Infection in bacterial or viral meningitis
- Xanthochromia in subarachnoid haemorrhage
- Cell count in suspected ventriculitis via EVD.

Pressure – diagnostic and treatment
Suspected raised intracranial pressure. **Note that this must never be performed for this indication unless CT reveals widely patent perimesencephalic cisterns and no obvious mass effect. Inappropriate use of the technique in these cases can lead to coning and death.**

Technique

- Aseptic technique
- Skin preparation and drape
- Local anaesthetic infiltration 1 per cent lidocaine
- **Midline approach** usually at **L3–4, L4–5 or L5–S1 interspace**; spinal needle directed at a cranial angle of 10–20°
- 'Pop' is often felt as the **ligamentum flavum** is traversed
- Remove stylet in spinal needle
- Allow CSF to drip from the needle – **never aspirate**
- Quickly place manometer on spinal needle and read off pressure on column of CSF (**normal opening pressure 5–10 cmH$_2$O**)
- Remove manometer and replace stylet once sufficient CSF has been expressed
- Remove spinal needle
- Patient should remain flat for at least 30 min to prevent a low pressure headache.

↑ **Example viva question**

What structures are traversed by the spinal needle during lumbar puncture (from skin to deep)?

- Skin
- Subcutaneous tissue
- Fat
- Supraspinous ligament
- Interspinous ligament
- Ligamentum flavum
- Epidural fat
- Dura
- Arachnoid into subarachnoid space

---

27 Carotid endarterectomy

Possible viva questions related to this topic

→ What are the indications for performing a carotid endarterectomy (CEA)?
→ Are you aware of any trials that support CEA?
→ Which preoperative imaging modalities are commonly employed to establish the diagnosis of carotid stenosis?
→ How do you perform a CEA?
→ What is a shunt and when is it used?
→ What are the potential complications of performing a CEA?
→ Which cranial nerves may be injured during a CEA?
→ How is the patient monitored perioperatively? What is transcranial Doppler (TCD)?

Related topics

Topic	Chapter	Page
Atherosclerosis	49	177
Brain-stem death and transplantation	106	423

INDICATIONS

Large randomized trials have now provided reliable data identifying who should undergo surgery.

Several thousand patients are randomized to **surgery with appropriate medical therapy** or **medical therapy alone.**

North American Symptomatic Carotid Endarterectomy Trial (NASCET)
- CEA beneficial to patients with a symptomatic carotid stenosis with 70–99 per cent (but not occlusion)
- Follow-up: 2-year risk of ipsilateral stroke reduced by CEA from 26 per cent to 9 per cent ($P < 0.001$)
- 30-day perioperative stroke and death rate was 5.8 per cent
- Numbers needed to treat (NNT) to prevent one ipsilateral stroke in 2 years = 6.

European Carotid Surgery Trial (ECST) – mirrored NASCET findings
- CEA reduced absolute stroke risk and death over 3 years from 21.9 per cent to 12.3 per cent ($P < 0.01$)
- 30-day perioperative stroke and death rate was 7.5 per cent.

Recent data also suggest that maximum benefit is gained if CEA is done within 2 weeks of symptoms.

Asymptomatic patients (no focal symptoms within 6 months)

The Asymptomatic Carotid Atherosclerosis Study (ACAS)
- Recruited patients with **60–99 per cent stenosis**
- **5-year rate** of **ipsilateral stroke** and **death** twice as high in the control group (11 per cent versus 5.1 per cent for CEA patients)
- 67 patients needed to have CEA to prevent one disabling stroke or death in 2 years!

Asymptomatic Carotid Surgery Trial (ACST)
- Patients allocated **immediate** versus **delayed CEA**
- **Immediate CEA halved the net 5-year stroke risk from 12 to 6 per cent,** including the 3 per cent perioperative hazard, in **asymptomatic patients aged less than 75 years** with a **carotid stenosis of 70 per cent** or more.

The trialists cautioned that, despite trial recommendations, either an inappropriate selection of patients or technically poor surgery with a higher than 3 per cent complication rate will obviate any benefit to the patient from intervention. CEA in a selected subpopulation of asymptomatic patients should be considered as a long-term (> 5 years) stroke prevention strategy.

Example viva question

Which patients benefit from CEA?

- Symptomatic patients with a > 70 per cent carotid artery stenosis
- Asymptomatic patients aged less than 75 years with at least 70 per cent carotid stenosis
- Other indications include lesser degrees of stenosis in symptomatic individuals, who may have a dominant hemisphere largely supplied by that artery and whose contralateral vessel is occluded

---

SURGICAL (CONVENTIONAL) TECHNIQUE

Preoperative considerations

- **Preoperative assessment** should include an up-to-date (< 2 weeks) **carotid duplex. Digital subtraction angiography** (DSA) can also be done

- Today, a **magnetic resonance angiogram** (MRA) is routinely performed
- **Appropriate management** of other **co-morbidities**: half deaths after CEA are the result of cardiac disease
- **Preoperative check** of **recurrent laryngeal** and **hypoglossal nerve** function if patient has undergone a previous CEA or thyroidectomy. Bilateral injury of either nerve is fatal
- Symptomatic patients should also have a **preoperative head CT** or **MRI** because < 2 per cent patients have other **significant brain pathology**, including malignant tumours (dangerous to operate on).

Procedure

- Usually performed under **general anaesthetic**
- **Loupe magnification**
- **Head** is **extended** and **turned away** from the side of operation and placed on a **rubber ring** slightly head up
- **Incision**: centred over the **anterior border of sternocleidomastoid** muscle from ear lobe to sternal notch, angling behind the ear if necessary for a high bifurcation
- Dissection continued down to the **carotid bifurcation**
- Dividing the **common facial vein** may be necessary for exposure
- Retract **internal jugular vein** laterally. **Carotid vessels** are **controlled with slings**, although the authors do not subscribe to slinging the internal carotid artery (ICA) because of the potential of dislodging thrombus
- **Infiltrate carotid sinus** with **1 per cent lidocaine** to prevent reflex hypotension and bradycardia
- Mobilize ICA 1 cm beyond the upper limit of the plaque
- **Identify** and **conserve** principal cranial nerves:
  - ○ vagus (X)
  - ○ hypoglossal (XII)
  - ○ glossopharyngeal (IX) – only with high dissections
- **Systemic heparinization** (5000 units)
- **Apply soft clamps** to **distal ICA, common carotid artery** (CCA) and **external carotid artery** (ECA) in that order
- Make a **longitudinal arteriotomy** from the distal CCA across the plaque and into the ICA beyond the stenosis using a no. 11 blade and Pott's scissors
- A shunt may be required at this point if there is any evidence under local anaesthetic of neurological hemispherical symptoms, or under general anaesthetic of inadequate cross-flow on transcranial Doppler (TCD) or other measures of cerebral blood flow.
- Enter **endarterectomy plane** using a Watson–Cheyne dissector
- It is conventional to divide the plaque first at the CCA aspect and then carefully mobilize it up to the ICA, where it is cut **transversely** using micro-scissors to **avoid leaving an intimal flap**

- **Tack down** any **intimal flaps** using fine interrupted Prolene sutures (6/0 or 7/0)
- Remove all loose intimal fragments
- **Close arteriotomy** either:
  - **primarily**: running 6/0 Prolene suture
  - **patch** (prosthetic or long saphenous vein)
- Before final couple of sutures flush with **heparin saline**
- **Restore flow**: ECA before ICA to minimize chances of embolization of any loose material within the lumen or clot proximal to the CCA clamp.

Postoperatively

- Check for any neurological deficit
- Patient should be further monitored in a high dependency setting.

Perioperative monitoring

The **principle of monitoring** is to correct and/or prevent cerebral ischaemia before onset of permanent neurological injury.

Transcranial Doppler is the most versatile and practical of available methods. It can:

- Anticipate requirement and urgency for shunting
- Diagnose intraoperative embolization, thereby permitting early ICA clamping in patients with unstable plaques
- Ensure optimal shunt function
- Can also detect **postoperative hyperperfusion** and **monitor treatment response**.

TCD uses a **low frequency (2 MHz) pulsed-wave ultrasound beam** directed through the **thin temporal bone**. This permits **insonation** of the middle cerebral artery (MCA), which receives **80 per cent of the ICA inflow**.

The quality of the signal depends on the thickness of the cranium. An **inaccessible window** is present in about **10 per cent of patients**.

Neurological activity can be evaluated directly by performing a CEA under **local anaesthetic**. This is a sensitive method of detecting **clamp ischaemia** and is the gold standard in determining who needs a shunt, although it will **not prevent thromboembolic complications**.

Shunt

This is a **conduit**, usually made of **plastic**, which **diverts blood flow** around the surgically opened carotid artery **while the endarterectomy** is **performed**. A shunt is used to **ensure adequate cerebral perfusion**.

- **Routine** versus **selective** use

Decision to use a shunt:

- **Intraoperative assessment**: temporary clamping of ICA under local anaesthetic
- **Stump pressure measurement** (back pressure of ICA after clamping): used to assess the adequacy of cerebral perfusion (about 40 mmHg)
- **TCD or other methods of cerebral blood flow monitoring**.

SURGICAL COMPLICATIONS

Intraoperative

Cerebral ischaemia leading to **neurological deficits** in **about 2 per cent**.

- Embolization of debris during vessel manipulation
- Poor flushing technique after arteriotomy closure
- Hypotension or poor protection during cross-clamping.

Cranial nerve injuries
- Hypoglossal (XII)
- Vagus (X)
- Mandibular branch of the facial nerve (V_e)
- Spinal accessory nerve
- Glossopharyngeal nerve (IX) – more common after high carotid artery dissections
- Superior laryngeal nerve (branch of vagus).

Overall rate of **cranial nerve injury 8.6 per cent**, although **92 per cent** are **transient** (NASCET findings).

Early

Thirty-day perioperative stroke and death rates between **5.8 and 7.3 per cent** in symptomatic individuals (NASCET + ECST data).

Asymptomatic patients − 2–4 per cent.

Medical problems
NASCET reported that **about 10 per cent** of surgical patients suffered a medical complication **within 30 days** of the operation; **70 per cent** were of **short duration** and resulted in only **2.7 per cent of patients** having **prolonged stays**.

Severe medical complications included:

- Myocardial infarction
- Arrhythmia
- Congestive cardiac failure
- Severe hypertension
- Severe hypotension.

Wound haematoma – large or rapidly expanding haematomas require urgent re-exploration, because there is a risk of airway obstruction.

Hyperperfusion syndrome

- Uncommon but dangerous
- Hyperaemic cerebral perfusion can cause cerebral oedema and haemorrhagic stroke
- Patients complains of a severe headache that improves with blood pressure control.

Wound infection

Late

- False aneurysm formation
- **Re-stenosis** (wide range of 2–36!) – found to be lower if **patch angioplasty** is employed to close arteriotomy.

28 Carpal tunnel decompression

Possible viva questions related to this topic

→ What are the signs and symptoms of carpal tunnel syndrome?
→ What are the risk factors for developing carpal tunnel syndrome?
→ What other conditions should be excluded and what investigations would you perform to establish a diagnosis?
→ What is the flexor retinaculum and what are its attachments?
→ What structures lie within the carpal tunnel?
→ What are the surgical options?
→ Where would you place your incision for carpal tunnel decompression?
→ Describe the surgical approach to carpal tunnel decompression.
→ How do you differentiate the median nerve from the flexor tendons?
→ How would you minimize sensory loss over the thenar eminence?
→ What are the possible surgical complications?
→ What is the predicted outcome?

The **carpal tunnel** is a space on the **ventral surface** of the **wrist** between the bony gutter of the concave carpus and the overlying flexor retinaculum.

Carpal tunnel syndrome occurs when there is an **increase** in **pressure** within this tunnel, leading to **compression** of the **median nerve**.

↑ **Example viva question**

What is the flexor retinaculum and what are its attachments?

The **flexor retinaculum** is a **strong band of fibrous tissue** attached to four bony points on the **volar** aspect of the wrist. Its attachments are:

Laterally (radial): scaphoid tubercle, ridge of trapezium
Medially (ulnar): pisiform and hook of hamate

Contents of the carpal tunnel: think **11** structures – **10** tendons and **1** nerve:

- Median nerve (most **superficial** structure)
- Flexor digitorum superficialis $\times$ 4
- Flexor digitorum profundus $\times$ 4
- Flexor pollicis longus
- Flexor carpi radialis

RISK FACTORS

- Idiopathic (common)
- Obesity
- Rheumatoid arthritis
- Diabetes mellitus
- Thyroid dysfunction
- Acromegaly
- Amyloid (infiltration of the flexor retinaculum)
- Pregnancy
- Ganglion
- Repetitive use of vibrating tools
- Tight bandaging and plaster immobilization – especially when the wrist is immobilized in extreme flexion after a fracture
- Trauma – distal radius fractures.

SYMPTOMS AND SIGNS

- Patient typically wakes at **night** with **burning pain, numbness** or **tingling** in the **hand**, typically relieved by hanging the arm out of bed and shaking it
- **Pain** and **paraesthesiae** in the distribution of the median nerve
- **Wasting** of the **thenar** muscles
- **Signs**: positive **Tinel's** (tapping over the median nerve at the wrist reproduces the tingling sensation) and **Phalen's** (maximal flexion of wrist for 1 minute exacerbates the symptoms, which are promptly relieved when the flexion is

discontinued). This is more important in clinical practice. Time to symptoms is inversely proportional to the severity
- **Preserved sensation** over the thenar eminence.

DIFFERENTIAL DIAGNOSIS AND INVESTIGATIONS

- Symptoms and signs may mimic a C6–7 cervical spondylosis
- Cervical spine radiographs or magnetic resonance imaging (MRI) may demonstrate degenerative changes, causing confusion
- Nerve conduction studies:
  - sensory nerve velocities most helpful
  - compare with ulnar nerve velocities
- MRI may be useful in identifying soft-tissue space-occupying lesions in the tunnel.

TREATMENT OPTIONS

Non-surgical

- Wrist splintage at night
- Hydrocortisone injections into the carpal tunnel, diuretics
- Correctable causes investigated and appropriately treated.

Surgical

- Carpal tunnel decompression:
  - open
  - endoscopic (Chow's method) using a two-port technique. Thought to minimize scarring, lower incidence of wound complications and allow earlier return to work.

SURGICAL PROCEDURE

Use an **anterior (volar)** approach.

Preoperative

- This operation can be done under a local (Bier's block) anaesthetic, direct local anaesthetic into the palm or general anaesthetic
- A tourniquet on the upper arm is mandatory for a bloodless operative field
- Arm is laid supine on the side table.
- Clean the forearm and fingers and drape the limb, but leave fingers and hand exposed.

Perioperative

- **Incision: longitudinal** from **distal flexor crease** to **transverse palmar crease**. This is in line with the radial border of the ring finger, avoiding damage to the palmar cutaneous branch of the median nerve.

- Incision is deepened down through the longitudinal fibres of the palmar aponeurosis to expose the transverse fibres of the flexor retinaculum.
- A small self-retaining retractor is placed.
- A **MacDonald dissector** is placed under the flexor retinaculum, which is then incised longitudinally with a scalpel down to the retinaculum. This exposes the median nerve.
- **Inadequate decompression** and persistent symptoms can be a problem if the proximal part of the retinaculum has not been adequately released where it disappears under the skin in the proximal aspect of the wound. This should be released with the Macdonald dissector along the surface of the median nerve
- In **rheumatoid arthritis** there may be an associated hypertrophic synovium affecting the flexor tendons. Therefore, perform a **flexor synovectomy** by stripping the synovium with a pair of fine bone nibblers.

Closure

- Deflate tourniquet
- Achieve meticulous haemostasis
- Close skin with interrupted Prolene sutures
- Apply compression bandaging
- Should be replaced with an adhesive dressing in 24 hours
- Elevation of hand recommended
- Early finger exercises encouraged
- Remove sutures at 10 days.

SURGICAL COMPLICATIONS

- **Infection**
- **Haemorrhage**
- **Scar tenderness** – can occur in up to 40 per cent of patients
- **Nerve damage**
  - median nerve itself
  - recurrent motor branch of the median nerve; this innervates the thenar muscles. Division will cause wasting of these muscles and impede fine movements of the hand
  - palmar cutaneous branch of the median nerve; this supplies sensation to the skin over the thenar eminence. Division will result in paraesthesiae
- **Recurrent symptoms** caused by inadequate decompression
- **Scar formation** – this is a high-risk area for keloid or hypertrophic scars
- **Reflex sympathetic dystrophy** (RSD).

PREDICTED OUTCOME

- Improvement in symptoms in **85 per cent of patients**
- Thenar muscle wasting may resolve.

29 Circumcision

Possible viva questions related to this topic

→ What are the indications for a circumcision?
→ What are the causes of a phimosis?
→ Describe your method of performing the operation.
→ Is there an alternative method in infants?
→ What methods of postoperative pain relief can be useful after circumcision?
→ What are the risks and complications of performing a circumcision?

↑ **Example viva question**

What are the indications for a circumcision?

Medical versus religious.

Medical
- Phimosis
- Senile
- Balanitis xerotica obliterans (BXO)
- Squamous cell carcinoma of the prepuce
- Paraphimosis (irreducible)
- Recurrent urinary tract infections
- Recurrent balanitis

PHIMOSIS

- **Congenital**: as a result of congenital adhesions between the glans and foreskin; it is not normally possible to retract the foreskin in the first year of life
- **Acquired**: commonly the result of BXO; can also be senile.

PROCEDURE

- Patient laid **supine** under **general** anaesthetic.
- The surgery is covered with **intravenous antibiotics** if there has been **any evidence of infection**, e.g. balanitis.

- **Penile block** performed.
- External genitalia prepared with aqueous antiseptic and draped accordingly.
- **Prepuce** retracted and glans beneath cleaned. **Preputial adhesions** freed using a **silver probe** or **artery forceps**. If foreskin too tight to retract, a dorsal slit may need to be performed.
- Two straight artery forceps placed side by side on the **dorsum** of the foreskin and scissors used to divide the foreskin between the two clips to a level about **5 mm** below the **corona**.
- The incision then carefully continued **circumferentially** by a **freehand** technique in either direction around the penis, keeping about 5 mm *below* the corona until the incisions meet at the frenulum.
- **Frenulum** picked up with another artery forceps and redundant skin excised.
- **Frenulum** and its **artery transfixed** or a **box stitch** used to create haemostasis. Bleeding vessels along the way either clipped and tied with an **undyed dissolvable suture** such as 3/0 Vicryl or coagulated with **bipolar diathermy**.
- After obtaining careful haemostasis, **ridge of skin below the corona and free edge** of the foreskin remaining down the shaft **opposed** with **interrupted absorbable suture** – in the authors' experience Vicryl Rapide.
- **Topical lidocaine** (2 per cent) gel applied to the distal end of the penis.
- Penis loosely dressed in **paraffin gauze** and then dry gauze.
- Postoperative instructions would include a **daily bath** with good amount of analgesia.
- In **sexually active** men, they should be warned to **refrain** from **intercourse** until the wound is fully healed, which will take least **2–3 weeks**.
- The foreskin should be sent for **histology** if **BXO** or **carcinoma** is suspected.

Postoperative analgesia

- All circumcisions should be performed with either a **caudal** or a **penile block** *in situ*. This makes the postoperative period more comfortable.
- Insertion of a **non-steroidal anti-inflammatory** suppository just before the end of the general anaesthetic will also give good analgesia for the first 12 hours.
- Oral analgesia can be used thereafter. Patients should not need an epidural or patient-controlled analgesia (PCA).

INFANTS

Commercial devices such as the **Plastibell (Hollister)** instrument have been used but have proved to be generally unsuccessful. The foreskin is freed and retracted. The Plastibell is slipped over the glans penis and the foreskin ligated and divided in the groove of the instrument. The foreskin is cut and removed.

↑ **Example viva question**

What are the complications?

- Infection
- Bleeding
- Haematoma
- Excision of too much skin
- Injury to the glans penis, degloving injury
- Breakdown of wound
- Urinary retention
- Psychological morbidity
- Urethrocutaneous fistula
- Meatal stenosis
- Ischaemia and necrosis of the distal part of the penis
- Need to repeat circumcision

30 Emergency splenectomy

FUNCTIONS OF THE SPLEEN

- **Fetus**: major site for **haematopoiesis**
- **Childhood**: produces **Immunoglobulin M (IgM)**
- **Adult**: acts as a **filter** – allows **resident macrophages** to remove **abnormal erythrocytes, cellular debris** and **encapsulated poorly opsonized bacteria**.

INDICATIONS FOR EMERGENCY SPLENECTOMY

- **Traumatic rupture**: normally following road traffic accident (RTA) or violent falls
  - ○ **mechanism of injury**: direct blunt force; deceleration and compression injuries to the left side of the abdomen
- **Spontaneous rupture**: in enlargement.

SIGNS AND SYMPTOMS OF SPLENIC INJURY

- **Left upper quadrant pain** (stretching of the splenic capsule)
- **Peritonitis** (from extravasated blood)
- **Kehr's sign**: referred left shoulder tip pain resulting from diaphragmatic irritation by extravasated blood
- **Associated injuries,** e.g. left-sided lower rib fractures and bruising.

INDICATIONS FOR OPERATIVE MANAGEMENT

Conservative management

May be possible in **minor injury** (grades I–III) and where there is no evidence of haemodynamic instability.

Surgery indicated in:

- **Haemodynamic instability** or **peritonitis**
- **Persistent coagulopathy and bleeding**
- **Additional intra-abdominal injury** requiring surgical intervention
- **Confounding injury**: an additional injury that interferes with patient's monitoring, e.g. pelvic fracture with continuing bleeding
- **Worsening pain** and **tenderness**
- **Severe splenic injury**: grades **IV + V**.

PROCEDURE

- Patient is laid **supine**.
- **Anaesthetic** is **general**.
- Prepared and draped from **nipple** to **groin**.
- Intravenous **penicillin** (or suitable alternative in allergic individuals) given at induction.
- A **nasogastric tube** should be placed because of the risk of **acute gastric distension** after the procedure.
- **Upper midline incision** ($\pm$T-shaped extension).
- Check that spleen is the cause of the bleed and, if so, proceed with splenectomy before inspecting the rest of the abdomen.
- Mobilize spleen and deliver it into the abdominal wound by dividing the **lienorenal ligament**.
- **Compress vascular pedicle** between the finger and thumb.
- Enter **lesser sac** by dividing the greater omentum between ligatures.
- Palpate the **splenic artery**, which lies superior to the pancreas. Mobilize and then ligate it with 0 Vicryl ties.

- Free the **left colic flexure** from the spleen.
- Free **attachments** to the **diaphragm**.
- Ligate and divide the **gastrosplenic ligament** along with the **short gastric vessels**.
- Double ligate and divide the splenic vessels but **beware** of the **tail of the pancreas**.
- **Pack** the **splenic bed** and achieve haemostasis.
- A **drain** should be placed in the splenic bed and secured.
- Mass closure with looped 1/0 nylon or PDS.

COMPLICATIONS

- **Chest infection**
- **Subphrenic abscess**
- **Bleeding**
- **Damage to adjacent structures**:
  - stomach
  - splenic flexure of colon
  - diaphragm
  - pancreas: pancreatic fistula (damage to the pancreatic tail during ligation of splenic vessels), so will be beneficial to drain – analyse drain fluid for grossly elevated amylase
- **Overwhelming post-splenectomy sepsis (OPSS)**: see below
- **Small bowel obstruction**: loops of small bowel may adhere to a raw area underneath the diaphragm on the left side
- **Acute gastric dilatation**: hence importance of a nasogastric tube
- **Development of splenunculi**: splenic tissue shed during the operation may undergo hypertrophy – no bad thing in the trauma setting!
- **Infections**: more prone to certain infections (see 'Prophylaxis' below)
- **Malaria**: more susceptible to the effects of malaria. Post-splenectomy patients no longer have a spleen to sequester infected red blood cells and therefore harbour a higher parasite load. These people should be advised not to visit malaria endemic zones
- **Thrombocytosis**: usually after splenectomy for **hypersplenism** occurring in the **first 48 hours**. There is usually a **rise** in **white cell** and **platelet counts**, often confused with a picture of sepsis.

Overwhelming post-splenectomy sepsis (OPSS)

- Typically caused by **encapsulated bacteria**, the most common being:
  - pneumococcal (50 per cent)
  - meningococcal
  - *Escherichia coli*
  - *Haemophilus influenzae*

- Symptoms and signs are a flu-like prodromal illness followed by headache, fever, malaise, coma, adrenal haemorrhage and circulatory collapse
- Affects 2 per cent of trauma splenectomies – OPSS is greatest if splenectomy performed during infancy
- Occurs usually within 2 years of operation
- Mortality rate is high: 50–90 per cent
- Prevented primarily by immunization (see below).

PROPHYLAXIS

All elective and emergency patients undergoing splenectomy should receive **prophylactic immunization** against:

- *Haemophilus influenzae*: **Hibivax**
- *Streptococcus pneumoniae*: **Pneumovax**
- *Neisseria meningitidis* strain C: **Meningiovax**.

In the **emergency scenario** this should be given **postoperatively** but **not** while the patient is **haemodynamically unstable** because this can lead to further compromise.

Penicillin prophylaxis (or suitable alternative if allergic) should also be prescribed. **Duration** is **debatable**. Some surgeons advocate lifelong prophylaxis whereas others suggest a shorter interval of around 2 years, with a low threshold for antibiotic treatment in the advent of any infection. **Infants** are recommended to continue to take it until adulthood.

SUCCESSFUL CONSERVATIVE TREATMENT

Most patients who fail conservative management do so within **5 days**.

If initial management is successful, obtain a **follow-up ultrasound scan** at **5 days** to document non-progression of splenic injury. A **post-discharge CT scan** is advised **6 weeks** after injury to **confirm complete healing**. The patient should be advised to refrain from **contact sports** for **3 months**.

31 Femoral and brachial embolectomy

Possible viva questions related to this topic

→ How do you perform a femoral embolectomy?
→ What surface landmarks are used to locate the femoral artery?
→ What are the boundaries of the femoral triangle?
→ What are the contents of the femoral triangle and their relationships?
→ What are the contents of the femoral canal and what are its borders?
→ When is a femoral embolectomy indicated?
→ What are the presenting features of acute critical ischaemia of the limb?
→ What are the causes of this problem?
→ How is thrombus distinguished from embolus in acute ischaemia?
→ How would you manage a patient with acute critical ischaemia of the lower limb?
→ What are the complications associated with the vertical groin incision?
→ How would you approach performing a brachial embolectomy?

Related topics

Topic	Chapter	Page
Femoral hernia repair	32	102
The femoral triangle	8	24

ACUTE CRITICAL LIMB ISCHAEMIA

↑ **MRCS viva**

What are the clinical features of acute critical limb ischaemia?

Learn the six 'Ps'.

Sudden onset of:

Pain
Pallor
Pulselessness
Paraesthesiae
Paralysis
Perishing cold (poikilothermia)

Causes

- **Embolic**: most commonly arise from the following sites:
  - ○ **heart,** either from **left ventricular** mural **thrombus** following an acute **myocardial infarction** and **congestive cardiac failure,** or from the **left atrium** in **atrial fibrillation**
  - ○ **peripheral blood vessels**: **aortic** or **popliteal aneurysm, iliofemoral stenoses**
- **Acute thrombosis** of an already atherosclerotic segment of artery.

It is often **difficult** to make the **distinction** between **thrombosis** and an **embolus** in the **lower limb**.

Findings suggestive of **embolus** include:

- No prior history of vascular disease
- Normal contralateral leg circulation
- History of cardiac arrhythmia or recent myocardial infarction
- Patients with **embolic disease** who frequently have **profound leg ischaemia** caused by the **proximal nature** of the occlusion (aortic or femoral bifurcation) and the **absence** of **developed collaterals**
- Angiography is usually required to distinguish between the two.

Principles of management

- **Medical treatment** – liaise with medical colleagues
- Treat **atrial fibrillation**, e.g. with **digoxin** after confirmation with an ECG
- Treatment of arterial embolism – intravenous **analgesia** and **heparinization**
- Emergency **angiogram + thrombolysis** (with streptokinase or tissue plasminogen activator) if there are the facilities to do so
- This should be followed by **heparinization** and commencement of **warfarin** for at least **6 months**
- Further cardiac investigations such as an **echocardiogram**
- **Surgical** option would be **femoral embolectomy**.

The choice between the two therapies depends on the **degree** of the ischaemia.

Patients who have developed **paralysis** or **paraesthesiae** of the limb should proceed **promptly** to **embolectomy** irrespective of the aetiology, because there may be significant delay to reperfusion when the time that it takes for angiography and thrombolysis is taken into account.

Embolectomy is indicated in:

- Common femoral artery proximal to groin
- Brachial and axillary arteries.

More **distal emboli** can be treated by **thrombolysis**.

A non-viable limb should not be re-vascularized.

Patient should give **consent** for **bypass grafting** and **amputation** in case the leg becomes unsalvageable.

FEMORAL EMBOLECTOMY

- Patient is fully **heparinized**.
- The **anaesthetic** is either **local** or **general**. **Local** is usually **preferred** considering the likely number of other co-morbidities that the patient will have.
- The leg is cleaned and draped as appropriate but with the foot put into a **transparent sterile bag** so that reperfusion can be assessed later.
- **Vertical incision** centred over the midpoint at the groin crease is made directly over the artery. **Landmarks**: femoral artery lies at the **midinguinal point** – midway between the **anterior superior iliac spine** and the **pubic symphysis**.
- Deepen incision over the artery by cutting through subcutaneous fat and staying **medial** to sartorius. Expose **femoral sheath**. Incise it longitudinally to expose the femoral artery.
- Pass a Lahey retractor **posteriorly and sling the artery with sloupes such that both proximal and distal control** are achieved. The **profunda femoris** should also be exposed and slung.
- A suitable size of **Fogarty catheter** is selected (size **3F** or **4F** femoral catheters) and the **balloon tested** with saline.
- **Arteriotomy** is performed over the origin of the profunda – ideally **transverse** because it **reduces** the risk of **stenosis** on closure.
- The **uninflated** catheter is passed proximally through the vessel beyond the site of the clot. The **balloon** is **inflated** and the catheter withdrawn slowly until the catheter is pulled out through the arteriotomy and the embolus recovered.
- The assistant is asked to pull on the sloupes for haemostasis.
- This procedure is repeated **proximally** and **distally** until no further clot is retrieved.
- The proximal and distal artery are flushed with **heparinized saline**.
- The arteriotomy is closed **transversely** with **4/0 Prolene sutures**.
- A suction drain can be placed within the wound upon closure.

Complications associated with the vertical groin incision

- Wound infection
- Haematoma
- Lymphocoele/persistent lymph leak
- Flap necrosis and/or scarring.

↑ **Key learning points**

Brachial embolectomy

The brachial artery may have to be exposed in order to **dislodge** an **embolus** or for exploration after **trauma**.

Similar principles and procedure as a femoral embolectomy.

Medial approach

Incision made in the line of the artery along the **medial edge** of **biceps muscle**. The **basilic vein** and the **medial cutaneous nerve** of the forearm are **superficial** to the deep fascia at this level.

The **deep fascia** is **divided** and the inner fibres of the **biceps muscle** are **retracted upwards**. The brachial artery should then be found **lying** on the **triceps muscle** with the **median nerve anterior** to it.

Lying with the brachial artery are two **venae comitantes**.

Anterior (antecubital fossa) approach

Useful when it is deemed necessary to **embolectomize** the **radial** and **ulnar arteries** separately. However, the brachial artery may bifurcate high in the arm.

Sigmoid-shaped incision.

The distal end of the brachial artery lies in the antecubital fossa. By dividing the **bicipital aponeurosis** the brachial artery is exposed, with the **medial cubital vein** crossing it obliquely. The **median nerve** lies medial to the **brachial artery** and the **radial nerve** lies inferior to the **brachioradialis** muscle.

Close the brachial artery with a **vein patch** or use a **transverse incision**.

32 Femoral hernia repair

Related topics

Topic	Chapter	Page
Femoral and brachial embolectomy	31	98
Inguinal hernia repair	33	106
The femoral triangle	8	24

Example viva question

What are the boundaries of the femoral canal?

Medial: lacunar ligament
Lateral: femoral vein
Anterior: inguinal ligament
Posterior: pectineal ligament

- Generally a **femoral hernia**, if present, should be **repaired promptly** because it has a **narrow neck** and is more likely to **obstruct** or **strangulate** than an **inguinal hernia. Exceptions** can be made if the patient is **frail and elderly** and the hernia has been an **incidental finding**

- Fifty per cent strangulate within 1 month.
- More common in females because:
  - the inguinal ligament makes **wider angle** with pubis in females
  - **enlargement of fat** in middle age stretches the canal and this fat atrophies later, leaving a larger canal
  - **pregnancy** stretches **transversalis fascia**.

Example viva question

What are the differences between an inguinal and a femoral hernia?

	Inguinal hernia	Femoral hernia
Incidence	In males and females more common than femoral hernias	More common in females than males (4:1)
Obstruction and strangulation		See above. Furthermore a femoral hernia is more likely to strangulate without obstructing (**Richter's hernia**)
Position relative to the pubic tubercle	Superior and medial	Inferior and lateral
Palpation	Soft	Firm
Percussion	May be resonant	Dull
Auscultation	Bowel sounds commonly heard	Bowel sounds rarely heard

---

APPROACHES

Three approaches to the femoral canal have been described:

1. **Low (Lockwood) used for elective repair:**
   - appropriate for **non-strangulated** hernias
   - incision is 8–10 cm long in **groin crease, below medial half** of inguinal ligament.
2. **Transinguinal/high (Lotheissen):**
   Rarely used today but is **suitable** for **strangulated hernias**, because it affords suitable **access** for **bowel resection** but there is a **risk** of subsequent **inguinal hernia**. Incision as for **inguinal hernia**, then expose inguinal canal and dislocate spermatic cord laterally. Incise **transversalis fascia** as described in McEvedy's approach (below).
3. **Extraperitoneal (McEvedy)** – used for emergency repair.

Irrespective of approach, the following **principles** apply:

- **Dissection** and **mobilization** of the **femoral sac**
- **Inspection** and **reduction** of the **sac contents**
- **Ligation** of femoral sac
- **Femoral hernia repair**, which includes either **approximation** of the **inguinal** and **pectineal ligaments** or insertion of a **mesh plug** into the femoral canal.

STRANGULATED FEMORAL HERNIA REPAIR

An **extraperitoneal** or **McEvedy** approach should be used because it gives better **control** and **access** to inspect the affected loop of bowel and makes a **bowel resection** and **anastomosis easier** to **perform** if necessary.

Incision: **vertical** incision placed **2 cm** above the medial third of the inguinal ligament and extended proximally.

Go through:

- Skin
- Subcutaneous tissue
- Rectus sheath
- Rectus abdominis
- Transversalis fascia
- Peritoneum.

Divide **inferior epigastric vessels**:

- Hernia sac is held with two artery forceps and incised
- Bowel within hernia sac: bowel is drawn **downwards** and the **ligamentous margins** of the sac neck are **dilated** with two fingers forming a wedge
- **Bowel viability** is then assessed
- Pay due attention to the **constriction ring**
- If there is doubt about bowel wall viability (see below), cover it with a **warm saline-soaked pack** and re-examine in **5 mins**. If the bowel is not viable after this time, the affected segment is **resected** and **anastomosed** end to end with a one-layer extramucosal technique
- If, at any stage, access were **difficult** or the affected loop of bowel were to fall back into the abdomen and **not be recoverable**, you would perform a **laparotomy through a lower midline incision**
- Return the sac contents into the abdomen
- **Sac closed** with an **absorbable** suture (2/0 Vicryl) and excised 1 cm distal to the ligature
- Perform hernia repair by: **approximating inguinal and pectineal ligaments** using interrupted **non-absorbable monofilamentous suture (1/0 nylon)**. **Three** sutures

will usually suffice to narrow femoral ring. While this is done, care is taken to **protect** and **avoid constriction** of the laterally placed **femoral vein**. The authors personally **dissect out** the femoral vein before any repair because visualizing it prevents injury and problems with compression
- An alternative method of repair is to fill the femoral canal with a plug of **rolled mesh**, which may then be secured with sutures
- Closure:
  ○ subcutaneous tissue with 2/0 Vicryl
  ○ skin with 3/0 Monocryl.

Assessment of bowel viability

- **Viable bowel** = pink, visible peristalsis and **mesenteric pulsation, sheen** to bowel wall
- **Gangrenous bowel** = green, black or purple colour with a **malodour. There is no visible mesenteric pulsation** and the bowel wall would have lost its sheen.

In general, if there is **any doubt** about viability, it is best to **resect** it.

↑ Key learning points

The accessory obturator artery

Present in **50 per cent** of patients.

In **50 per cent** it has an **aberrant medial course** running **posterior** to the lacunar ligament.

Avoid dividing the **lacunar ligament** (the Hay–Groves manoeuvre) to dilate the femoral canal in cases where you need more access to perform a bowel resection. The authors would have a low threshold to converting to a laparotomy if this were the case.

---

33 Inguinal hernia repair

↑ **Key learning point**

Definition

A **hernia** is the **abnormal protrusion** of a **viscus** or **part** of a **viscus** through an **opening** in the **walls** of its **containing cavity** into **another body compartment**.

TYPES

- Indirect (60 per cent) (lies **lateral** to the **inferior epigastric artery**)
- Direct (35 per cent) (lies **medial** to **inferior epigastric artery**)
- Pantaloon (5 per cent) (combined).

SLIDING HERNIA

A **sliding hernia** is formed when a **retroperitoneal organ** protrudes outside the abdominal cavity in such a manner that the **organ itself** and a **peritoneal surface** constitute the **hernia sac**.

Organs that can be found **within** a sliding hernia include:

- Colon
- Caecum
- Appendix
- Ovary
- Bladder
- Fallopian tubes and uterus (rare).

INDICATIONS FOR INGUINAL HERNIA REPAIR

- Symptomatic
- Incarcerated
- Strangulated.

↑ **Example viva question**

What is the anatomy of the inguinal canal?

- **4 cm tunnel** in the lower abdominal muscles
- Runs **inferomedially** between the **deep** and **superficial** inguinal rings

Boundaries
Anterior wall: external oblique + internal oblique for lateral third
Roof: conjoint tendon
Floor: inguinal ligament
Posterior wall: transversalis fascia and conjoint tendon

Contents
Male: spermatic cord
Female: round ligament

↑ **Example viva question**

What is the spermatic cord?

Spermatic cord: extends from the deep inguinal ring to the posterosuperior border of the testicle.

Contents

Think of **12 structures!**

- **Coverings:**
  - external spermatic fascia
  - cremasteric fascia
  - internal spermatic fascia
- **Arteries:**
  - testicular
  - artery to vas
  - cremasteric
- **Vas deferens**
- **Veins:**
  - pampiniform plexus
- **Lymphatic vessels**
- **Nerves:**
  - **genital** branch of the **genitofemoral** nerve
  - **sympathetics**
- **Processus vaginalis.**

The **Royal College of Surgeons' guidelines** on hernia management suggest the **Liechtenstein repair** or **Shouldice technique** for primary uncomplicated inguinal hernias.

OPEN LIECHTENSTEIN REPAIR

- History and examination
- Exclude other causes of pain
- Gain informed consent
- Mark side
- Prophylactic antibiotics (particularly in an incarcerated hernia)
- Usually one shot of a broad-spectrum antibiotic, e.g. cefuroxime, at induction will suffice
- **General** or **local** anaesthetic can be used

- Shave pubic hair and prepare skin and drape appropriately
- **Incision: inguinal** or **skin crease**
- Identify **anterosuperior iliac spine** (ASIS) and **pubic tubercle**
- Place inguinal incision **2 cm above** and **along medial two-thirds** of **inguinal ligament**. Do not incise skin lower than mid-inguinal point (surface marking of deep inguinal ring)
- Ligate any large vessels with 2/0 Vicryl ties
- Divide Scarpa's fascia and deepen incision to the external oblique aponeurosis. Identify **inguinal ligament** and **superficial inguinal ring**
- Make a short fenestration in the line of the external oblique fibres. Beware: **do not** make split **too low**, otherwise there will be difficulty in closing the aponeurosis at the end of the operation
- Insert the scissors to separate the canal contents from the aponeurosis. This reduces risk of damage to the **ilioinguinal nerve**
- Now enlarge the slit medially and laterally to open the inguinal canal to include the **superficial ring**
- Apply forceps to each edge of the aponeurosis
- Apply self-retaining retractors
- Create 'pockets' above and below
- **Identify** and **conserve** the **ilioinguinal nerve** on the anterior aspect of the cord
- Mobilize the cord by dividing the mesentery just above and lateral to the pubic tubercle (blunt dissection)
- Apply a **hernia ring** or piece of tape
- Move the cord **downwards** and **laterally** and divide the coverings along a line just superior to it. This exposes the site of a direct hernia (**medial to the epigastric vessels**) in the **transversalis fascia**
- **Always exclude an indirect sac**: open the spermatic fascia covering the cord. Identify the sac and isolate it to the **level of the deep ring**
- **Identify** and **conserve** the **vas deferens**
- **Open** the **sac** and release the contents into the abdominal cavity. Beware of a sliding hernia. **Transfix** (with 2/0 Vicryl) and **divide** the hernia sac
- Apply a **polypropylene mesh** – cut into a 'fish' shape to repair and reinforce the **weakened posterior wall**
- The authors use a **2/0 Prolene suture on a J-shaped needle**; the mesh should be anchored to the **pubic tubercle**, the lower edge sutured to the **inguinal ligament** – avoid including any **external oblique fibres**
- **Overlap** the **lateral borders** ('fishtail') around the **cord** (reconstruction of the deep ring). Leave a slight gap of approximately **5 mm** around the spermatic cord
- Suture the **lateral** and **superior borders** of the mesh in place to the **underlying muscle** using interrupted 2/0 Prolene. This should be **'tension free'**; otherwise perform a **Tanner slide**

- **Closure**: infiltrate the wound in layers with **local anaesthetic** (make an effort to block the ilioinguinal nerve – thought to reduce postoperative pain):
  - 1/0 Vicryl to external oblique fascia
  - 2/0 Vicryl to Scarpa's fascia
  - 3/0 Monocryl to skin; Steri-Strips
- **Check ipsilateral testicle** is drawn down to the bottom of the scrotum
- **Postoperative advice**: avoid **heavy lifting for 6–8 weeks.**

↑ **Key learning point**

Hernia recurrence

Most commonplace is **medial recurrence**. Therefore, it is important to get mesh **far enough over** to the **midline**.

Direct hernias often recur at the **pubic tubercle** and **indirect hernias** recur at the **internal ring**.

Causes:

- Poorly placed or insufficient stitches
- Infection
- Poor tissue
- Poor collagen formation
- Surgical tension

SHOULDICE REPAIR

This was popularized at the **Shouldice Clinic** (Toronto) and is useful if **repairing a strangulated hernia when insertion of a mesh is not recommended as a result of high risk of infection**. This method **double breasts** the **transversalis fascia** and conjoint **tendon** with four continuous lines of non-absorbable suture to **reinforce** the **posterior wall** of the inguinal canal. The suture tract runs from the pubic tubercle to a new internal ring and results in layered approximation of the conjoint tendon to the inguinal ligament. In experienced hands, the reported incidence of recurrence is **1 per cent** – lowest rate of recurrence for non-mesh repairs.

LAPAROSCOPIC REPAIR

This is indicated in **bilateral inguinal hernias** and **recurrent hernias**. The mesh is stapled between the peritoneum and the fascia transversalis. The laparoscopic approach is either **transperitoneal (TAP)** or **total extraperitoneal (TEP)**.

COMPLICATIONS

General versus specific

Specific
- **Wound:**
  - bruising and haematoma
  - infection
  - sinus formation
- **Scrotal**:
  - ischaemic orchitis
  - testicular atrophy
  - hydrocoele
  - damage to vas deferens – infertility
- **Operation failure:**
  - recurrence (aim for 0.5 per cent 5-year recurrence rate)
  - missed hernia (usually indirect)
  - dehiscence
- **Nerve injuries**
- Must warn patient of risk of **postoperative chronic pain** (up to **30 per cent**).

34 Laparoscopic cholecystectomy and laparoscopy

Possible viva questions related to this topic

→ What are the contraindications to performing a laparoscopic cholecystectomy?

→ What important risks should be explained to the patient in obtaining consent for laparoscopic cholecystectomy?

→ What is Calot's triangle and why it is important to identify this landmark?

→ What are the important steps in performing a laparoscopic cholecystectomy? How many ports will you use?

→ How can you ensure that you are dividing the cystic artery rather than the right hepatic artery?

→ When would you perform an intraoperative cholangiogram? Why should it be encouraged?

→ How do you establish a pneumoperitoneum for laparoscopy?

→ What are the reported advantages of laparoscopic surgery over open surgery? What are some of the disadvantages?

Related topics		
Topic	Chapter	Page
DVT prophylaxis and coagulation in surgery	73	297
Functions of the liver	96	384
Biliary tree and gallbladder	5	17
Liver	10	28
Abdominal incisions	64	259

Currently in the **UK 90 per cent** of cholecystectomies are performed **laparoscopically**.

INFORMED CONSENT

Important risks associated with laparoscopic cholecystectomy include:

• Pain
• Haemorrhage
• Infection
• Common bile duct injury and possibility of jaundice
• Bowel injury requiring laparotomy
• Possibility of conversion to an open procedure (usually 1/40 – higher if previous abdominal surgery because of adhesions).

CONTRAINDICATIONS

Absolute

- Carcinoma of the gallbladder
- Severe chronic obstructive pulmonary disease (COPD)
- Bleeding diathesis
- Intraoperative:
  - unexpected pathology, e.g. severe cholecystitis, portal varices
  - inability to delineate anatomy safely
  - uncontrollable bleeding
  - adjacent organ damage.

Relative

- Liver: cirrhosis with portal hypertension
- Pregnancy
- Morbid obesity
- Previous abdominal surgery – adhesions causing difficult laparoscopic access and progress
- Acute cholecystitis.

CALOT'S TRIANGLE

Borders are:

- **Superiorly**: inferior surface of the liver
- **Laterally**: cystic duct
- **Medially**: common hepatic duct.

Contents are:

- **cystic artery** – this is a branch of the right hepatic artery
- cystic lymph node.

It is important to identify and dissect out Calot's triangle in order clearly to visualize the **cystic duct** and **artery** so that both structures can be clipped and divided safely.

PRINCIPLES OF SURGERY

Preparation

- Warn patient of risks (above)
- **Deep vein thrombosis (DVT) prophylaxis** – venous stasis can be induced by the **reverse Trendelenburg position** (see 'DVT prophylaxis and coagulation in surgery', Chapter 73, page 297)

- Single-dose **antibiotic prophylaxis** has been shown to **reduce wound infections** after cholecystectomy
- **Anaesthetic** is general
- Place patient on a **radiolucent operating table** in case an on-table cholangiogram is required
- **Skin preparation**: nipple to suprapubic region
- **Check** and **arrange leads** and **equipment**
- **Local anaesthetic** is administered to the skin where the port sites are made.

Access

- **Open Hasson technique** is advocated by the surgical Royal Colleges because **closed Veress needle** insertion is **blind** and thought to be **less safe**
- **Infraumbilical** incision
- Identify **umbilical cicatrix** and follow it down to the **junction** with the **linea alba** and make an incision
- Insert a pair of McIndoe's scissors and open the peritoneum. Introduce **10 mm camera port without the sharp trocar** under **direct vision**
- Create **pneumoperitoneum** by insufflating with **carbon dioxide. Low pressure** and **high flow** indicate correct positioning of the port in the peritoneal cavity. Aim for a pressure of **12–14 mmHg** but this varies according to the body habitus of the patient.

Dangers associated with high insufflation pressures

Respiratory
- Splinting of diaphragm leading to impaired gaseous exchange
- ↑ Risk spontaneous pneumothorax after higher inflation pressures by anaesthetist to compensate for this.

Cardiovascular
- Reduced venous return leading to reduced cardiac output
- Reduced venous return increases risk of DVT (venous stasis).

Assessment

- Examine whole of abdominal cavity methodically
- Decide whether laparoscopic approach is feasible
- If so, insert the three remaining ports under direct vision:
  - **10 mm epigastric** (subxiphisternal) port – just to the right of the midline
  - **5 mm midclavicular** line port
  - **5 mm anterior axillary line** (5 cm below costal margin) port – parallel to umbilicus
- Tilt head upwards (**reverse Trendelenburg's position**) and patient is rolled **towards** operator (left side)

- Grasp **fundus** of gallbladder using a **tissue-holding forceps** via the most lateral port and retract it in a **cephalad** direction over the liver. Ask the assistant to hold. This minimizes the fold in the gallbladder infundibulum and brings **Calot's triangle** more clearly into view
- Pull gallbladder away from the liver by **inferolateral traction** on **Hartmann's pouch**. This aids identification of the cystic and common bile ducts by pulling them out of alignment
- Start **dissecting high** on the **neck** of the gallbladder and proceed in a **lateral to medial direction**, keeping close to the gallbladder until the anatomy is well defined. The **cystic duct node** usually provides a useful starting point for the dissection
- **Define** and dissect out **Calot's triangle** and its contents. **Skeletonize** the **cystic duct**
- **Double clip** the **cystic duct** and **artery** using a **multiple clip applicator** and divide them. **Follow cystic artery to the gallbladder wall to ensure that you have not divided the right hepatic artery**
- Obtain a **cholangiogram** as indicated:
  - jaundice
  - preoperative deranged liver function tests (LFTs)
  - dilated common bile duct on preoperative ultrasonography
- Perform **diathermy dissection** of gallbladder off hepatic bed, keeping gallbladder always on the stretch
- Remove gallbladder via the **infraumbilical** port ± BERT bag (for the endoscopic retrieval of tissue)
- **Lavage liver bed** with **warm physiological (0.9%) saline**
- Secure haemostasis with hook or ball diathermy
- Consider drain
- Release pneumoperitoneum and watch the instruments carefully as you withdraw them from the abdominal cavity
- **0 Vicryl stitch** on a J needle to close **umbilical** and **epigastric** port sites
- Absorbable suture to skin.

OPERATIVE CHOLANGIOGRAPHY

Not all surgeons perform routine intraoperative cholangiography, although there are **good reasons** why it should be **encouraged**. It can help:

- Define the anatomy
- Detect the presence of common bile duct stones
- Avoid further morbidity because ductal stones can be extracted using a choledochoscope during the same operation. This **avoids** the need for a **postoperative ERCP** (endoscopic retrograde cholangiopancreatography), which has its own inherent risks including 1 per cent mortality rate
- Identify an injury.

LAPAROSCOPIC VERSUS OPEN SURGERY

Advantages

- Less traumatic for patients
- Reduced postoperative pain
- Improved cosmesis
- Faster postoperative recovery
- Reduced adhesion formation
- Shorter stay in hospital and quicker return to normal daily life.

Disadvantages

- Steep learning curve
- Inadvertent damage to surrounding structures as a result of limited field, e.g. visceral injury.

35 Long saphenous varicose vein surgery

Possible viva questions related to this topic

→ What are the indications for performing varicose vein surgery?
→ What tributaries of the long saphenous vein would you encounter during a Trendelenburg procedure?
→ What is the course of the long saphenous vein in the lower leg?
→ How is the stripping of the long saphenous vein carried out?
→ What incision would you make to gain access to the saphenofemoral junction during Trendelenburg's operation?
→ How do you perform multiple phlebectomies of varicose veins?
→ What are the main complications of varicose veins?

Related topics		
Topic	**Chapter**	**Page**
Femoral hernia repair	32	102

DEFINITION

Varicose veins are **dilated tortuous superficial veins** affecting the **lower limb**. Found in distribution of the:

• long saphenous vein (most common)
• short saphenous vein.

AETIOLOGY

This is **uncertain** but an underlying **weakness** of the **vein wall** is likely.

INDICATIONS

The indications for varicose vein surgery are to **prevent** the **complications** from developing or progressing. These are:

• Varicose eczema, lipodermatosclerosis and ulceration
• Bleeding

- Superficial thrombophlebitis
- Pain
- Calcification and periostitis
- Psychological complications
- Cosmetic reasons.

In most cases, do not operate if there is **deep venous obstruction** or **incompetence**.

It is **mandatory** to obtain a **venous duplex scan** preoperatively to map out the venous incompetence.

LONG SAPHENOUS VARICOSE VEIN SURGERY

- Accurate marking of varicosities is essential before the operation. Come to an agreement with the patient on which ones are to be removed.
- Place patient **supine** in the **Trendelenburg position** (30° head-down tilt). **Legs** are placed **straight** but **abducted**, with both feet resting on the edges of a **long board** at the lower end of the table.
- Make an **oblique incision** parallel to and below the inguinal ligament in the **groin crease** over the **saphenofemoral junction (SFJ)**. This is located **2 cm lateral** and **below** the **pubic tubercle**.
- Deepen incision through Scarpa's fascia and insert a West self-retaining retractor. The subcutaneous fatty tissue can be swept away with a swab to expose the long saphenous vein (LSV) and its tributaries.
- Dissect out the LSV and follow it up to the **SFJ.**
- Dissect out and **ligate** all **tributaries.**
- It is important to **display** the **femoral vein** 1 cm above and below the SFJ in order to prevent accidental division of it rather than the LSV.
- A **double tie** is used to ligate the LSV with **0 Vicryl** flush with the SFJ, and divide it such that there is a tuft of vein left at the SFJ to prevent the sutures from falling off.
- Introduce a **stripper** distally and feed it down to a **hand's breath below** the **knee**.
- Make an **incision** over the tip of the stripper, deliver the vein, and tie and ligate the distal LSV. Strip out the proximal part of the vein with gentle traction along the long axis of the leg, applying some pressure over the tunnel as the stripper is withdrawn. In the authors' experience, this reduces the risk of haematoma and bruising postoperatively.
- Perform **multiple phlebectomies** as agreed preoperatively with the patient:
  - small vertical stab incisions are made over the varicosities; a loop of vein is brought out through the stab incision by blunt dissection with an artery forceps or a special fishhook
  - the loop of vein is divided between two artery forceps

- using traction and rotation, the vein is pulled until it breaks
- bleeding is controlled by local pressure
- you may have to ask the anaesthetist to put the patient's head down further to reduce venous bleeding.
- Achieve haemostasis.
- Close the groin wound so that the SFJ is buried under opposed Scarpa's fascia.
- The authors use a subcuticular skin closure in the groin wound and Steri-Strips across the phlebectomy sites.
- A **pressure dressing** with **wool crepe band** or **Velband** is placed over the limb.
- **One** postoperative dose of **subcutaneous heparin** is given to reduce the risk of a **DVT**.
- Patient is sent home, usually the same day, with usual varicose vein surgery advice, including changing the dressing for a thromboembolic stocking on day 5. The patients should be advised to keep this on for around 2 weeks.
- No follow-up is necessary.

↑ Example viva question

What are the surface markings of the long saphenous vein?

Drains **medial end** of **dorsal venous arch** in the **foot.**

Passes **anterior** to the **medial malleolus** and ascends in company with the **saphenous nerve** in the **superficial fascia** over the **medial side** of the **leg.**

Behind the knee, the LSV lies **one hand's breadth** behind the medial aspect of the **patella.**

It then passes along the **medial aspect** of the thigh through the lower part of the saphenous opening in the **cribiform fascia** to join the **femoral vein 2 cm below** and **lateral** to the **pubic tubercle** (SFJ).

TRIBUTARIES OF THE LSV

There are commonly **six:**

1. Superficial inferior epigastric vein
2. Superficial external pudendal vein
3. Deep external pudendal vein
4. Superficial circumflex iliac vein
5. Anterolateral thigh vein
6. Posteromedial thigh vein.

36 Mastectomy, axillary dissection and breast reconstruction

Possible viva questions related to this topic

→ What is a mastectomy?
→ When would you perform a mastectomy?
→ What types of mastectomy do you know about?
→ What types of axillary clearance are there?
→ How would you perform an axillary dissection?
→ What is breast reconstruction?
→ What can be used to reconstruct a breast?
→ When should drains be removed post-mastectomy?

Related topics

Topic	Chapter	Page
Breast cancer	50	182
Wound healing, scarring and reconstruction	83	342
Skin grafting and flap reconstruction	78	320
Drains in surgery	72	295

↑ Key learning point

Definitions

- **Mastectomy**: the surgical removal of all breast tissue of one breast
- **Axillary clearance**: the surgical excision of all axillary lymph nodes up to a predetermined level
- **Breast reconstruction**: the use of material, either prosthetic or living, to create a new breast mound

TYPES OF MASTECTOMY

- **Subcutaneous**: all breast tissue is removed but the **overlying skin** including the nipple–areolar complex **remains**.
- **Skin sparing**: all breast tissue and the **nipple–areolar** complex are **removed** but the **overlying skin remains**.

- **Simple (or total)**: **all breast** tissue and overlying skin is **removed**.
- **Modified radical**: **all breast** tissue, overlying skin and axillary **lymph nodes** are **removed**.
- **Radical**: all breast tissue, overlying skin, pectoralis muscles and axillary lymph nodes are removed. This is very rarely used any more.

INDICATIONS FOR MASTECTOMY

Therapeutic mastectomy for carcinoma of the breast

- Two or more tumours in separate areas of the breast
- Widespread DCIS (ductal carcinoma *in situ*)
- Subareolar tumour
- Large tumour relative to breast size
- High risk of further disease (*BRCA*-1/-2 positive)
- Previous irradiation to breast
- When irradiation is contraindicated (e.g. early pregnancy)
- Patient preference.

Prophylactic mastectomy

- Strong family history for breast carcinoma
- To obtain optimal symmetry for reconstruction
- For peace of mind after mastectomy for carcinoma of the contralateral breast.

AXILLARY CLEARANCE LEVELS

The axilla is divided into **three levels**. These levels are defined by the inferior and superior borders of **pectoralis minor**:

1. **Level 1**: axillary contents **below** pectoralis minor
2. **Level 2**: axillary contents up to **upper border** of pectoralis minor
3. **Level 3**: axillary contents to the **outer border** of the first rib.

A **level 2** axillary clearance will take all nodes from **levels 1 and 2**. A level 3 clearance will take nodes from levels 1, 2 and 3. **Level 2** is most commonly performed and is **adequate clearance** in almost all cases unless large apical nodes are present when level 3 would be needed. Some surgeons will perform a level 3 clearance in the case of metastatic melanoma (see 'Malignant melanoma', Chapter 60, page 232).

MODIFIED RADICAL MASTECTOMY

Preoperative considerations and management

- Check that a **biopsy-proven diagnosis** has been reached and that the **side is confirmed** and marked

- **Reconstruction** should be offered to all women undergoing mastectomy
- The **breast care nurse** should have seen the patient preoperatively
- **Multidisciplinary** team (MDT) approach
- Group and save and routine preoperative bloods
- Careful, **informed consent**.

Mastectomy operation

- Place patient **supine** with the ipsilateral arm secured to an arm board
- **Mark** the limits of **the breast**
- Mark a **transverse ellipse** encompassing the nipple–areolar complex and the lump and **ensure** that these wound edges will **approximate**
- Make a skin incision along the marked ellipse
- Elevate superior and inferior skin flaps between **subcutaneous fat** and **breast fat** to the extents of the breast, as previously marked:
  - ensure the **flap thickness** is adequate for skin viability but that no breast fat is included in the flap
  - handle the skin **gently** and use **non-crushing** instruments (e.g. skin hooks) to avoid skin flap necrosis
  - check the flap thickness regularly to avoid 'buttonholing'
- At the upper and lower extents of the breast, dissect down towards the chest wall to **pectoralis fascia**
- Dissect along the chest wall in the **plane** between **pectoralis fascia** and **breast tissue** from medial to lateral in order to lift the breast from the chest wall. Leave the axillary tail attached:
  - ensure that large **perforating vessels** are **ligated** or cauterized before they are cut to avoid **retraction** of cut vessels
- Identify the border of **pectoralis major** and clear the axillary tail
- **Mark** the specimen at the **axillary tail** and **anteriorly**
- **Wash** the cavity with water to eliminate any solitary tumour cells and unvascularized **fat globules**
- Pack the cavity with saline-soaked gauze and change gloves.

Axillary clearance

- Extend the incision superolaterally to the **anterior** border of **latissimus dorsi**
- Identify the **lateral** border of **pectoralis major** and the **anterior** border of **latissimus dorsi**, which form the **anterior** and **posterior** boundaries of the clearance
- Dissect around the lateral border of pectoralis major to reach **pectoralis minor** and retract this medially to visualize the **level 2** axillary contents
- Continue your dissection superiorly to identify the **axillary vein**, the **upper boundary** of the clearance. Dissect along and visualize the inferior border of this vein along its whole length

- Gently dissect the axillary contents away from the chest wall identifying:
  - **intercostobrachial nerve(s)**: these can be cut if necessary to facilitate clearance but will result in numbness of the medial arm
  - **nerve to serratus anterior** (posterior to the midaxillary line)
  - **nerve to latissimus dorsi**
  - subscapular vessels
- When all vessels and nerves have been identified, the axillary contents can be removed
- Mark the specimen at the **apex**
- Insert two drains – one for the mastectomy flaps and one for the axilla
- Close the skin ensuring that any length discrepancy between the skin edges is evenly distributed to avoid '**dog ears**'.

Postoperative

- **Check Hb the next day**
- **Inspection of skin flaps for evidence of necrosis**
- **Drain management**:
  - a chart of **daily drainage** should be kept
  - there is **no consensus** between specialties as to **when** drains should be **removed** postoperatively. Many breast surgeons will remove drains when the **drain effluent becomes serous** with little weight placed on volume of drainage. This is in contrast to **plastic surgeons** who will often leave drains until < 30 mL **drainage** in a **24-hour** period. The type of operation will obviously have an impact on this decision with immediate reconstruction requiring more cautious drain management.

RECONSTRUCTION

All women undergoing mastectomy **should be offered** breast **reconstruction**, the goal of which is to create a mound to **match the remaining natural breast**.

There are **three main types** of reconstruction – **prosthetic, autologous** and a **combination** of the two. Any of these can be performed at the same time as mastectomy (**immediate reconstruction**) or during a separate operation (**delayed reconstruction**).

Prosthetic reconstruction involves inserting an **implant** between the chest wall and the pectoralis muscles, which can be either a **fixed-volume** silicone implant or an **expandable** saline-filled implant, depending on the nature of the overlying skin and the size of the desired reconstruction. **Expanders** are gradually filled with **saline** over 3–6 months and then removed and replaced with permanent fixed-volume implants. A relatively recent development is a permanent **expandable implant**, which has an outer fixed-volume silicone chamber and an inner expandable saline chamber. This allows for tissue expansion and reconstruction in a **one-stage procedure**.

Autologous reconstruction involves moving tissue from elsewhere to the breast to create a breast mound. Common donor sites are:

- **The back** (latissimus dorsi – muscle and skin)
- **The abdomen** (TRAM [transverse rectus abdominus myocutaneous] – muscle, fat and skin; DIEP [deep inferior epigastric perforator] – fat and skin)
- **The buttock** (SGAP/IGAP [superior gluteal artery perforator/inferior gluteal artery perforator] – fat and skin)

Combination reconstruction is generally used with a latissimus dorsi flap, when the bulk of the muscle itself would not create an adequate mound to match the remaining breast. An **implant** is inserted between the pectoralis muscles and transposed latissimus dorsi to increase the **volume** of the breast while overlying **latissimus dorsi** and its skin paddle create a better **texture and shape** than prosthetic reconstruction alone.

37 Open appendicectomy

Possible viva questions related to this topic

→ How would you prepare a patient for an open appendicectomy?
→ Why do you give intravenous antibiotics?
→ How would you perform an open appendicectomy?
→ What are the complications of an appendicectomy?
→ Where would you make your incision for an appendicectomy? What layers do you go through to reach the peritoneum?
→ Do you bury the appendix stump?
→ When do you expect a difficult appendicectomy? What methods would you employ before calling a senior colleague for help?
→ What would you do if the appendix were normal?
→ How would you manage an appendix mass? When would you operate?

Related topics		
Topic	**Chapter**	**Page**
Abdominal incisions	64	259
Abscess and pus	44	158

PREPARATION

- Full **history** and **examination**. Investigations: **full blood count** (FBC) and **C-reactive protein** (CRP) ± **imaging** (ultrasonography or CT)

Prepare patient for theatre:

- Obtain **informed consent** including **risk** of wound infection, **intra-abdominal abscess/collection** and possibility of a **normal appendix**
- Patient is **kept nil by mouth**, given **intravenous fluids** and **antibiotics**, the latter ideally in the anaesthetic room **before** surgery
- Use **cefuroxime** (broad-spectrum) and **metronidazole** (anaerobic cover)
- **Prophylactic antibiotics** should be routinely given because the **incidence** of **wound** and **intra-abdominal infections** is high after appendicitis
- Under **general anaesthetic** with an **endotracheal tube**, patient is placed **supine** on the table. **Abdomen** is examined under anaesthetic – is there a **mass**? This may help determine the best place for the incision
- The entire abdomen should be **cleaned** and **draped** to **expose** the **right lower quadrant** including the right ASIS, umbilicus and midline.

PROCEDURE

- **Incision: Lanz** – centred over **McBurney's point** (⅓ way from the ASIS to the umbilicus) in Langer's lines (better **cosmesis**). **Gridiron** is less good cosmetically but enables **easier extension** of the wound
- Commence incision 1–2 cm medial to ASIS and continue it transversely
- A **midline** incision should be employed if the patient were **elderly** and there may be a possibility of a **caecal carcinoma**
- Introduce a **Norfolk and Norwich** self-retaining **retractor**
- Peritoneum held up with two artery forceps and divided with a scalpel
- Care is taken not to damage any underlying loops of bowel
- **Microbiology swab** is taken of any peritoneal fluid for **microscopy**, **culture** and **sensitivity**
- **Inspect**:
  - ○ **caecum** and **small bowel** for any other pathology, e.g. **caecal neoplasm** or **Meckel's diverticulum**
  - ○ in **women** inspect the **ovaries** and **fallopian tubes** – rule out **pelvic inflammation**, **pelvic abscess** or even an **ectopic pregnancy** (a preoperative β-hCG [human chorionic gonadotrophin] should have been checked!)
  - ○ if all normal, proceed and **mobilize caecum** (most lateral structure in the peritoneum). Locate appendix by following the taenia to the base of the appendix. If possible **deliver appendix** into the wound.

↑ **Example viva question**

What layers do you go through to reach the peritoneum?

Layered incision through:

- Skin
- Fat
- Scarpa's fascia
- Fat
- External oblique aponeurosis
- Internal oblique (muscle splitting incision with Langenbeck retractors)
- Transverse abdominis (muscle splitting incision with retractors)
- Transversalis fascia and peritoneum, which are fused

- Position:
  - ○ retrocaecal 62 per cent
  - ○ pelvic 34 per cent
  - ○ medial pre-ileal 1 per cent; post-ileal 0.5 per cent.

- **Confirm diagnosis** and begin **mobilization of appendix.** Hold appendix with a pair of **Babcock's forceps** and avoid perforating it
- The **mesoappendix** is divided between artery forceps and secured with 2/0 Vicryl ties to **skeletonize the appendix** and free it to its **base**
- A **straight crushing clamp** is applied across the base and replaced **5 mm distally**. After applying a **0 Vicryl tie** in the form of a **surgeon's knot** to the base, divide the appendix flush to the clamp using a **scalpel**
- Diathermy is applied to the **pouting mucosa** of the appendix base to **prevent mucocele formation** and **reduce** the **bacterial load**
- Ensure that the instruments used to divide the appendix are not used again so as to **avoid contamination**
- The authors **do not routinely** apply a **purse-string** (in the form of a 'Z' stitch or **purse-string**) to **bury the stump**. There is no evidence to suggest that routinely burying the stump of the appendix reduces **intra-abdominal infection, faecal fistula formation** or **stump blow-out**
- The abdomen is then **washed out** with **warm saline** and **10 per cent betadine**
- If there is a **pelvic collection**, have a **low threshold** for inserting a **drain** and carrying out a **full pelvic lavage**
- Achieve **haemostasis**

↑ **Key learning points**

How to take out a difficult appendix

Commonly asked not only in the MRCS viva but also at general surgical registrar interviews!

Expect a **difficult operation** if the **history** is **long** and if an **appendix mass** is present.

The appendix is usually in a **retrocaecal** or **pelvic** position. Consider:

- Using your **index finger** of your dominant hand **gradually** to 'winkle' out the appendix
- Removing the appendix **retrogradely** (base first)
- In a true retrocaecal appendix, the **caecum** can be **mobilized** by **dividing** its **lateral peritoneal attachments** as for a right hemicolectomy
- **Enlarging** the **incision** by cutting the muscle. Don't be afraid to do this
- Getting a **good assistant** to help retract for you
- In the presence of an **abscess** and **being unable to find** the appendix, placing a **large size Robinson drain** into the abscess, **washing out** the abdomen with saline and closing it

- **Wound** is **closed** in layers using **absorbable sutures**
- The authors use continuous **1/0 Vicryl** to **peritoneum** and **muscular layers** with **2/0 Vicryl** to the **subcutaneous layer** and **3/0 Monocryl** to the **skin**
- If the patient had a **perforated appendicitis** he or she should continue to have **5 days** of **intravenous antibiotics** postoperatively
- If the appendix were only **inflamed** (pre-perforation) **one further dose** should suffice
- The appendix is routinely sent for **histological confirmation** (to exclude carcinoid and carcinoma). Sometimes the appendix looks normal but microscopically may be inflamed. The specimen should always be sent for histological confirmation.

↑ **Example viva question**

What would you do if the appendix were normal?

If the appendix were **normal looking**, I would need to search for other possible causes:

- In a **woman**, look at the **right fallopian tube and ovary**
- Inspect the **terminal ileum** and palpate for any thickening. This might indicate **Crohn's ileitis** or **tuberculous ileitis** depending on background
- The **small bowel** is run to examine for a **Meckel's diverticulum** or for any **inflamed mesenteric lymph nodes (mesenteric adenitis)**
- Palpate posterior abdominal wall, ascending colon, liver edge and gall-bladder fundus (for **cholecystitis**). Look for **bile-stained fluid** suggesting a **perforated duodenal ulcer**
- Inspect the large bowel (**sigmoid diverticulitis**)
- If there were an **inflamed Meckel's diverticulum** this would need to be resected with a short segment of adjacent normal bowel, and a primary interrupted extramucosal anastomosis performed

---

COMPLICATIONS

General versus specific

Specific complications include:

- Wound infection
- Wound abscess
- Bleeding and haematoma
- Pelvic abscess and collection

- Peritonitis
- Keloid scar formation
- Peritoneal adhesions
- Increased incidence of right inguinal hernia (damage to ilioinguinal nerve)
- Incisional hernia (rare)
- Damage to other structures, e.g. small bowel, caecum (caecal fistula) and fallopian tubes
- Normal appendix!

↑ **Example viva question**

How do you manage an appendix mass?

An **appendix mass** is usually treated **conservatively** with **bed rest** and **intravenous antibiotics**. **Serial examination** to monitor the patient's progress carefully is important. An **interval appendicectomy** is usually performed at **6 weeks**.

Indications for **surgical intervention** are:

- The **mass** becomes **tender** or **enlarges**
- The patient becomes **toxic** with a **swinging pyrexia** and **tachycardia** and increasing **white cell count (WCC and C-Reactive Protein (CRP))**
- The patient develops signs of **peritonitis**, **obstruction** or **paralytic ileus**

---

38 Orthopaedic related approaches and procedures

REDUCTION OF A COLLES' FRACTURE

A **Colles' fracture** is a **distal fracture** of the **radius** that occurs in **elderly, osteoporotic** patients. It usually results from a **fall** on to the **outstretched hand** and results in the **'dinner fork'** deformity.

The fracture is:

• dorsally angulated
• impacted
• radially deviated
• associated with an avulsion of the ulnar styloid.

Complications

• Malunion
• Subluxation of the radioulnar joint
• Extensor pollicis longus tendon rupture

- Joint stiffness
- Carpal tunnel syndrome
- Sudeck's atrophy.

Reduction

- **Disimpact** the **fracture** by **pulling** and **flexing** the **wrist dorsally**
- **Reduce** the **fracture** by **pushing** the **distal fracture** in a **volar direction** with **ulnar deviation**
- Set in plaster of Paris (POP).

OPEN REDUCTION AND INTERNAL FIXATION (ORIF) OF SCAPHOID FRACTURE

Indications for surgery

- Non-union
- Freshly displaced fracture
- Trans-scaphoid perilunate dislocation.

Procedure

- Dorsal longitudinal incision
- Preserve radial artery
- Appraise need for a bone graft; if required harvest from iliac crest
- From distal to proximal:
  - guide pilot drill
  - use image intensifier (I/I) to view position
  - Herbert screw fixation
- I/I to confirm position
- Set in POP.

↑ **Example viva question**

What is the anatomical snuffbox?

Lateral border: two tendons
- abductor pollicis longus
- extensor pollicis brevis

Medial border: extensor pollicis longus

Floor: scaphoid bone

Contents: radial artery and nerve

Clinical significance

The **scaphoid** bone can be palpated in the **snuffbox** and is at risk in injuries that involve **force** applied to the **palmar surface** of the outstretched hand. The scaphoid is at risk of **proximal avascular necrosis** in fractures affecting the **waist** of the scaphoid as a result of its **end-arterial blood supply.**

Any **tenderness** elicited in the **snuffbox** with the typical background history should arouse suspicions of a scaphoid fracture and appropriate **scaphoid radiological views** requested.

SURGICAL APPROACHES TO THE HIP

Anterior (Smith–Petersen) approach

Internervous plane between tensor fascia lata (superior gluteal nerve) and sartorius (femoral nerve), then divide rectus femoris and anterior third of gluteus medius.

Used commonly in paediatric orthopaedic surgery to correct congenital dislocation of the hip.

Lateral (Hardinge) approach

Patient is placed **laterally** on the table. A **longitudinal incision** is made 10 cm below the greater trochanter and curved posteriorly.

Split **tensor fascia lata, gluteus medius** and **minimus** or detach them from the greater trochanter.

Incision is then extended through **vastus lateralis** on to the anterior aspect of the femur, which should expose the capsule of the hip joint.

Beware of the **superior gluteal nerve.**

Posterior approach

Skin incision is centred on the **posterior** part of the **greater trochanter.** Proximally it is curved towards the **posterosuperior iliac spine.** After the subcutaneous tissue, this involves splitting **gluteus maximus** and detaching **piriformis, obturator internus** and **gemelli** from the femur. This achieves access to the **posterior capsule** of the hip joint.

Beware of the **sciatic nerve.**

DYNAMIC HIP SCREW (DHS) INSERTION

- **General** or **spinal** anaesthetic
- **Broad-spectrum intravenous antibiotics** at induction
- Patient placed **supine** on an **orthopaedic traction table**
- **Reduce fracture** by **traction, abduction** and **internal rotation**, and hold in place using the traction table
- Check **adequate reduction** by using **image intensifier**
- Area is prepared and draped with a **transparent polythene sheet**
- Make a **15 cm longitudinal incision** from **greater trochanter** down the thigh
- **Layers traversed**:
  - skin
  - subcutaneous fat
  - fascia lata
  - vastus lateralis to expose upper lateral femur
- **Guidewire** is passed across the fracture into the femoral head
- Use the **jig** to achieve an angle of **135°** to the femoral shaft. Use the image intensifier in **two planes** to check **adequate placement**
- Distance the screw needs to travel is measured accordingly and the path is **drilled** over the guidewire
- The drill hole is **tapped** before the screw is inserted over the guidewire
- Use the image intensifier to check for a satisfactory position in the femoral head (screw tip should abut the subchondral bone)
- **Remove wire**. Use the **periosteal elevator** to clear the lateral femur before applying a **five-hole buttress plate** over the end of the DHS
- The plate is secured with screws through both cortices
- A **check radiograph** is performed before closing the wound in layers
- A **suction drain** should also be used.

APPROACH TO THE KNEE JOINT

Anteromedial approach

Longitudinal incision centred over the **medial border** of the **quadriceps tendon**. Start 8 cm proximal to the patella and extend distally.

Curve incision to the **medial aspect** of the **patella** and then return to midline inferiorly. Lower limit should be the **tibial tuberosity.**

The **plane of dissection** should be between **vastus medialis** and the **quadriceps tendon.**

Expose capsule of joint by dividing the fascia.

Patella is reflected laterally and the knee flexed to obtain optimal views.

Lateral parapatellar approach

Incision parallel to the lateral edge of the patella 1–2 cm from it.

Divide extensor expansion, capsule and synovial membrane.

Avoid infrapatellar branch of **saphenous nerve**.

39 Perforated duodenal ulcer and exploratory laparotomy

Possible viva questions related to this topic

→ How would you perform an open repair of a perforated peptic ulcer?
→ What would your postoperative management be?
→ What is the differential diagnosis with the same clinical presentation?
→ Name four features of pneumoperitoneum on plain radiographs
→ What is the most common cause of free intra-abdominal gas?
→ Does the absence of air under the diaphragm on an erect chest radiograph exclude a perforated peptic ulcer?
→ What conditions may mimic the appearance of a pneumoperitoneum?
→ How much free gas needs to be present to be detected on plain erect chest radiograph?
→ What are the typical presenting features of a perforated peptic ulcer?
→ What do you understand by the term 'right paracolic gutter phenomenon'?
→ How do you perform an exploratory laparotomy?

Related topics		
Topic	Chapter	Page
GORD and Barrett's oesophagus	56	214

CLINICAL FEATURES

Typically, perforated duodenal ulcers produce **acute onset epigastric pain** followed by more **generalized abdominal pain**.

Sometimes **right iliac fossa** pain occurs as a result of duodenal–gastric contents accumulating at this site under gravity. This can sometimes be confused with acute appendicitis – '**right paracolic phenomenon**'.

The patient may also complain of **right shoulder tip** pain caused by **referred pain** from diaphragmatic irritation.

Nausea is **common** but vomiting is uncommon.

The patient lies perfectly still with **frequent shallow respirations**. The diagnosis can be made from the end of the bed.

Examination reveals a **distended** and **'board-like'** abdomen as a result of involuntary contraction of rectus abdominis. There is a paucity/absence of bowel sounds.

Systemic signs include **pyrexia**, **tachycardia**, **tachypnoea** and a **dry tongue**.

↑ **Key learning points**

Common topic to be asked alongside being shown **erect chest** and **supine abdominal radiographs**.

Example

This erect chest radiograph and supine abdominal film were taken of a 34-year-old man with a 24-hour history of sudden-onset worsening generalized abdominal pain.

What do these radiographs show?
Free air under the diaphragm
Visible **falciform ligament**

Rigler's sign: both sides of the bowel wall are seen since air outside the wall (free intraperitoneal air) acts as a contrast medium as it does physiologically when inside the bowel.

What is the most likely diagnosis?

In a man of this age and with this history, the most likely diagnosis is a **perforated duodenal ulcer**.

PREDISPOSING FACTORS

- Young men below the age of 50 years
- Smokers
- Drinking excess alcohol
- Steroids
- NSAID use.

Twenty per cent of cases have **no prior history** of peptic ulcer disease.

DIFFERENTIAL DIAGNOSIS

- Acute pancreatitis
- Acute cholecystitis
- Acute appendicitis
- Leaking abdominal aortic aneurysm
- Myocardial infarction.

CONDITIONS THAT MIMIC THE APPEARANCE OF A PNEUMOPERITONEUM

- **Chilaiditi's sign** – presence of intestine (colon) between the liver and diaphragm
- Subphrenic abscess
- Basal atelectasis that mimics the contour of the hemidiaphragm
- Subdiaphragmatic fat
- Cysts in pneumatosis coli.

Pneumoperitoneum

The **most common pathological cause** of **free intraperitoneal gas** is a perforated peptic ulcer.

It is possible to detect **1 mL** of free air on an erect chest radiograph or decubitus view.

Features on a **plain radiograph** include:

- Free air under the diaphragm (erect chest radiograph)
- The falciform ligament of the liver
- The lateral wall of the large bowel – **Rigler's sign**
- Air around the liver
- Free air in triangular shapes between loops of bowel.

The **absence** of subdiaphragmatic air on an erect chest radiograph **does not** exclude a perforated peptic ulcer.

Approximately **10–30 per cent** of cases do not demonstrate free intra-abdominal gas. If in doubt request a **lateral decubitus view** because this is more sensitive at picking up free air.

OTHER COMMON CAUSES OF VISCUS PERFORATION

- **Perforated diverticular disease** – normally free air is not detected because the perforation gets sealed off and there is less air in the colon
- **Appendix**
- Malignant **colonic tumour**
- **Gallbladder**
- **Small bowel** (in obstruction).

PERFORATED PEPTIC ULCER REPAIR

If patient is **aged over 60 years** with **multiple co-morbidities** and a **systolic blood pressure** < 100 mmHg, consider conservative management with a **strict nil-by-mouth** regimen and **nasogastric tube** insertion.

- **Preoperative preparation** includes **fluid resuscitation**, **urinary catheter insertion** for strict input/output assessment, **good pain control**, **broad-spectrum antibiotics**, strictly **nil-by-mouth** regimen with placement of a **nasogastric tube**
- Under **general anaesthetic** (endotracheal intubation) patient is placed **supine** on the table. Skin preparation includes the whole of the abdomen, as a perforated colonic lesion cannot be ruled out
- **Upper midline incision** made from xiphisternum to umbilicus initially – can be extended later if necessary
- **Wound retraction** using a self-retaining retractor or an assistant if required
- **Careful assessment** of **stomach** (especially lesser curvature) and **duodenum** is made
- The **perforated ulcer** is **identified**. If **gastric** in nature, **biopsy** from edge is taken and sent to histology to **rule out malignancy**
- Closure of the ulcer is made using an **omental patch** and interrupted parallel absorbable sutures. The authors believe that **primary closure** of the ulcer is **technically** unacceptable because there is bound to be **tension** on already friable tissue and therefore technical failure ensues. The omental patch is positioned so that it is placed right down into the ulcer cavity
- **Peritoneal lavage** is performed with warm physiological saline to include the **subphrenic spaces, paracolic gutters** and **pelvis**
- The authors' practice is to place a drain near the patch site, although this is controversial
- **Definitive treatment** for the **ulcer** in the form of a truncal vagotomy and drainage or partial gastrectomy is **no longer performed**
- **Broad-spectrum antibiotics** should be **continued** postoperatively for **at least 5 days** and then reviewed.

Variant scenarios

- If at laparotomy the surgeon cannot find a perforated peptic ulcer he would explore all abdominal organs including the gallbladder and sigmoid colon. Other causes for an acute abdomen should be excluded.
- For a **bleeding perforated gastric ulcer**, **distal gastrectomy** should be performed.
- In a perforated anterior duodenal ulcer with a coexisting bleeding posterior duodenal ulcer ('**kissing ulcers**'), the author would insert non-absorbable sutures at the base of the bleeding ulcer and close the anterior gastroduodenotomy as a pyloroplasty.

Example viva question

How do you perform an exploratory laparotomy?

Methodical approach
Inspect and palpate:

1. Right lobe of liver, gallbladder, left lobe of liver, spleen
2. Diaphragmatic hiatus, abdominal oesophagus, stomach, duodenal bulb
3. Bile duct, right kidney, duodenal loop and transverse colon
4. Body and tail of pancreas, left kidney
5. Mesenteric root, superior mesenteric vessels, middle colic artery, aorta, inferior mesenteric artery
6. Appendix, caecum, colon, rectum
7. Pelvis, uterus, fallopian tubes, bladder
8. Hernial orifices, iliac vessels

40 Renal transplantation

Possible viva questions related to this topic

→ What are the indications for performing a renal transplantation?
→ What are the most common causes of end-stage renal failure?
→ What types of renal donors have you heard of?
→ What are the principles of preparing a patient for renal transplantation?
→ How would you perform a renal transplant?
→ What are the operative principles of renal transplantation in adults?
→ What anastomoses are performed in a renal transplantation?
→ What are the possible complications?
→ How might you be aware that transplant rejection is occurring?
→ Outline the three main types of allograft rejection.
→ What are the indications for renal replacement therapy?
→ How can this be achieved?

Related topics

Topic	Chapter	Page
Brain-stem death	106	423
Kidney	9	26
Oliguria and renal replacement	116	482
Anastomosis and anastomotic leak	66	270
Abdominal incisions	64	250

INDICATIONS

Renal transplantation has become a **cost-effective, safe mode of treatment** for **end-stage renal failure. Quality of life** is improved considerably. The **most common reasons in the UK** are:

• Diabetes mellitus
• Hypertensive renal disease
• Glomerulonephritis
• Polycystic kidney disease
• Reflux pyelonephritis
• Congenital obstructive uropathies.

DONOR TYPES

- **Cadaveric** (most common) **or deceased donors.** These can be divided into **brain-stem death donors** who will become **heart-beating** donors (90 per cent of solid organ donors) and donors who do not fulfil the **brain-stem death criteria (non-heart-beating cadavers)**
- **Living** who can be **related** or **unrelated** to the recipient.

PREPARATION

- Careful consent
- Donor kidney retrieval – **limit** ischaemic time
- Antibiotics – usually co-amoxiclav (Augmentin)
- Immunosuppression (methylprednisolone) + calcineurin inhibitor
- Mannitol
- Cytotoxic cross-match
- Blood available (type matched) – usually for 2 units
- Work patients up for contraindications:
  - cancer
  - infections, e.g. need a urinary tract free of sepsis
  - anatomical urological problems
- Correct metabolic abnormalities, e.g. hyperkalaemia
- Does the patient require dialysis preoperatively?
- Truly multidisciplinary approach.

PROCEDURE

- **Prepare donor kidney** under **sterile** conditions (usually at 4°C in theatre). This involves assessment for damage, cleaning off excess fat and **preparing renal vein** and artery for prompt anastomosis
- **Lanz** or **hockey-stick** incision (usually contralateral iliac fossa to the side where the donor organ originated – heterotopic transplantation)
- Divide anterior abdominal wall muscles.

Extraperitoneal approach

- Identify and **mobilize external iliac artery** and **vein** and control with **sloupes.** These vessels are **clamped** before anastomosis. Minimize disturbing the surrounding lymphatic vessels – there is a risk of developing a postoperative lymphocoele
- Remove the prepared donor artery from ice.

- *Perform*:
  - **end-to-side anastomosis** between **donor renal artery** and **external iliac artery** or **internal iliac artery** with **5/0 Prolene**
  - **end-to-side anastomosis** between **donor renal vein** and **external iliac vein**
- Remove clamps
- Secure haemostasis
- Fill **bladder** with **physiological saline**
- **Spatulate** end of **ureter** and anastomose to the **dome of the bladder** using **4/0 PDS** and a **submucosal tunnelling technique** to prevent **urinary reflux**. Test the anastomosis by **refilling** the **bladder** with saline
- When the three anastomoses have been performed, the **renal pelvis** is the most **anterior structure**, then **artery** and the **vein** most **posterior**
- Take a **renal biopsy** (time 0 biopsy) for future **baseline comparisons**
- Wound closure in layers leaving a large silicone tube drain *in situ*.

POSTOPERATIVE CONSIDERATIONS

- Administer **immunosuppressive regimen**, e.g. steroids, ciclosporin, azathioprine
- Careful monitoring of urine output and fluid administration are essential in the early postoperative period: the patient may be anuric, polyuric or producing urine in a manner appropriate to the fluid balance.

COMPLICATIONS

- Bleeding
- Haematoma
- Delayed graft function – 20–30 per cent because of acute tubular necrosis
- Infection:
  - immunosuppression increases susceptibility
  - bacterial pathogens complicating any surgery
  - opportunistic infections, e.g. cytomegalovirus (CMV)
- Ureteric leakage or stenosis
- Renal vein thrombosis
- Lymphocoele around kidney
- Rejection (see below)
- Increased risk of malignancy (lymphoma) because of immunosuppression.

FEATURES OF REJECTION

- **Pyrexia**
- **Tenderness** over the graft
- **Reduction** in **urine output**

- Weight gain
- Rising creatinine.

TYPES OF REJECTION

Hyperacute rejection

Recipient's serum has preformed antibodies against the donor kidney's antigens. Antibodies adhere to the endothelium of the graft causing graft thrombosis and infarction. This type of rejection is rapid – within minutes of surgery – and is prevented by ABO matching and cross-matching tests. It is treated by graft nephrectomy.

Acute rejection

This is a **T cell-mediated** attack on the graft involving **CD4 cells**. It usually presents **within 3 months** of transplantation and causes **graft dysfunction**. The diagnosis is confirmed with a **biopsy** of the graft and is **treated by a short course of high-dose immunosuppression** with **steroids** or **anti-lymphocyte antibodies**.

Chronic rejection

This occurs usually **> 6 months** after renal transplantation. It involves both the **humoral** and **cell-mediated** arm of the immune response. Characteristic histological features include **glomerulosclerosis** and **intimal thickening** of **small arteries**.

Non-immunological factors are also implicated including **viral infection** and **drug toxicity.** Unfortunately it is **not treatable** or **reversible**.

Graft survival rates		
Donor type	**1-year survival rate (%)**	**5-year survival rate (%)**
Cadaveric	85	65
Living related	90	80

41 Thyroidectomy

Related topics		
Topic	**Chapter**	**Page**
Hyperparathyroidism	58	224
Thyroid gland and parathyroid glands	18	49
Thyroid cancer	62	244
Triangles of the neck	20	53

INDICATIONS

- **Malignancy**: except anaplastic tumour or lymphoma
- **Adenomas** (fine-needle aspiration cannot often differentiate benign from malignant)
- **Thyrotoxicosis** (failed medical management)
- **Pressure symptoms**: dyspnoea or dysphagia
- **Cosmesis**: large multinodular goitre.

PREOPERATIVE

- **Vocal cord check** with **indirect laryngoscopy** must be performed even if there is no suspicion of recurrent laryngeal nerve (RLN) palsy

- Render thyrotoxic patients **euthyroid** with **carbimazole** and **propranolol**
- **Informed consent** (including hypothyroidism, risk to parathyroids and RLN)
- General anaesthetic
- Patient positioned **supine** with **neck extended. Head ring** and **sandbags** placed in the **interscapular region**
- The neck is prepared and draped appropriately
- **Transverse collar incision 2 cm** above the **sternal notch** in Langer's lines
- **Extend incision** as far **laterally** as the **medial border** of **sternocleidomastoid** and deepen it through **subcutaneous tissue** and **platysma**
- Raise **superior** and **inferior subplatysmal flaps** above strap muscles using Allis tissue forceps and a combination of sharp and blunt dissection. This process should be continued **superiorly** to the upper border of the **thyroid cartilage** and **inferiorly** to the **sternal notch**
- Position **Joll's self-retractor** such that its clips are at the midpoint of the incision
- Identify the **midline raphe** between the strap muscles, incise the **deep cervical fascia**, and extend incision superiorly and inferiorly to expose the thyroid gland. Mobilize the **medial border** of **sternocleidomastoid.**

↑ **Example viva question**

What layers are traversed in your approach to the thyroid gland?

- Skin
- Subcutaneous fat
- Platysma
- Deep investing fascia
- Strap muscles (sternohyoid and sternothyroid)
- Pretracheal fascia
- False sheath of connective tissue overlying the thyroid
- Isthmus of the thyroid gland

- Begin dissecting the **plane** between the **strap muscles** and the **thyroid,** working out to the lateral lobe.
- Identify the **middle thyroid vein**; ligate and divide it with 2/0 Vicryl ties. Use this to enable you to **dislocate** the **lobe medially.**
- Open the space between the **thyroid gland, oesophagus** and **posterolateral neck tissues** (including vertebrae) to **identify** the recurrent laryngeal nerve (**RLN**). The **inferior thyroid artery** often acts as a **marker.**
- Follow the RLN upwards to its point of entry close to the larynx. Now move your body to face the patient's head and **draw the thyroid gland downwards** to aid identification of the **superior pole vessels.**

- It is advisable to **secure the upper pole vessels initially** because this will facilitate delivery of the gland into the surgical field.
- Sweep sternothyroid away with a pledget and find the medial space between the larynx and medial edge of the upper lobe. Make a **window** for entry here and pass a **Kocher's grooved director** through. **Clip vessels individually** using a **Lahey**, staying **close** to the **upper pole** of the thyroid gland. This reduces the risk of damage to the **superior laryngeal nerve**.
- Remember that the right upper pole is usually higher than the left. Now turn towards the patient's feet to deal with the **inferior thyroid vein**.
- Keep the **RLN in view at all times**. Isolate the **inferior thyroid vessels**, clip and tie **close to the thyroid gland** to avoid damaging the **parathyroid glands** or their **blood supply** from the **inferior thyroid artery**.
- Dissect the thyroid gland off the front of the trachea. **Divide** the **ligament of Berry**, which is a strong ligament that attaches the posterior aspect of the thyroid gland to the trachea.
- For a **thyroid lobectomy**, apply a heavy pair of forceps to the thyroid in the midline, divide the thyroid and **oversew** the **remaining lobe** with an **absorbable suture**. This **removes** the **isthmus** with the specimen.
- For a **subtotal thyroidectomy**, perform a similar mobilization of the other lobe, divide the isthmus and work **laterally**, freeing the lobe from the trachea. Apply a **series of forceps** to the lateral portions of the gland with the aim of **leaving** $5\,cm^3$. Excise the thyroid with a scalpel and oversew the remnants with a **continuous absorbable suture** (1/0 Vicryl) and **attach it** to the **pretracheal fascia**.
- **Secure haemostasis** using **ligatures** and **ties** (**avoid diathermy** – minimizes damage to the laryngeal nerves and parathyroid glands) and insert a **small suction drain** into the thyroid bed.
- Bring it out between the strap muscles. If the strap muscles were divided (usually for a large goitre) repair them with an interrupted absorbable suture (1/0 Vicryl).
- Close the platysma with continuous 1/0 Vicryl.
- Use a **subcuticular Prolene** to skin (with beads) – **reduces** incidence of **keloid** and **hypertrophic scar** formation compared with metal clips.

COMPLICATIONS

- **Haemorrhage** – potential for airway compromise
- Wound infection
- RLN palsy
- Superior laryngeal nerve palsy
- Hypothyroidism
- Hypocalcaemia secondary to parathyroid bruising or inadvertent removal
- Keloid scar
- Stitch granuloma.

↑ **Example viva question**

What should be next to the patient's bedside postoperatively? Under what circumstance is this used and if this were to occur what else must you do?

Always have a pair of **suture cutting scissors** or **clip removers** by the **bedside** in case the patient develops a **haematoma** causing a **respiratory obstruction**. If this were to happen, the **dressings** should be **removed** and, if a haematoma is seen, the **sutures and clips** should be **removed immediately**. Once the haematoma has been decompressed, the patient should be taken back to theatre for formal exploration and closure of the wound. The **hospital cardiac arrest team** should also be **alerted** promptly in case urgent intubation is required.

42 Tracheostomy

Possible viva questions related to this topic

→ What are the indications for a tracheostomy?
→ What types of tracheostomy have you heard of?
→ How do you perform a tracheostomy?
→ What layers do you go through to perform a tracheostomy?
→ What are the potential complications of performing a tracheostomy?
→ What is your postoperative management?
→ Which anatomical structure is at high risk of damage when performing a tracheostomy on a child?

TYPES

Elective versus emergency tracheostomy

Tracheostomy is **not usually** performed as an **emergency** procedure because it cannot be performed as **quickly** and **safely** as a **cricothyroidotomy**.

Percutaneous tracheostomy

This **avoids** the need for the patient to go to **theatre** and be operated upon by a surgeon. This can be done in the **intensive care setting** under **local anaesthetic** whereby a **14G cannula** is inserted with a **guidewire** with subsequent **serial dilatation**. The **advantages** include avoiding **patient transfer** and supposedly **reduced incidence of** **haemorrhage** and **infection**.

Mini-tracheostomy

A **small tracheostomy tube** is placed through the **cricothyroid membrane** to aid bronchial toileting and aspiration of secretions. This is **not a definitive airway**, because the **tube** is **not cuffed**.

INDICATIONS

Airway obstruction

- **Congenital,** e.g. laryngeal cysts, tracheo-oesophageal anomalies
- **Trauma** to larynx
- **Infection:** acute epiglottitis
- **Head and neck tumours**: tongue, larynx, pharynx and thyroid
- Facial fractures
- **Bilateral vocal cord paralysis**
- Sleep apnoea syndrome.

Respiratory insufficiency

- **Long-term management** of a **ventilated patient** (most common reason)
- **Failed extubation** in intensive care
- Chest injury (flail chest)
- Pulmonary disease.

Tracheostomy reduces upper airway dead space by 70 per cent.

Tracheobronchial tree protection

Temporary versus **permanent**.

- **Trauma**: burns to head and neck
- **Coma**: head injury, drug overdose
- **Neurological problems**: myasthenia gravis, multiple sclerosis
- **Head and neck surgery**: supraglottic laryngectomy.

(EMERGENCY) TRACHEOSTOMY

- Lie patient **supine** with **neck extended**
- Perform under general anaesthetic and intubation (elective cases)
- In emergency situations, give oxygen and inject local anaesthetic if there is time
- **Vertical incision** – from lower border of the thyroid cartilage in the midline to the suprasternal notch (**transverse incision** 2 cm below cricoid cartilage in **elective** cases)
- Deepen incision and extend between **strap muscles**
- Retract or divide **thyroid isthmus**
- **Recheck size** of **cuffed tube** to be placed
- Feel for **first tracheal ring**
- Try to identify the **innominate vein**. This structure is at **high risk** of damage when performing a tracheostomy on a **child**, because it **lies high** on the **trachea**

- Vertical incision through the second and third tracheal rings. Do not remove the trachea cartilage in children because this can lead to tracheal collapse. Damage to first tracheal ring may result in subglottic stenosis; lower placement risks tracheo-innominate fistula
- The anaesthetist should be asked to withdraw the endotracheal tube to above the incision and be ready to change the ventilator to the tracheostomy and then withdraw the endotracheal tube
- Aspirate trachea
- Insert tracheal dilator or cuffed tube to secure airway
- Closure: skin edges closed loosely, tapes to secure tube.

POSTOPERATIVE MANAGEMENT

- Nurse upright
- Regular suction
- Humidified oxygen with 5–7 per cent carbon dioxide to prevent apnoea
- Mucolytic agents are sometimes employed
- Leave tube in place for 1 week before replacing it.

↑ **Example viva question**

What layers do you go through when performing a tracheostomy?

Structures encountered (superficial inwards):

- Skin
- Superficial fascia
- Platysma
- Investing layer of cervical fascia (surrounds strap muscles)
- Pre-tracheal fascia
- Thyroid isthmus
- Trachea

Example viva question

What are the potential complications of performing a tracheostomy?

Complications
Immediate
- Asphyxia
- Pneumothorax
- Haemorrhage or haematoma
- Cricoid cartilage injury
- Damage to the oesophagus

Early
- Aspiration
- Obstruction
- Cellulitis
- Tracheitis
- Mucus plugging
- Malpositioned tube
- Creation of a false track
- Subcutaneous emphysema

Late
- **Delayed haemorrhage** – usually **secondary** to **tracheo-innominate fistula** occurs **>48 hours** postoperatively
- Vocal cord palsy
- Atelectasis and bronchopneumonia
- Tracheocutaneous or tracheo-oesophageal fistula
- Subglottic stenosis
- Tracheomalacia
- Tracheal stenosis
- Difficult decannulation

APPLIED SURGICAL PATHOLOGY

43 Pathology definitions: helpful A–Z guide

Abscess	Localized collection of pus, surrounded by a pyogenic membrane
Adenoma	Benign glandular neoplasm
Aneurysm	Abnormal permanent dilatation of a blood vessel or part of a heart chamber
Apoptosis	Programmed cell death
Atrophy	Pathological or physiological reduction in size or number or both of an organ or tissue
Carcinoma	A malignant epithelial neoplasm
Cirrhosis	Combination of widespread fibrosis and regenerative nodule formation following necrosis of hepatic cells
Cyst	Cavity with an epithelial lining and containing fluid or other material
Cytokine	Substances produced by one cell that influence the behaviour of another, affecting intercellular communication
Cytotoxic	Causing cell injury but not necessarily lethal
Differentiation	*Embryological*: process by which a cell develops special characteristics *Pathological*: degree of morphological resemblance of a neoplasm to its parent tissue
Diverticulum	Abnormal hollow pouch communicating with the lumen of the structure(s) from which it has arisen
Dysplasia	Abnormal growth and differentiation of a tissue in epithelia – often a feature of the early stages of neoplasia
Dystrophy	Abnormal development or degeneration of a tissue
Ectasia	Abnormal dilatation
Ectopic	Tissue or substance in or from an inappropriate site (not metastasis)
Effusion	Abnormal collection of fluid in a body cavity
Embolus	Fluid or solid mass mobile within a blood vessel and capable of blocking its lumen
Empyema	Cavity filled with pus
Endocrine	Characteristic of cells producing hormones secreted into the blood with distant effects
Endotoxin	Toxin derived from disruption of the outer membrane of Gram-negative bacteria
Erosion	Loss of superficial layer or surface
Exophytic	Tumour growing outwards from a surface usually because it lacks invasive properties
Exotoxin	Toxin secreted by living bacteria
Exudate	Extravascular accumulation of protein-rich fluid as a result of increased vascular permeability
Fibrosis	Process of depositing excess collagen into tissue in attempted repair
Fistula	Abnormal connection between two epithelial-lined surfaces

Gangrene	Bulk tissue necrosis. Dry = sterile; wet = bacterial putrefaction
Grade	Degree of malignancy of a neoplasm (well, moderately or poorly differentiated)
Granulation tissue	Newly formed connective tissue often found at the edge or base of ulcers and wounds, made up of capillaries, fibroblasts, myofibroblasts and inflammatory cells embedded in mucin-rich ground substance during healing
Granuloma	An aggregate of epithelioid macrophages often including giant cells
Haematoma	Localized collection of blood or blood clot, usually within solid tissue
Hamartoma	Congenital tumour-like malformation comprising two or more mature tissue elements normally present in the organ in which it arises
Hernia	Abnormal protrusion of an organ or part of it from one body compartment to another
Hyperplasia	Enlargement of an organ or tissue as a result of increased cell numbers
Hypertrophy	Enlargement of an organ or part of it as a result of increased cell size
Infarction	Death of a tissue as a result of insufficient blood supply
Ischaemia	Inadequate blood supply to, or to part of, an organ
Malignant	Condition with risk of morbidity and mortality, usually applied to tumours
Metaplasia	Reversible change in the character of a tissue from one mature cell type to another
Metastasis	Process by which a primary malignant neoplasm gives rise to secondary tumours at distant sites, usually by lymphatic, vascular or transcoelomic spread
Mucocele	Mucus-filled cyst or hollow organ
Mutation	Irreversible alteration in the base sequence of DNA, which may occur spontaneously or in response to a mutagenic agent; may result in the synthesis of an abnormal protein product
Necrosis	Pathological cell or tissue death within a living organism irrespective of cause
Neoplasm	Abnormal or uncoordinated tissue growth persisting after withdrawal of the initiating cause
Oedema	Abnormal collection of fluid within or between cells
Oncogene	A gene inappropriately, abnormally or excessively expressed in tumours, the product of which is responsible for their autonomous growth
Opsonin	Factor which enhances the efficiency of phagocytosis because it is recognized by receptor(s) on leukocytes; two major opsonins are the Fc fragment of immunoglobulin G and a product of complement, C3b

Organization	Natural process of tissue repair
Papilloma	Benign neoplasm of non-glandular epithelium
Papillary	Surface of a lesion characterized by numerous folds, fronds or villous projections
Paracrine	Characteristic of neighbouring cells of different types influencing each other by secretion of cytokines, growth factors or hormones
Pleomorphism	Variation in size and shape, usually of nuclei and characteristic of malignant neoplasms
Polymorphic	Consisting of more than one cell type
Polyp	Sessile or pedunculated protrusion from a body surface
Pseudocyst	Cavity with a distinct wall but lacking an epithelial lining containing fluid
Pseudomembrane	False membrane consisting of inflammatory exudate rather than epithelium
Putrefaction	Decomposition or rotting of dead tissue as a result of bacterial action, often accompanied by unpleasant odours
Repair	Healing with replacement of lost tissue not necessarily by similar tissue
Resolution	Restoration of normality
Sarcoma	Malignant connective tissue neoplasm
Sclerosis	Hardening of a tissue often caused by excess deposition of excess collagen
Serous	Containing serum or a fluid resembling it
Sinus	Blind-ending tract communicating with an epithelial surface – can be normal or abnormal
Stenosis	Narrowing of a lumen
Stoma	Any normal, pathological or surgically constructed opening between one hollow structure and another or the skin
Stroma	Non-neoplastic reactive connective tissue within a neoplasm
Telangiectasia	Dilated small blood vessels
Thrombus	Solid mass of coagulated blood formed within the circulation
Ulcer	Breach in epithelial surface with tissue loss

44 Abscess and pus

Possible viva questions related to this topic

→ What is an abscess?
→ Give surgical examples of abscesses.
→ What tissue is the wall of an abscess characteristically composed of?
→ What is pus?
→ What are the possible sequelae of an abscess?

Example viva question

What is an abscess?

This is a common starting question, and it is important to get the definition right because examiners can trip you up from the start. It is a good route into a viva on abscesses, acute or chronic inflammation.

An abscess is a **localized collection of pus** surrounded by a **pyogenic membrane**, which may occur as a consequence of acute inflammation.

This can lead to 'what's acute inflammation?' (see 'Acute inflammation', Chapter 45, page 161), or 'tell me what the membrane consists of? Or 'what's pus?'.

The pyogenic membrane consists of fibrin, neutrophils, capillaries and occasional fibroblasts.

Pus contains a mixture of dead and dying neutrophils and pathogens, cellular debris and globules of lipid.

The stimulus to acute inflammation is persistent, and often an infective agent such as *Staphylococcus aureus* or *Streptococcus pyogenes*.

EXAMPLES OF ABSCESSES AND CAUSATIVE ORGANISMS (THIS LIST IS NOT EXHAUSTIVE)

Pilonidal abscess

Arises from infection of a **pre-existing** pilonidal sinus. **Gram-negative** anaerobic organisms and *Bacteroides fragilis* are often the cause.

Perianal abscess

Infection of **hair follicles** caused by *Staphylococcus aureus*. This organism is often responsible for abscess formation wherever it causes disease; examples include lung abscesses, psoas abscesses (see below), meningitis and brain abscesses, etc.

Appendix mass

A sequela of acute appendicitis. Caused by coliforms.

Liver abscess

May be caused by **amoebae** or **coliforms**.

Breast abscess

Caused by **skin** organisms such as *S. aureus*.

Psoas abscess

Caused by *S. aureus*, tuberculosis (TB) and other rarer causes.

Tuberculous abscess

This is a 'cold' abscess.

Subphrenic abscess

Usually **post-abdominal surgery** or **perforated** intra-abdominal **viscus**. Presents with spiking temperature.

Perinephric abscess

A sequela of acute pyelonephritis.

Sterile abscess

Absence of micro-organisms. Causes include:

• Intramuscular injection of irritant agents such as paraldehyde (historical)
• Sterilization of a septic abscess by antimicrobials.

TREATMENT AND SEQUELAE

The appropriate treatment of most abscesses is **surgical drainage**. Antibiotics are not effective because they **do not penetrate** the abscess, and antibiotic treatment may lead to a **chronic abscess**.

Natural history of an abscess is to **discharge itself** through a line of **least resistance**. Often abscesses **point** and then burst. This is seen in perianal abscesses that are not drained surgically.

If incised and drained, an abscess may form **a sinus tract** (connection between the abscess and the skin or a mucosal surface lined by epithelium). If the tract connects **two epithelial surfaces**, a **fistula** results (see definitions in 'Pathology definitions: helpful A–Z guide', Chapter 43, page 155).

Metastatic abscesses can result from **haematogenous spread** of the causative micro-organism. An example includes liver abscesses secondary to appendicitis.

45 Acute inflammation

Possible viva questions related to this topic

→ Define acute inflammation?
→ What cell types are involved in acute inflammation and at what times?
→ What triggers acute inflammation?
→ What are the beneficial and harmful effects of acute inflammation?
→ What are the clinical features of acute inflammation?
→ What are neutrophils for?
→ What are the major differences between acute and chronic inflammation?
→ What is complement? What does it do? What is its role in acute inflammation?
→ What is a cytokine? What is a chemokine? What do they do?

Related topics		
Topic	Chapter	Page
Chronic inflammation	53	197
Abscess and pus	44	158

DEFINITION

- The cellular and vascular response to injury
- Short in duration
- Cellular and chemical components.

CAUSES

Injury by:

- Pathogens: bacteria, viruses, parasites
- Chemical agents: acids, alkalis
- Physical agents: heat, trauma, radiation
- Tissue death: infarction.

> ↑ **Key learning point**
>
> A viva on abscesses is an easy way into a discussion of acute inflammation and vice versa, because an abscess is a sequela of acute inflammation (see below).

STAGES OF ACUTE INFLAMMATION

- **Dilatation** of local capillaries
- Increase in **endothelial permeability**
- Leakage of protein-rich **fluid** into the interstitial space, including fibrinogen
- Fibrinogen converted to **fibrin,** which forms a meshwork of fibrinous exudate
- **Leukocyte** margination to peripheries of capillaries and migration into the interstitial space; mostly neutrophils
- Acute inflammation is mediated by **chemicals,** such as interleukins and histamine, and **proteins,** such as the complement cascade (see below)
- Later on **lymphocytes** appear
- **Lymphatics** become dilated and carry the oedema fluid with pathogens to **lymph nodes,** where lymphocytes contribute to the immune response.

> ↑ **Example viva question**
>
> ### What is complement? What is its role in acute inflammation?
>
> Complement is a component of the **innate** immune system. It consists of a cascade of proteins that result in the formation of a membrane attack complex, which can **destroy invading bacteria** or **recruit other cells** to the inflammatory response such as neutrophils (below). Their proteins can also act as **opsonins** (see definition on page 156).
>
> There are two main activating arms of the complement cascade. The classic pathway consists of **antigen–antibody complexes.** The alternative pathway is activated by contact with **micro-organisms.**

ROLE OF THE NEUTROPHIL

The predominant cell involved in acute inflammation is the **leukocyte.** Appears **early** – the first cellular component to appear.

Attracted to the site of inflammation by inflammatory mediators (chemotaxis). They can move. When they are recruited from blood vessels, they **marginate,** by adhering to the vascular endothelium (the endothelium expresses more adhesion molecules in response to cytokines), **roll,** pass between endothelial cells and emigrate into the interstitial inflammatory exudate.

Phagocytosis of micro-organisms, with lysosomal and free radical degradation of pathogens.

CHEMICAL MESSENGERS IN ACUTE INFLAMMATION

Acute inflammation requires several chemical messengers to enable cells to communicate with each other and mediate the immune response. **Cytokines** are soluble, biologically active molecules secreted by cells that have a variety of effects on the function of target cells. **Chemokines** cause the direct migration of target cells to the site of release.

Examples of cytokines include (non-exhaustive):

- **Interleukin 1** (IL-1): neutrophil adhesion and vascular adhesion molecules
- **Interleukin 2** (IL-2): proliferation, differentiation of B cells and natural killer (NK) cells
- Tumour necrosis factor (TNF): causes fever and promotes inflammatory response, neutrophil adhesion
- Interferon: activation of macrophages, NK cells
- Histamine: released early, vasodilatation and increased permeability.

MACROSCOPIC/CLINICAL FEATURES

Formulated by Celsus and summarized in Latin words:

- **Rubor** (redness), caused by increased flow in dilated capillaries
- **Dolor** (pain), caused by distortion of the local architecture and local release of chemical mediators such as prostaglandins, which induce pain
- **Calor** (heat), caused by local vasodilatation
- **Tumor** (swelling), caused by extravasation of fluid
- **Loss of function**: caused by pain and swelling.

General features include **fever**, caused by chemical mediators such as interleukins which change the set point for temperature homoeostasis.

BENEFICIAL EFFECTS OF ACUTE INFLAMMATION

- **Dilution** of bacterial toxin.
- Defence mechanisms are brought to the pathogen, such as **neutrophils**, which can phagocytose, **complement**, which can cause cell lysis, and **antibodies**, which facilitate cellular defence. **Drugs** and **nutrients** (for neutrophils) are also delivered.
- Increased drainage into the **lymphatic system** where antigens reach lymph nodes to stimulate the immune response.
- **Fibrin** traps the pathogen in one place, where it can be attacked by the above inflammatory components.

HARMFUL EFFECTS OF ACUTE INFLAMMATION

- **Destruction** of normal tissue (see below), particularly in autoimmune disease such as rheumatoid arthritis
- The acute inflammatory response in certain parts of the body can cause lethal **swelling**, e.g. acute epiglottitis and loss of the airway
- **Hypersensitivity reactions** (e.g. anaphylaxis and asthma).

OUTCOMES OF ACUTE INFLAMMATION

- **Resolution:** tissues restored to normal
- **Chronic inflammation:** if the causative agent is not removed
- **Pus** and **abscess** formation: a mixture of dead bacteria and neutrophils within the affected tissues (see 'Abscess and pus', Chapter 44, page 158)
- **Organization:** tissues are replaced by granulation tissue.

46 Aneurysms

Possible viva questions related to this topic

→ What is the definition of an aneurysm?
→ How would you classify aneurysms?
→ Where do they commonly occur?
→ How do aneurysms present?
→ What are their complications?
→ What are the important factors in deciding when to operate electively on an abdominal aortic aneurysm?
→ How would you manage a patient who presented with a ruptured abdominal aortic aneurysm?
→ Is screening for abdominal aortic aneurysms effective? Have you heard of the MASS Trial?

Related topics

Topic	Chapter	Page
Screening in surgery	77	316

Key learning point

Definition: **dilatation** of part of an **artery vessel** or **heart chamber** by at least **100 per cent** (> 50 per cent = arteriomegaly).

CLASSIFICATION

- **False**: as a result of a traumatic breach of the wall with the sac made up from the compressed surrounding tissue
- **True**: dilatation involving all layers of the wall.

By shape

- **Fusiform**: spindle shaped, involving whole of the circumference
- **Saccular**: small segment of wall ballooning as a result of localized weakness.

By cause

Acquired versus congenital

- **Acquired**: normally caused by atherosclerosis
- **Traumatic**: e.g. popliteal artery aneurysms in horse-riders!
- **Inflammatory**: these rupture at a smaller diameter and can be very challenging at surgery
- **Mycotic**: infective, e.g. caused by endocarditis; syphilis – typically saccular and affecting the thoracic part of the aorta
- **Connective tissue disorders**: e.g. Marfan's and Ehlers–Danlos syndromes.

The most common site is the abdominal aorta (2 per cent finding at postmortem examination).

Abdominal aortic aneurysms (AAAs) often associated with aneurysmal dilatation of the **iliac, femoral and popliteal** vessels.

Popliteal aneurysms: most common peripheral aneurysm and second most common type of aneurysm.

Splenic artery aneurysms: $<1/10\,000$; four times more common in women, especially at child-bearing years. 25 per cent rupture, especially in the third trimester. Associated with pancreatitis.

Intracranial 'berry' aneurysms: found at the junction of the limbs in the circle of Willis.

Charcot–Bouchard aneurysms: microaneurysms in the brain as a result of hypertension.

EPIDEMIOLOGY

- **Incidence**: increases with age, 5 per cent of over-50s; 15 per cent of over-80s
- **Sex**: male:female = 6:1
- **Family history**: 12-fold risk for first-degree relatives affected
- **Distribution**: aneurysms caused by atherosclerosis found in the abdominal aorta; 30 per cent have iliac disease; 95 per cent **infrarenal**.

CLINICAL FEATURES

This depends on **site. Seventy-five per cent are asymptomatic**. Incidental finding during screening or investigation of other problems

Berry aneurysms: rupture causes **subarachnoid haemorrhage**.

AAA: abdominal pain referred to the back (can be acute or chronic).

COMPLICATIONS OF AAA

- **Rupture**
- **Thrombosis** (causing lower limb ischaemia)
- **Embolism**
- **Fistulation** to bowel (aorto-enteric), to vena cava, renal vein
- **Pressure effects** on adjacent organs
- **Death**.

INVESTIGATIONS

- **Chest radiograph** (thoracic extension)
- **ECG**
- **Echocardiogram:** to aid in assessment of perioperative risk
- **ESR (erythrocyte sedimentation rate):** is there an inflammatory component?
- **Urea and electrolytes (U+Es):** preoperative renal failure is associated with a poorer prognosis
- **Ultrasonography:** size
- **Computed tomography (CT):** to look at juxtarenal anatomy. Need to avoid suprarenal clamping if at all possible. Also look at the distal extent of the aneurysm – directs need for a bifurcated graft if iliac arteries are involved? Key modality to diagnose rupture.
- May require a 'stenting' CT if endovascular repair considered
- **Arteriography:** multiple, rare aneurysms occurring with aberrant anatomy such as horse-shoe kidneys. No longer used for assessment of aneurysm diameter.

MANAGEMENT ISSUES

Most important factor is the **size** of the aneurysm: repair all above **5.5 cm in diameter (UK Small Aneurysm Trial)**.

Some surgeons would advocate repair at **6 cm in women** because they are less prone to rupture.

No benefit to repair of those sized 4–5.5 cm – operative mortality outweighs risk of rupture. These patients should be enrolled on an **annual ultrasonography screening programme** and operated on when they attain the requisite size:

- 5-year rupture rate: 25 per cent for > 5 cm
- Age limit for cut-off for surgery: 85 years, but need to consider patient on an individual basis.
- Elective mortality rate: 1–5 per cent in regional centres
- Emergency mortality rate: up to 80 per cent!

> ↑ **Example viva question**
>
> ### *Emergency question: the leaking aneurysm*
>
> **Assess** and **resuscitate** patient simultaneously – to stabilize patient
>
> ABC protocol
> **Two large-bore cannulae** into antecubital fossa veins – not central line
> Intravenous fluids **judiciously** – maintain BP around 90–100 mmHg
>
> *Intravenous analgesia*
> **Urinary catheter** – with a **urometer bag**. Measure hourly urine outputs
> because this is the **most sensitive marker** of tissue perfusion
> **Blood tests**: FBC (full blood count), U+Es (urea and electrolytes), glucose,
> amylase, LFTs (liver function tests), clotting screen
> **Cross-match** 10 units of packed red blood cells + 4 units of fresh frozen
> plasma (FFP)
> Contact senior member of surgical team
> If patient **stable**, CT to confirm diagnosis
> If any signs of being **unstable**, theatre
> Contact **anaesthetist** and theatre staff ahead. Book an intensive care bed
> Speak to the patient and relatives

SCREENING ISSUES

MASS Trial

Screening in AAAs is effective in certain groups of patients.

There is a definite survival benefit after screening for AAAs in **men** aged **> 65 years**. Below this age the data are less clear.

Screening in women **does not** seem to be effective.

47 Asbestos

Possible viva questions related to this topic

→ What are the different forms of asbestos? Which one is the most common?
→ What types of asbestos cause disease?
→ What is the most important factor in the development of asbestosis?
→ In which occupations are people particular exposed to asbestos?
→ What happens to the asbestos fibres when they are inhaled?
→ What lung-related problems do asbestos cause?
→ Which type of asbestos is associated with the development of mesothelioma? Why is this type of asbestos more pathogenic than the other types?

Related topics		
Topic	Chapter	Page
Respiratory failure and respiratory function tests	119	495

Asbestos is a family of **fibrous silicates**.

It is used for insulation and the manufacture of brake linings and other friction materials.

There are over **50 types**. Only **three** are important in **human disease**, as follows.

Chrysotile

• **Curled flexible serpentine** mineral (**long woolly** fibres)
• **White asbestos** – accounts for 95 per cent of asbestos used in industry
• Associated with **pulmonary fibrosis**.

Crocidolite

• **Brittle straight amphibole** mineral (**straight short** fibres)
• **Blue asbestos**
• Associated with **pulmonary fibrosis** and **malignant mesothelioma**.

Amosite

- **Brittle straight amphibole** mineral (**straight long** fibres)
- **Brown asbestos**
- Associated with **pulmonary fibrosis.**

AT-RISK OCCUPATIONS

- Shipworkers
- Laggers and industrial plumbers
- Builders
- Workers in old institutions such as hospitals that had insulation installed more than 50 years ago.

DISEASES CAUSED BY ASBESTOS

Malignant

- **Mesothelioma** of pleura, pericardium and peritoneum
- **Bronchogenic carcinoma**: usually bronchioloalveolar cell carcinoma; squamous cell and adenocarcinoma also associated

Benign

- Asbestosis: **fibrosing lung disease**
- **Pleural plaques:** these can be mistaken for malignancy
- Pleural effusion.

PATHOGENESIS

- Important determining factor for the development of asbestosis is the **amount of dust inhaled**
- **Inhaled fibres** that reach the **alveoli** are ingested by alveolar **macrophages,** stimulating release of **C5a** and other **chemoattractants**
- **Amphibole fibres**, which are **short** and **stiff**, penetrate more **deeply** into the lungs than the longer fibres of the other types of asbestos and hence are **more pathogenic**
- Most of the inhaled asbestos is **cleared** by the **macrophages**; the rest reaches the lung and lymphatics
- Some ingested fibres are coated by **haemosiderin** and **glycoproteins** to form characteristic beaded, dumbbell-shaped, **asbestos bodies.**

Lung injury-related mechanisms and subsequent pulmonary fibrosis include:

- Release of **lysozymes** or **toxic free radicals** by macrophages recruited to the site of the asbestos deposition

- Release of **fibrogenic cytokines** and **growth factors** by alveolar macrophages after phagocytosis of the fibres
- Direct stimulation of **fibroblast collagen synthesis** by asbestos.

In addition to pulmonary fibrosis, asbestos induces **pleural reaction** manifested by:

- **Benign effusions**
- **Fibrous pleural** and **fibrocalcific plaques**.

This leads to **alveolar obliteration** with **compensatory dilatation** of intact bronchioles.

48 Ascites

Possible viva questions related to this topic

→ What are the causes of ascites?
→ What signs can be elicited in the patient?
→ What is ascites?
→ How is ascites formed?
→ How do you classify ascites?
→ Based on your understanding, how might liver cirrhosis cause ascites?
→ What tumours are particularly associated with malignant ascites?
→ What investigations can be carried out on ascitic fluid to ascertain the cause of the ascites?
→ How would you perform an ascitic tap? What layers do you traverse?
→ What are the indications for the use of a shunt in the management of ascites?

↑ **Example viva question**

What is ascites?

Ascites is an **abnormal** accumulation of fluid in the **peritoneal cavity**.

CLASSIFICATION AND CAUSES

Cirrhotic versus **malignant** versus **pancreatic** versus **chylous**.

Transudate (protein content $< 30\,g/L$) versus **exudate** (protein content $> 30\,g/L$).

Transudate

Hydrostatic changes
This leads to **increase** in **portal venous pressure**:

- **Cirrhosis**: the **transudate** fluid mainly escapes through the capsule of the liver
- **Right-sided cardiac failure**
- **Constrictive pericarditis**
- **Budd–Chiari syndrome**
- **Thoracic duct obstruction.**

Plasma oncotic changes
- **Liver failure** with **hypoproteinaemia**
- **Protein-losing enteropathy**
- **Starvation**, cachexia
- **Nephritic** and **nephrotic syndromes**, renal failure.

Metabolic or endocrine changes
- **Hypothyroidism**
- **Secondary hyperaldosteronism** (though not in Conn's syndrome).

Exudate

Inflammatory causes
These causes result in **protein leakage**:

- Peritonitis: bacterial and tuberculous
- Post-irradiation
- **Talc granulomata**
- **Pseudomyxoma**
- **Peritoneal infiltration by carcinoma**
- Severe uraemia
- Pancreatitis.

Iatrogenic
- **Operative abdominal surgery**: excess free fluid
- **Continuous ambulatory peritoneal dialysis** (CAPD).

FORMATION OF ASCITES

Fluid accumulation within the peritoneal cavity is dependent on regulating the **inflow** and **outflow** of fluid. The most important factors are the **inflow pressure**, **capillary permeability**, **colloid osmotic pressure** and **lymphatic outflow capacity** (see 'Starling forces in the capillaries/oedema', Chapter 101, page 401).

Inflow is governed by **venous pressure**. There is a **pressure gradient** for **peritoneal fluid absorption**, which is created by **negative intrathoracic pressure** generated during the **respiratory cycle**. **Outflow fluid** is controlled primarily by the **lymphatics**. Ascites forms where there is an **imbalance** of fluid movements. In ascites, **raised venous pressure** is the cause of the **inflow problem** to the peritoneal cavity (portal hypertension) and **blocked lymphatics** are the cause of the **outflow problem**.

Cirrhosis produces ascites by **increasing** both **portal vascular resistance** and **splanchnic blood flow**. These two factors act to create **portal hypertension**, which in turn leads to **increased visceral lymph formation**. This increase in lymph production exceeds absorption capacity and hence fluid accumulates in the peritoneal space. The **extracellular fluid (ECF) volume falls**. The **kidney** responds by stimulating the **renin–aldosterone** axis, leading to an increase in the ECF. This in turn leads to further lymph formation and exacerbates the ascites.

INVESTIGATIONS ON ASCITIC FLUID

- **Microscopy** for bacteria, white cells and red cells
- **Culture and sensitivity** for **TB and other bacteria**
- **Cytology** for:
  - involvement by metastatic or primary carcinoma
  - involvement by lymphoma
- **Biochemistry** for:
  - protein content
  - amylase if pancreatitis is suspected
- **Cytogenetics** where appropriate.

TUMOURS ASSOCIATED WITH MALIGNANT ASCITES

- Ovary
- Breast
- Colon
- Pancreas
- Stomach
- Liver
- Lymphoma.

SPECIFIC TESTS FOR ASCITES

- Shifting dullness within the abdomen
- Fluid thrill
- Flank dullness within the abdomen.

ASCITIC TAP

- Perform under sterile conditions
- If ascites not clinically apparent or easy to locate, this procedure should be done under **ultrasound guidance** to prevent visceral injuries
- Local anaesthetic infiltrated and site marked
- A narrow-gauge needle should be introduced first to check position before a larger-gauge cannula is inserted into the abdomen
- **Seldinger technique**
- When in position a plastic tube can be connected to a urine bag in order to collect the ascitic fluid.

↑ **Example viva question**

What layers do you traverse when performing an ascitic tap?

Layers traversed:

- Skin
- Superficial fascia
- Scarpa's fascia
- External oblique
- Internal oblique
- Transversalis fascia
- Extraperitoneal fat
- Parietal and visceral peritoneum

TREATMENT

- Mainstay of treatment of ascites is to **treat** the **underlying cause**
- Patient placed on a **weight reduction programme**
- Judicious use of **diuretics**
- **Low-sodium, high-protein diet**.

In **diuretic-resistant ascites**, **shunting** can be performed in a number of ways:

- **Peritoneovenous shunting** (Le Veen shunt): a subcutaneous Silastic catheter is used to drain the fluid into the jugular vein.
- **Denver shunt**: this is a modification, adding a small subcutaneous pump that can be compressed externally.

- **Transjugular intrahepatic portosystemic stent shunt (TIPSS)**: this is a side-to-side shunt stenting a channel between a branch of the portal vein and hepatic vein.

Radiological techniques have now widely replaced the difficult surgically formed shunt operations, e.g. selective splenorenal (Warren) shunt – anastomosis of the distal (splenic side) splenic vein into the left renal vein with ligation of the left gastric vein.

49 Atherosclerosis

DEFINITION

A **pathological process** of the vasculature beginning with **endothelial dysfunction,** resulting in **migration of macrophages** across the endothelium, formation of **foam cells** and a **necrotic lipid core**, and migration of **vascular smooth muscle cells** to form a **fibrous cap**. This process ultimately results in **stenosis** of the vessel and **rupture of the cap** can lead to **thrombosis** and possible infarction of the supplied tissue.

MECHANISMS OF PLAQUE FORMATION

- **Endothelial dysfunction** as a result of:
  - loss of laminar blood flow in turbulent areas around bifurcations leading to **decreased wall sheer stress** and direct endothelial cell changes.
  - **oxidative stress**, e.g. free radicals from smoking
  - possible **infective cause**: ? *Chlamydia* implicated

- **Low-density lipoprotein** (LDL) becomes oxidized (ox-LDL) and damages endothelium further – tight junctions are disrupted
- **Macrophages** migrate across endothelium by the interaction with selectins, integrins and intercellular adhesion molecules (ICAMs)
- Macrophages **ingest ox-LDL** and become activated
- Some macrophages become **foam cells** and migrate to **form a lipid core**
- Plaque is stabilized by migration of **vascular smooth muscle cells** to form a fibrous cap. **Endothelial progenitor cells** have also been shown to play an important role in the formation of the cap. They are derived from the **bone marrow**.

MECHANISMS OF PLAQUE RUPTURE

- **Macrophages** secrete **enzymes** to break down the collagen within the fibrous cap (matrix metalloproteases or **MMPs**)
- Increased rate of **apoptotic cell death** within the cap, weakening it further
- Flow across a thinned fibrous cap causes **biomechanical stress**, which ultimately leads to plaque rupture
- **Lipid core is exposed** to flowing blood
- Platelets adhere and the **clotting cascade** activated, causing a **thrombosis** (see 'DVT prophylaxis and coagulation in surgery', Chapter 73, page 297).

RISK FACTORS

- Smoking
- Hypertension
- Diabetes mellitus types 1 and 2
- Family history of atherosclerotic disease
- Increased cholesterol (specifically increased LDL and decreased high-density lipoprotein or HDL).

Sites, symptoms and complications

Site	Symptoms	Complications
Aorta	Pain from expanding aneurysm Claudication from occlusive aortoiliac disease Distal embolic disease 'trash foot' – particularly post-AAA repair Can be asymptomatic	Aneurysm rupture Critical or acute limb ischaemia
Coronary arteries	Angina	Myocardial infarction Coronary dissection — rare but can occur after angioplasty ± stenting
Carotid arteries and cerebral vasculature	Can be asymptomatic Transient ischaemic attacks (TIAs)	Cerebrovascular accident (stroke) Carotid aneurysm Hypoperfusion syndrome with bilateral disease (rare)
Popliteal and lower limb vasculature	Claudication Distal embolization – painful gangrenous toes *In situ* thrombosis (particularly popliteal)	Ulceration and critical limb ischaemia – may lead to amputation Distal embolization may lead to gangrene of the toes Thrombosis of a popliteal aneurysm may cause acute limb ischaemia

↑ **Key learning point**

Any question relating to the therapeutic options of atheroma is obviously wide ranging. Try to **structure and categorize your answer** – this gives you a few moments to think and also gives the examiner the impression that you're not about to reel off a badly constructed list of surgical options, missing key medical points!

THERAPEUTIC OPTIONS

These depend on site and type of disease process (occlusive or aneurysmal) and can be split into medical, surgical and radiological.

Occlusive disease

Medical
Secondary prevention

- Diet and pharmacological manipulation of LDL (e.g. statins) – recent **ASTEROID trial** shows approximately 7 per cent reduction in atheroma volume over 12 months in the high-dose statin group)
- Antihypertensives (especially angiotensin-converting enzyme inhibitors or ACEIs and angiotensin II antagonists)
- Management of diabetes and strict blood sugar control
- Stop smoking and lifestyle modification.

Acute treatment

- High-dose aspirin (300 mg) for acute myocardial infarction (MI)
- Intravenous thrombolysis (e.g. streptokinase, tissue plasminogen activator or tPA, recombinant tPA) for MI and cerebrovascular accident (CVA)
- Acute β blocker and statin therapy for MI.

Symptom relief

For example, sympathectomy for foot pain in critical limb ischaemia.

Surgical (depends on site)
Lower limb/aorta

- Bypass grafting: anatomical versus extra-anatomical. Conduit can be vein, artery or synthetic (e.g. Dacron for aorto-bifemoral, PTFE (polytetrafluoroethylene) for femoral–distal bypass)
- Acute embolectomy for lower leg embolus.

Coronary arteries

Coronary artery bypass grafting (CABG).

Carotid arteries

Carotid endarterectomy (see 'Carotid endarterectomy', Chapter 27, page 81).

Radiological/cardiological intervention
Lower limb/aorta

- Angioplasty ± stenting (can be subintimal for complete occlusion)
- Intra-arterial thrombolysis for acute thrombus in lower limb/upper limb vasculature.

Coronary arteries

Angioplasty ± stenting (sirolimus-eluting stents now used to prevent re-stenosis).

Carotid arteries

Angioplasty + stenting – relatively new treatment, no long-term follow-up.

Aneurysmal disease

Medical
Secondary prevention

- **Low-dose aspirin** (anti-platelet) and **statins** (the **Heart Protection Study** and many studies since have shown a significant risk reduction in atheroma-related ischaemic events after the administration of a long-term statin)
- **Diet** and pharmacological manipulation of LDL (e.g. statins)
- **Antihypertensives** (especially ACEs and angiotensin II antagonists)
- Management of **diabetes** and **strict blood sugar control**
- **Smoking cessation** and lifestyle modification.

Surgical and radiological
Aorta

- Surgery: AAA repair with Dacron graft
- Radiology: AAA stent.

Popliteal

- Surgery: bypass grafting and ligation of aneurysm
- Radiology: covered stent.

50 Breast cancer

Possible viva questions related to this topic

→ What do you understand by the term 'ductal carcinoma *in situ*' or 'DCIS'? How is it treated?
→ What would you do if you saw a patient with a breast lump in clinic?
→ What are the risk factors for breast carcinoma?
→ What is the management strategy for breast carcinoma?
→ What staging systems do you know?
→ How does breast cancer spread?
→ What adjuvant treatment is available for breast carcinoma and for whom is it suitable?
→ What is the prognosis of the various types of breast cancer?
→ What is the Nottingham prognostic index?
→ What do you understand about Herceptin? What is its action?

DUCTAL CARCINOMA *IN SITU*

DCIS is a **non-invasive precancerous** process. It occurs most commonly in the **40 to 60 year olds** and presents with a **nipple discharge** and/or **mass**. DCIS is **usually unilateral** and, if left untreated, **proceeds to invasive ductal carcinoma**. There is a **25–50 per cent risk of breast cancer at 10–15 years**. When DCIS recurs, 50 per cent will be invasive tumours.

Example viva question

What are the risk factors for breast carcinoma?

Breast cancer represents 20 per cent of all cancers in women. It is the most common cause of death in women aged 35–55 years and there is a linear increase in risk with an increase in age. One in seven women will eventually develop breast carcinoma.

Risk factors
- **Age:** linear increase with age so older people more at risk
- **Female** sex (remember it can occur in men)
- **Oestrogen exposure:** early menarche, late menopause, oral contraceptive pill
- **Nulliparous** (early pregnancy is protective as is multiparity)
- **Weight** (in patients aged >55 years)
- **Family history** and genetic factors:
  - *BRCA*-1 (2 per cent of all breast carcinomas) and *BRCA*-2
  - relative risk × 5 if multiple relatives affected
  - relative risk × 9 if first-degree relative with bilateral cancer
  - Li–Fraumeni syndrome (increased risk of multiple primary cancers)
- **Geography:** high in North America and Europe, low in Africa and south-east Asia
- **Atypical hyperplasia**
- **Upper class** > lower class
- **Unmarried** > married
- Jewish individuals and nuns have higher risk

LOBULAR CARCINOMA *IN SITU*

Lobular carcinoma *in situ* (LCIS) is found predominantly in **premenopausal women.** It does not present as a mass and is often seen in biopsies. It is also often associated with an infiltrating tumour, although not necessarily lobular carcinoma.

CLINICAL FEATURES AND ON EXAMINATION

- **Painless breast lump: hard** and **irregular, fixed** to underlying tissues (although small T1a tumours are impalpable)
- **Nipple discharge:** blood-stained
- **Pain** is **less common** as is skin ulceration
- **Nipple retraction**, skin tethering
- **Lymphadenopathy**, limb oedema, satellite nodules

- **Skin infiltration** (chest, back and neck)
- Localized skin oedema (**peau d'orange**)
- **Metastatic symptoms and signs**: cachexia, ascites, jaundice, pathological fractures, central nervous system (CNS) symptoms.

METHODS OF STAGING

There are **three major clinical systems for staging**: UICC (Union Internationale Contre Le Cancer), Manchester and Columbia.

The **UICC is the most comprehensive** and relates to **primary tumour, nodal disease** and **systemic disease**.

⇡ **Key learning point**

UICC system

T0 – subclinical
T1 – ≤ 2 cm
T2 – > 2 cm but < 5 cm
T3 – > 5 cm
T4 – any size with chest wall or skin invasion
N0 – no nodal disease
N1 – ipsilateral, mobile axillary node involvement
N2 – ipsilateral, fixed axillary node involvement
N3 – ipsilateral internal mammary node involvement
M0 – no distant metastases
M1 – distant metastases

PREDICTORS OF POOR OUTCOME

- **Tumour size**: the bigger the tumour, the worse the prognosis
- **Tumour grade: Bloom and Richardson** grading system based on histological architecture – from grade 1 (well differentiated) to grade 3 (poorly differentiated)
- **Nodal involvement: five or more positive nodes** on sampling; **< 20 per cent 5-year survival rate**
- Vascular invasion in primary tumour (tumour spreads haematogenously and via the lymphatics)
- **Multicentricity** of primary tumour
- **Oestrogen receptor positivity** (predicts response to tamoxifen; negative is worse prognosis).

↑ **Example viva question**

How is a lump assessed in clinic?

Examination and investigation of a lump in the clinic

Triple assessment:

1 **Clinical examination**
2 **Radiological assessment** (mammography > 35 and ultrasonography < 35 years)
3 **Pathological** (cytology or histology).

After a full examination, either fine-needle aspiration cytology (**FNAC**) should be performed or a core biopsy (**Trucut**) taken. These investigations have a preoperative diagnostic **sensitivity of > 95 per cent**.

Tissue or cells are graded as below:

FNAC (cytology)	Trucut (histology)
C1 inadequate	B1 normal
C2 benign	B2 benign
C3 equivocal	B3 equivocal
C4 suspicious	B4 suspicious
C5 malignant	B5 malignant

NOTTINGHAM PROGNOSTIC INDEX (NPI)

This is based on **tumour size** (in centimetres), **tumour grade** (1–3) and **nodal disease** status (1 = no nodal involvement, 2 = one to three nodes, 3 = more than four nodes or apical node)

$$NPI = size \times 0.2 + stage + grade$$

If NPI < 3.4, 15-year survival rate is 90 per cent
If NPI > 5.4, 15-year survival rate is 8 per cent.

MANAGEMENT OF BREAST CANCER

- **Multidisciplinary** approach
- Treat **local disease** and **axillary disease**
- Can be **split into surgical management** of the **breast and the axilla** and **systemic medical management** including hormonal therapy, chemotherapy and radiotherapy.

Surgical management of the breast

- **Breast-conserving operations** are the norm where possible (wide local excision or WLE instead of mastectomy)
- **Clear resection margins** of $> 5\,mm$ are required histologically
- Incomplete excision requires a further WLE or mastectomy
- **Whole-breast radiotherapy** is used for **local disease control** and to prevent local recurrence after WLE, provided that margins are clear; given if local recurrence risk is thought to be > 15 per cent
- **Reconstruction may be immediate or delayed**, depending on the tumour and patient choice: immediate skin-sparing mastectomy and prosthesis or a free or pedicled flap
- Delayed reconstruction with tissue expansion or a free or pedicled flap.

Management of the axilla

- Treated as a **separate entity** to the breast
- May be **sampled** or **cleared**
- **Sampling** provides **essential diagnostic information** although nodes may be missed
- **Clearance** can be split into **three different levels**:
  - **level 1**: below pectoralis minor
  - **level 2**: up to upper border of pectoralis minor
  - **level 3**: to the outer border of the first rib
- As levels of clearance increase, risk of postoperative lymphoedema increases
- **Sentinel node biopsy** is a new technique aimed at identifying the first or sentinel node draining the breast. It involves a combination of a radioactive isotope (technetium) and a blue dye. It is still experimental but shows great promise and will hopefully address the **60 per cent of women who are N0** and do not need sampling
- **Radiotherapy** is used on the **axilla** if positive nodes are found on sampling. An **alternative** is a **level 2 clearance**. If both radiotherapy and surgery are utilized, the risk of lymphoedema goes up dramatically.

Systemic treatment

Can be given as **primary** method of treatment, although **more usually** given as **adjuvant therapy**.

Split into **hormonal therapy** (e.g. tamoxifen) and **chemotherapy**. Specific chemotherapeutic regimens are beyond the scope of this topic and are unlikely to be asked for:

- **Adjuvant chemotherapy** reduces mortality – **absolute survival benefit rate** at 10 years is **approximately 8 per cent**
- **Chemotherapy reduces** annual **risk of death by 30 per cent** for 10 years

- Evidence to suggest that **goserelin (Zoladex)** in combination with tamoxifen is as effective as adjuvant chemotherapy in young women with poor prognosis disease that is oestrogen receptor positive.

↑ **Example viva question**

What do you understand about Herceptin? What is its action?

Herceptin or **trastuzumab** is a **monoclonal antibody** directed at human epidermal growth factor 2 receptor (**HER2**) and prevents epidermal growth factor from binding. Some breast tumours (about 20 per cent) express this protein and, in these, Herceptin treatment appears to **halt the growth** or **shrink tumours**. There is some evidence to suggest that it has a **synergistic effect** with the chemotherapeutic agent **paclitaxel** and, given 1 year after chemotherapy in HER2-positive tumours, **reduces the recurrence rate by half**.

Herceptin is **now licensed** for use in **early breast cancer** – the National Institute for Health and Clinical Excellence (NICE) reported early in June 2006 about this indication.

RECURRENT DISEASE

- **Local recurrence**: treated by further WLE and/or radiotherapy if appropriate
- **Regional recurrence**: spread to axilla, brachial plexus, supraclavicular nodes – axillary clearance/radiotherapy
- **Distant metastases**: bone, lungs, liver and brain. Can cause hypercalcaemia, pleural effusion, hepatocellular jaundice, epilepsy and neurological symptoms.

Note that treatment can be **palliative as well as curative**:

- **Bisphosphonates** for hypercalcaemia and bone pain
- **Analgesia**
- **Social** and **psychological** support
- **Palliative radiotherapy**
- **Blood transfusion** for anaemia of chronic disease
- **Resection** for skin-ulcerating tumour
- Aspiration of pleural effusions and **pleurodesis**.

MANAGEMENT OF DCIS

- **Of all cases of DCIS, 1 per cent is found to have positive nodal involvement** and therefore must represent small tumours not found at histology or screening.

- A third of all cases of DCIS go on to become invasive ductal carcinoma if left untreated
- DCIS makes up **25 per cent of all screening-detected cancers**
- **Good prognosis** in most cases but diffuse process and often requires total mastectomy (5-year survival rate of 98 per cent)
- **Localized DCIS (< 4 cm)**: treated by WLE ± radiotherapy and tamoxifen
- **Widespread and/or multifocal DCIS**: treated by mastectomy ± tamoxifen.

51 Carcinogenesis

Example viva question

What is carcinogenesis?

This is the process that results in the **transformation** of **normal cells** to **neoplastic cells**, caused by **permanent genetic alterations** or **mutations**. It applies only to **malignant tumours**.

Compare **oncogenesis**, which is the process that leads to the formation of **benign** or **malignant tumours**.

Factors implicated in carcinogenesis are broadly divided into **genetic** and **environmental**.

Carcinogen is an agent **known** to cause or **suspected** of causing cells to transform and start dividing uncontrollably without their normal inhibitions, eventually developing into **neoplasms**.

TYPES OF CARCINOGENS

Chemical carcinogens

- **Remote:** precursor of a carcinogenic agent that may be found in food, the environment, exposure to certain chemicals, infective organisms and physical agents
- **Proximate:** metabolite(s) of a remote carcinogen that has some carcinogenic potential but may be modified further in the body into an ultimate carcinogen
- **Ultimate:** active carcinogen that interacts with DNA and causes cancer.

Remote/proximate/ultimate carcinogen sequence: best example is **β-naphthylamine**.

Direct effect or after **metabolic conversion**. These carcinogens are usually hydrocarbons, which form charged molecules called epoxides. Epoxides then bind to DNA and RNA, causing a genetic mutation:

- **Polycyclic aromatic hydrocarbons** (tar) in **smoke** cause **lung cancer**
- **Aromatic amines** (**β-naphthylamine** – used in the **rubber** and **dye industry**): converted to a carcinogen in the liver and thought to cause bladder cancer
- **Nitrosamines:** used in **fertilizers**, causing **gastrointestinal tract cancers**
- **Azo dyes** – in **bladder** and **liver cancer**.

Viral carcinogens

Some DNA and RNA viruses are **oncogenic**.

Directly: their **integration** into the **host genome promotes** over-activity of **proto-oncogenes** (see below).

Indirectly: cause malignancy **through diseases** such as **chronic hepatitis**, which predispose to **hepatocellular carcinoma**.

DNA viruses
Human papillomavirus in cervical (HPV-16 and -18), anal and oesophageal cancers

These viruses are seen in **cervical intraepithelial neoplasia (CIN)**. The viral DNA is integrated into the host cell DNA leading to over-expression of E6 and E7 viral proteins. They bind to and inhibit *p53* and *Rb* (see below). The **transformation zone** (**labile** area where **columnar epithelium** undergoes **metaplasia** to **squamous** type) is at the **squamocolumnar junction**.

Epstein–Barr virus – in Burkitt's lymphoma and nasopharyngeal cancer (NPC)

This was discovered in **cell cultures** from **Burkitt's lymphoma**.

It usually causes **infectious mononucleosis** but with a **co-factor** is **oncogenic**. Epidemiological evidence suggests that the co-factor is **malaria**, which has a causal link with **NPC**.

Hepatitis B and C

Strong association with **hepatocellular carcinoma**.

RNA viruses

- **Human T-cell leukaemia virus (HTLV-1)**: in T-cell leukaemia and lymphoma
- **Human immunodeficiency virus (HIV)**: in Kaposi's sarcoma.

Bacterial carcinogens

- *Helicobacter pylori* linked to gastric lymphoma and carcinoma

Radiant energy

- **Non-ionizing radiation – ultraviolet (UV) light**: malignant melanoma
- **Ionizing radiation**: leukaemia, skin and thyroid cancer.

Biological agents

- **Hormones**: oestrogens in breast and endometrial cancers
- **Androgenic and anabolic steroids** in hepatocellular carcinoma
- **Mycotoxins**: *Aspergillus* species **(aflatoxin)** in hepatocellular carcinoma
- **Parasites:**
  - schistosomiasis in bladder cancer
  - liver fluke in cholangiocarcinoma.

Other carcinogens

Industrial dusts

Asbestos: **malignant mesothelioma** and **carcinoma of the lung** (see 'Asbestos', Chapter 47, page 169).

Metals

- Nickel: NPC and carcinoma of the lung
- Arsenic: skin cancer.

HOST FACTORS

- **Race**, e.g. breast cancer is less common in Africa
- **Diet,** e.g. fat and colorectal carcinoma
- Genetics
- Age
- Gender
- **Pre-malignant lesions**, e.g. polyps, chronic ulcerative colitis, hepatic cirrhosis
- **Transplacental exposure**, e.g. diethylstilbestrol and vaginal cancer in female babies.

MULTI-STEP THEORY OF CARCINOGENESIS

Initiation refers to the induction of certain irreversible changes (mutations) in the genome of the cells, which bestows neoplastic potential when appropriately stimulated by promoting agents. Initiated cells are not transformed cells; they do not have growth autonomy or unique phenotypic characteristics.

Promotion refers to the process of tumour induction in previously initiated cells by chemicals called **promoters**. This stimulates clonal proliferation of the initiated cell.

Persistence is clonal proliferation of tumour cells that **no longer** require the presence of initiators or promoters.

ONCOGENES

A **proto-oncogene** is a cellular gene involved in **normal regulation** and **differentiation** of **cell growth**. Most are **growth factors** or **receptors**. When they become **mutated** they have **altered** and **enhanced expression** and become known as **oncogenes**. Oncogenes are classified by the function of their gene products (**oncoproteins**).

Examples

- *Bcl-2*: involved with apoptosis
- *Ras*: signal transduction molecule involved in intracellular signalling
- *Myc*: nuclear binding protein involved in cell proliferation.

Mechanism of oncogene activation

- Translocation of an oncogene to a position adjacent to an actively translocated gene (8 → 14 in Burkitt's lymphoma)
- Point mutation
- Gene insertion resulting in the proximity of an oncogene to a promoter or enhancing gene (retrovirus).

Abnormalities in oncogene expression may account for an increased risk of carcinogenesis:

- Production of an excessive amount of oncoproteins
- Production of abnormally functioning oncoproteins
- Loss of usual growth inhibition – tumour suppressor genes.

Oncoproteins encourage cells to grow **autonomously**, have **increased motility** and **reduced cell–cell adhesion**, all **features** of **malignancy**.

TUMOUR SUPPRESSOR GENES

These are **recessive genes** that encode **proteins** that **inhibit cell proliferation**. If their function is disrupted, uncontrolled cell proliferation, and hence tumours, are more likely to occur.

Examples

The p53 *gene*

This is the most common gene to be altered in human cancers (70 per cent of colon cancers and one-third of breast cancers). It repairs damaged DNA before the S-phase of the cell cycle by arresting the cell cycle in G1 until the damage is repaired. If the damage cannot be repaired, it induces the cell to undergo apoptosis. Loss of function causes:

• Mutations
• Binding of normal p53 proteins to proteins encoded by oncogenic DNA viruses.

*Retinoblastoma (*Rb1 *gene)*

Patients with retinoblastoma usually have a hereditary germline mutation on chromosome 13. Therefore sporadic loss of the other gene as a result of mutation leads to tumour development – Knudson's 'two-hit' hypothesis. This states that both alleles of the tumour suppressor gene need to be deleted or damaged for malignant transformation to occur.

↑ Key learning point

It is worthwhile knowing several examples of both **tumour suppressor genes** and **oncogenes** because this question is frequently asked.

---

52 Cell cycle

Possible viva questions related to this topic

→ What is the cell cycle and can you draw it?
→ Name some factors that influence the progression of the cell cycle.
→ What cell growth factors are important in wound healing and/or inhibition?
→ What cell types are there?

DEFINITION

The **cell cycle** describes the progressive steps that a cell moves through in order that **DNA** may be synthesized and cells may **divide**. It is made up of the following **phases**:

G0: resting phase – stable cells are held in G0
G1: first gap phase:
• **main determinant** of the cell cycle
• **variable duration**
• **four options:**
 (1) recycle and embark on another round of DNA synthesis and mitosis
 (2) decycle and move to **G0** phase
 (3) decycle and commit to **terminal differentiation**
 (4) abort and undergo **apoptosis**.

If the cell cycle is permitted to advance beyond the **restriction point**, the cell must **complete** the cycle and undergo mitosis (Fig. 52.1).

S: synthetic phase – DNA synthesis
G2: second gap phase
M: mitosis phase – nuclear and cytoplasmic division

The S, G2 and M phases are usually of constant length. The G2 phase may vary between cell types and species.

Example viva questions

Draw the cell cycle

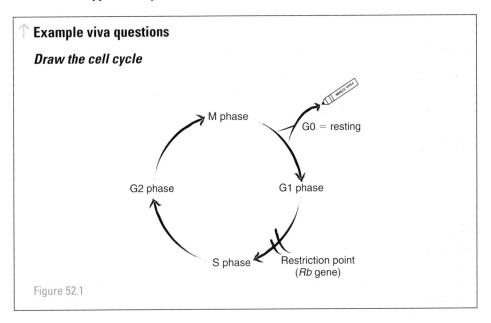

Figure 52.1

MOLECULAR CONTROLS

These regulate the passage of cells through specific phases of the cell cycle. There are **two types**: a cascade of **protein phosphorylation pathways** and **checkpoints**.

Cascade

The cascade involves **cyclins** and **cyclin-dependent kinases**. Cyclins are **regulatory proteins** with concentrations that rise and fall during the cell cycle. They form complexes with constitutively present **protein kinases** called cyclin-dependent kinases (CDKs). Different combinations of cyclins and CDKs are associated with each of the important transitions in the cell cycle.

Checkpoints

A set of **checkpoints** is present that monitor completion of the molecular events; if necessary they delay progression to the next phase of the cycle.

These checkpoints provide a **surveillance mechanism** for ensuring that critical transitions in the cell cycle occur in the **correct order** and that important events are completed with **fidelity**.

Examples

The gene *p53* is activated in response to **DNA damage** and **inhibits** further progression through the cell cycle by increasing expression of a **CDK inhibitor**.

Retinoblastoma (*Rb*) and related genes act at the **restriction point**, which **holds** the cell in the **G1 phase**.

Growth factors involved in stimulating inflammation and repair

These are important in **wound healing**:

- **Epidermal growth factor (EGF)** from epithelial cells
- **Fibroblast growth factor (FGF)**
- **Platelet-derived growth factor (PDGF)** from α granules in platelets and macrophages. It stimulates proliferation of epithelial cells in the epidermis with the help of EGF. It also stimulates proliferation of myofibroblasts in the dermis
- **Cytokines:** TNF
- **Transforming growth factor β (TGF-β)**: this stimulates the production of collagen and fibronectin from myofibroblasts.

Growth factors involved in inhibition of inflammation and repair

- Interferon-α
- Heparin
- Prostaglandin E_2.

Cell types

- **Permanent**: neurons, cardiac muscle
- **Stable**: liver, fibroblasts
- **Labile**: skin, blood, epithelium.

53 Chronic inflammation

Possible viva questions related to this topic

→ Define chronic inflammation.
→ What cell types are involved in chronic inflammation and at what times?
→ What are the beneficial and harmful effects of chronic inflammation?
→ What are the clinical features of chronic inflammation?
→ Give some examples of chronic inflammation.
→ What happens in chronic peptic ulceration?

Related topics

Topic	Chapter	Page
Acute inflammation	45	161
Abscess and pus	44	158

DEFINITION

• Tissue response to **persistent injury**
• **Long** in duration
• Cellular **components differ** from acute inflammation.

CAUSES

• **Foreign bodies** (granulomata): surgical sutures
• **Bacteria**: TB
• **Chronic abscess formation**: osteomyelitis
• **Transplant**: chronic rejection
• Inflammatory bowel disease
• Progression from acute inflammation.

↑ **Key learning point**

A viva on acute inflammation can easily lead into a viva on chronic inflammation and a viva on abscesses can lead into discussion of both types of inflammation.

HISTOLOGICAL AND CELLULAR FEATURES OF CHRONIC INFLAMMATION

Compare with acute inflammation ('Acute inflammation', Chapter 45, page 161):

- The histological pattern is **not as predictable** as in acute inflammation, and many of the features described below may coexist. There may be areas of ongoing acute inflammation.
- **Granulation tissue** may be present, as may fibrosis. These reflect the tissue's attempts at repair.
- **Lymphocytes** predominate – they are recruited by macrophages and cytokines.
- **Macrophages** are also present. In **granulomatous inflammation**, they fuse to form **multinucleate Langhan's giant cells**, the presence of which is microscopically diagnostic of graulomatous inflammation. They are important in phagocytosis and antigen presentation.
- **Plasma cells** are also present: derived from B lymphocytes that migrate into the area.

↑ **Example viva question**

Describe what happens in a chronic peptic ulcer.

A breach in the stomach mucosa occurs.

Acute inflammation continues in the part of the ulcer in contact with acid as the injury continues.

The base of the ulcer contains granulation tissue and fibrosis as attempts at repair occur.

Role of the macrophage

- Derived from **monocytes**
- Phagocytosis and killing of pathogens by lysosomes, scavenging of debris
- Attracted by chemotaxis and produces cytokines
- Antigen presentation
- Formation of Langhan's giant cells in granulomatous inflammation.

CLINICAL FEATURES

Fever is caused by the chemical mediators seen in acute inflammation, although it is not as severe.

The predominant leukocytes present at the site of inflammation can be measured in a **FBC** (lymphocytes, monocytes, eosinophils or neutrophils).

Weight loss may occur because of the high metabolic rate required to maintain cell division.

EFFECTS OF CHRONIC INFLAMMATION

- Secondary infection, e.g. in chronic epithelial injury
- Scarring
- Resolution (always some scarring)
- Secondary amyloidosis (rare) in rheumatoid arthritis and TB
- Local lymphadenopathy.

GRANULOMATOUS INFLAMMATION

↑ **Example viva question**

What is a granuloma?

This is a common opening question in a pathology viva. Granulomatous inflammation is commonly seen in surgical conditions – sutures, inflammatory bowel disease, etc. and is also a good route into a viva on inflammation.

A granuloma is a collection of **epithelioid (activated) macrophages**. Granulomatous inflammation is a form of chronic inflammation in which granulomata are seen histologically.

Histologically, **granulomatous inflammation** is characterized by the presence of **epithelioid macrophages**; these are so called because they resemble epithelial cells. These macrophages can fuse to form **multinucleate giant cells** (Langhan's cells), which are sometimes present in granulomatous inflammation.

Some causes

Infections	TB, leprosy
Chronic diseases	Sarcoidosis, Wegener's granulomatosis, inflammatory bowel disease (Crohn's disease)
Foreign bodies	Surgical sutures

54 Colorectal cancer

Possible viva questions related to this topic

→ How would you classify colonic tumours?
→ What are the risk factors for colorectal carcinoma?
→ What is the anatomical distribution of colorectal cancer?
→ How does colorectal carcinoma present clinically?
→ How is colorectal cancer staged?
→ What are the principles of management of colorectal cancer?
→ What is meant by the adenoma–carcinoma sequence?
→ What operations can be performed for colorectal cancer?
→ What is the prognosis after surgery for colorectal carcinoma?
→ What are the complications of surgery for colorectal carcinoma?
→ What are the advantages and disadvantages of pre- and postoperative radiotherapy?
→ What are the indications for chemotherapy in colorectal cancer?
→ What is the risk of malignant transformation in ongoing ulcerative colitis?

Related topics

Topic	Chapter	Page
Antibiotics in surgery	67	275
Bowel preparation	68	280
Cell cycle	52	194
Carcinogenesis	51	189
Anastomosis and anastomotic leak	66	270
Stomas	80	330
DVT prophylaxis and coagulation in surgery	73	297
Tumour markers	63	252
Diverticula	55	210

DISTRIBUTION AND RELATIVE INCIDENCE

- Rectal 38 per cent
- Sigmoid 28 per cent
- Caecal 12 per cent
- Transverse colon 5.5 per cent

- Ascending colon 5 per cent
- Descending colon 4 per cent
- Splenic flexure 3 per cent
- Hepatic flexure 2 per cent
- Anal 2 per cent
- Appendicular 0.5 per cent.

↑ **Example viva question**

What are the risk factors for colorectal carcinoma?

Colorectal carcinoma is the **second most common cancer** causing death in the UK with **20 000 new cases per year** in the UK – 40 per cent rectal and 60 per cent colonic.

Three per cent of patients present with more than one tumour (= synchronous tumours).

Risk factors
- **Family history** (although **75 per cent are sporadic**)
- **Adenomatous polyps** (see 'Adenoma–carcinoma sequence' below)
- Familial adenomatous polyposis coli (***FAP* gene** on chromosome 5q21)
- Hereditary non-polyposis colorectal carcinoma (**HNPCC**)
- **Diet**:
  - **low fibre** intake (decreases gut transit time, increasing the time that potential carcinogens are exposed to the gut mucosa)
  - **high carbohydrate and fat** intake (possibly favours bacteria that degrade bile salts into carcinogens)
  - **high protein** intake (particularly meat)
  - **low vitamin A, C and E** intake
- **Ulcerative colitis (UC)**: **1 per cent per year risk** of malignant transformation in ongoing colitis. After subtotal colectomy, the rectal stump still requires surveillance, leading to most UC sufferers opting for a modified panproctocolectomy and ileoanal pouch or end ileostomy
- Gardner's syndrome
- Other hereditary mutations of tumour suppressor genes or proto-oncogenes such as *p53* and *K-ras* (see 'Carcinogenesis', Chapter 51, page 189 and 'Cell cycle', Chapter 52, page 194)
- A **previous colonic neoplasm** increases the risk of a second tumour (metachronous tumour)

CLINICAL FEATURES

Many tumours can be asymptomatic, with **right-sided lesions** being more likely to be **clinically silent** than left-sided lesions.

Associated with primary tumour

- **Change in bowel habit**
- **Weight loss**
- Unexplained **microcytic anaemia** (iron deficiency)
- **Faecal occult blood (FOB) positive**
- **Obstruction**
- **Mucus or altered blood** per rectum (overt bleeding relatively uncommon in colonic tumours, more common in rectal tumours)
- **Tenesmus** (a feeling of incomplete evacuation)
- Can present with perforation and an acute abdomen
- Can present with colovesical/colovaginal fistula (uncommon).

Associated with metastatic disease

- Jaundice, ascites and hepatomegaly from liver metastases
- Pleural effusion, recurrent chest infections from lung metastases
- Bone pain from bone metastases
- Lymphadenopathy.

Note that **presentation** of the primary tumour is often **dependent on the site** of the tumour:

- **Right sided**: often clinically silent, iron deficiency anaemia, FOB positive, mass ± small bowel obstruction
- **Left sided**: fresh/altered blood and mucus per rectum, large bowel obstruction
- **Rectal**: tenesmus, incomplete evacuation, per rectum bleeding and mucus
- 30 per cent of cases present as an emergency and **20 per cent of all cases have metastases at presentation**.

PRINCIPLES OF MANAGEMENT

Diagnosis

- **Bloods**:
  - ○ FBC to look for microcytic anaemia
  - ○ U+Es and LFTs to look for any evidence of hepatic involvement or renal failure preoperatively
- Chest radiograph and ultrasonography of the liver ± CT of the abdomen and pelvis to **exclude metastasis**
- **Flexible sigmoidoscopy** can be used in elderly people, although a full **colonoscopy is the gold standard** for diagnosis + **biopsy**

Example viva question

How is colorectal cancer staged?

Classically colorectal tumours have been staged by the **modified Dukes' classification** although **TNM staging** of cancer is becoming more **standard** in the hands of specialist colorectal surgeons. The **tumour's stage** determines the **likely prognosis** for the patient, but tumours cannot be staged until the **histology of the specimen** has been performed. Thus, **all fit patients** with no evidence of metastasis should be offered **immediate surgery**.

Modified Dukes' classification

Based on the position of the tumour in relation to the muscularis propria (NOT the muscularis mucosa):

Class	Histology	5-year survival rate (%)
A	Limited to muscularis propria	90–100
B	Breaches the muscularis but does not involve lymph nodes	75
C1	Some nodes +ve, apical node −ve	30–40
C2	Apical node +ve	25
D	Evidence of metastases	<15

TNM classification

TX	Primary tumour cannot be assessed
T0	No primary tumour identified
Tis	Carcinoma *in situ* (tumour limited to mucosa)
T1	Involvement of submucosa, but no penetration through muscularis propria
T2	Invasion into, but not penetration through, muscularis propria
T3	Penetration through muscularis propria into subserosa (if present), or pericolic fat, but not into peritoneal cavity or other organs
T4	Invasion of other organs or involvement of free peritoneal cavity
NX	Nodal metastasis cannot be assessed
N0	No nodal metastasis
N1	One to three pericolic/perirectal nodes involved
N2	Four or more pericolic/perirectal nodes involved
MX	Distant metastasis cannot be assessed
M0	No distant metastases
M1	Distant metastases

You will not be asked to repeat the TNM staging but you should at least know Dukes' classification and be aware that there are other systems.

- **Barium enema** is also a gold standard for diagnosis (although this does not give a histological diagnosis, the classic 'apple-core' lesion appearance is diagnostic of colorectal carcinoma)
- In **frail patients** who would not withstand an invasive investigation or bowel preparation, **CT colonography** has been used, although this is not as sensitive or specific a test as either colonoscopy or barium enema
- **MRI of the pelvis** is particularly good for local **staging** of **rectal carcinoma** and **assessing** degree of **invasion** into the **mesorectal fat** surrounding the rectum.

SPREAD

- **Lymphatics**: these run with the blood supply and drain to regional lymph nodes, para-aortic nodes and then to the thoracic duct. Supraclavicular nodes can be involved in advanced carcinoma.
- **Blood borne**: portal vein drains metastases to the liver. Thirty per cent of patients have liver metastases at presentation. Lungs, adrenals, kidneys and bones are other sites of spread.
- **Transcoelomic**: seeding of carcinoma throughout the peritoneal cavity; occurs in 10 per cent of cases after resection. Spread to ovaries results in 'Krukenberg tumours'.

OPERATIONS FOR COLORECTAL CANCER

Principles of surgery

- **Bowel preparation** if not obstructed (see 'Bowel preparation', Chapter 68, page 280)
- Multidisciplinary approach: **stoma nurse** to counsel patient and site potential stomas preoperatively. It is good practice to obtain consent for a stoma and discuss the implications with the patient even in a planned primary anastomosis
- Full anaesthetic assessment
- **Epidural** for pain relief if possible
- **Prophylactic antibiotics** (see 'Antibiotics in surgery', Chapter 67, page 275)
- In potentially curable cases, aim for **wide resection margins** along with **regional lymphatics**. Rectal tumours should have a **total mesorectal excision** to decrease risk of recurrence
- In incurable cases, minimize surgery and aim to prevent or **treat obstruction**
- **Tension-free anastomosis** (see 'Anastomosis and anastomotic leak', Chapter 66, page 270)

↑ **Example viva question**

What is meant by the adenoma–carcinoma sequence and what is the evidence for it?

Most **colonic** carcinomas arise within adenomas and the accumulation of about 5–10 stepwise mutations in tumour suppressor genes or oncogenes over a lifetime results in cancer, e.g.

Tissue	Mutation
Normal colonic endothelium	*APC*
Small adenoma	*K-ras*
Large adenoma	*smad4*
Pre-malignant changes	*p53*
Colorectal carcinoma	E-cadherin – alters cell adhesion
Increasing aggressiveness and invasion	

Evidence
- Distribution of cancers is similar to polyps
- FAP always proceeds to cancer
- Adenocarcinoma is seen histologically in adenomatous polyps
- Systematic removal of polyps reduces lifetime cancer risk
- Age incidence peaks for polyps about 5 years before carcinoma

- If anastomosis looks oedematous or bowel edges do not bleed well, consider a **loop ileostomy** to allow the **anastomosis to heal**
- If primary anastomosis is not possible, consider a **staged procedure, raising a stoma** in the first instance with the option of reversing it later.

Specific operations

Elective operations for non-obstructed tumours

- **Right** colonic tumour: **right hemicolectomy** with primary anastomosis
- **Left** colonic tumour: **left hemicolectomy** with primary anastomosis
- **Transverse** colonic tumour: **extended** right or left **hemicolectomy**
- **Sigmoid** colonic tumour: **sigmoid colectomy**
- **High rectal** tumours: **anterior resection**
- **Low rectal** tumours: some can be treated by anterior resection but usually treated with an **abdominoperineal (AP)** excision and end-colostomy or ileostomy. For palliative resection and small tumours with liver metastases, **transanal excision** may be used.

Transanal stapling guns allow low primary anastomoses with only a small risk of anastomotic leak.

Operations for obstructed tumours

Right-sided tumours are often suitable for a **right hemicolectomy** or **extended right hemicolectomy** with **primary anastomosis**.

There are three approaches used for obstructed left-sided tumours.

Hartmann's operation

Resection with oversewing of the rectal stump and fashioning of an end-colostomy:

- Relieves obstruction and resects tumour
- No initial anastomosis
- Reversal possible but has 10 per cent mortality rate, so many patients end up with a permanent colostomy.
- Modification with formation of a mucous fistula can simplify the reversal operation and reduce the complication rate.

Primary resection and anastomosis

- Single procedure
- No stoma
- Anastomosis formed under suboptimal conditions – **higher incidence of anastomotic leak**
- Loop ileostomy can be fashioned to allow the primary anastomosis to heal. Reversal of this is a straightforward procedure
- On-table lavage and subtotal colectomy reduce incidence of sepsis.

Three-stage approach

Primary operation to relieve obstruction, second to resect tumour electively and third to close a colostomy:

- Out of favour with most colorectal surgeons
- Cumulative mortality rate is 20 per cent
- 50 per cent patients never have colostomy closed.

Palliative surgery

- **Resection of the primary tumour is the best palliation**, simultaneously curing obstruction and helping to prevent future obstruction.
- **Bypass procedures** many be of help in frail individuals with unresectable tumours to prevent obstruction.
- **Defunctioning colostomy**/ileostomy in frail/elderly patients can relieve obstruction.

- **Stenting of rectal tumours** can relieve low obstruction and is relatively **non-invasive.**
- Local transanal excision may be of help in low rectal cancers.
- Other techniques for rectal cancer include laser treatment, contact irradiation and electrocoagulation.
- **Radiotherapy in rectal tumours** and metastases (particularly bone) and chemotherapy may offer some short-term benefit.

COMPLICATIONS OF COLORECTAL CANCER SURGERY

These can be divided into general and specific, early and late.

General

- Anaesthetic complications
- Cardiorespiratory: myocardial infarction, pulmonary embolus
- **Deep vein thrombosis**: leg, mesenteric (see 'DVT prophylaxis and coagulation in surgery', Chapter 73, page 297)
- Postoperative **renal failure.**

Specific

Early
- **Wound infection** and/or **dehiscence**: reduced incidence with 'clean' operations and the use of bowel preparation, prophylactic antibiotics and a meticulous technique
- **Urinary retention**: cause by postoperative pain, denervation of the bladder or prostatic obstruction
- **Injury to ureters**: can lead to urinary fistulae, pyonephrosis
- **Injury to bladder**: denervation or direct trauma during anterior resection
- **Anastomotic leak**: the most feared complication of the colorectal surgeon and responsible for the major cause of postoperative morbidity and mortality along with cardiorespiratory complications. Increased risk in **low anastomoses** and emergency operations on **unprepared bowel**
- Postoperative ileus.

Late
- Anastomotic **stricture**
- **Sexual dysfunction** as a result of damage of the **splanchnic nerves** – more common in rectal surgery than colonic surgery
- 'Phantom rectum' – present in 50 per cent of AP resections (an unpleasant feeling of rectal discomfort despite the complete lack of the organ).

↑ **Example viva question**

What are the advantages and disadvantages of pre- and postoperative radiotherapy?

Radiotherapy
- **Neither preoperative nor postoperative** radiotherapy has been shown to **prolong survival** or reduce distant metastases
- **Both** forms **reduce local recurrence** rates

Preoperative
- Can be used to attempt to **downstage tumours**, increasing the chance of curative resection
- Compliance is high
- **Irradiated bowel** is **all resected** at surgery
- **Patients** may be included **who do not require it** and are found at laparotomy to have **earlier disease** than was first thought
- Makes **bowel friable** and **increases fibrosis** in the mesorectum in rectal surgery, making the planes more difficult to dissect and total mesorectal excision more difficult

Postoperative
- **Early disease excluded** as pathology known
- Does not delay surgery
- Small bowel more likely to be in the field
- Prolonged course
- May be delayed by surgical complications
- **Irradiated bowel is left in** and may result in **radiation colitis**
- Compliance is lower as a result of postoperative morbidity
- **Planes easier to dissect** in total mesorectal excision

CHEMOTHERAPY IN COLORECTAL CANCER

- **Improves survival** in **Dukes' C** tumours
- **Not indicated** in **Dukes' A** tumours
- **Controversy** about role in **Dukes' B** tumours
  - currently being investigated in the QUASAR (Quick and Simple and Reliable) trial
- QUASAR study to date has shown:
  - 5-fluorouracil (5FU) and folinic acid are effective as adjuvant therapy
  - high-dose folinic acid rescue confers no additional benefit
  - the use of levimasole confers no additional benefit.

PRINCIPLES OF FOLLOW-UP FOR COLORECTAL CANCER

- **Identification of recurrent disease:**
  - **regular surveillance colonoscopy** or barium enema to detect recurrence or metachronous tumours
  - carcinoembryonic antigen (**CEA**) is a tumour marker that can be used to predict recurrence (see 'Tumour markers', Chapter 63, page 252)
  - follow-ups with ultrasonography or CT of the liver and pelvis are helpful and have become standard level of care in many centres
- Check for postoperative complications
- **Ensure appropriate adjuvant therapy.**

55 Diverticula

Possible viva questions related to this topic

→ What is the definition of a diverticulum?
→ What is the difference between a true and a false diverticulum? Give examples.
→ What types of diverticula have you heard of?
→ What do you know about diverticular disease?
→ What are the complications of colonic diverticular disease?
→ How would you manage a patient who presents to the accident and
→ emergency department (A&E) with diverticulitis?
→ What is a Zenker's diverticulum? Describe the relevant anatomy.
→ What is a Meckel's diverticulum? How may it present?
→ What three surgical procedures may be used to deal with perforated diverticular disease?
→ Which has the lowest operative mortality rate?

↑ **Example viva question**

What is a diverticulum?

A diverticulum is an **abnormal outpouching** of a **hollow viscus** into the surrounding tissues.

CLASSIFICATION

1. **True diverticulum**: contains **all layers** of the wall of the viscus, e.g. Meckel's diverticulum
2. **False diverticulum**, only **some layers** present, e.g. colonic diverticulum (especially sigmoid colon).

Or classify by **aetiology**, so **congenital** (normally true in nature) versus **acquired**.

↑ **Key learning points**

Meckel's diverticulum

Rule of two: **2** per cent population; **2** inches long; **2** feet from the ileocaecal valve along the **antimesenteric** border; remnant of the **vitellointestinal duct**

Zenker's diverticulum

Pharyngeal pouch
Outpouching of pharyngeal mucosa through a gap between inferior constrictor and cricopharyngeus (**Killian's dehiscence**)

Dehiscence is in **midline** but **90 per cent present** on **left** side

Presentation: vomiting undigested food, halitosis and recurrent aspiration pneumonia

Diagnosis with **barium swallow**; danger with OGD (oesophagogastroduo-denoscopy) (perforation of pouch)

Surgery: laparoscopic versus open; staple off and invert pouch

---

DIVERTICULAR DISEASE

- Incidence: **60 per cent** of **80 year olds**
- Increasing in incidence (because of older population)
- **Developed countries**: associated with **low-fibre diet.**

Aetiology

Lack of fibre in the **diet** causes a **raised intraluminal pressure**, which in turn causes **outpouching** of the **colonic mucosa**. Normally occurs at **sites of weakness** where **mesenteric blood vessels** pass between **muscles** of the **taeniae coli.**

Distribution: **sigmoid colon** (45 per cent); sigmoid and descending colon (35 per cent); 10 per cent affect sigmoid, descending and transverse, 5 per cent pancolonic; caecum (5 per cent).

Presentation

Usually presents with its **complications**:

- **Diverticulosis**: asymptomatic, altered bowel habit or abdominal pain
- **Diverticulitis**: + inflammation
- **Per rectal (PR) bleeding** (usually in the absence of diverticulitis). Can be **localized**, usually with **mesenteric angiography**

- **Paracolic abscess**: pyrexia and abdominal mass
- **Peritonitis**: **faecal perforation** of one of the **diverticula**
- **Fistulae**: to **small bowel**, **large bowel**, **bladder** (colovesical) present with pneumaturia, faecaluria and chronic urinary tract infection or UTI (polymicrobial); **vagina** (colovaginal), **skin surface**
- **Stricture** ± obstruction.

Investigations in the acute setting

History
Left iliac fossa (LIF) pain, altered bowel habit, shivers/rigors, PR bleeding.

Examination
Pyrexia, dry, LIF tenderness.

Investigations
- **FBC** (raised WCC and neutrophilia)
- **Urine microscopy**: ?fistula; ?differential UTI
- **Erect chest radiograph**: **+ supine abdominal film** – perforation ± suspected obstruction
- **Rigid sigmoidoscopy**: to check that there is no tumour
- **Barium enema**: performed normally as an outpatient when pain has settled to confirm the diagnosis and look at severity and site
- **Ultrasonography**: can demonstrate thickened colon and useful to exclude localized collections
- **CT** is the investigation of choice if the pain does not settle. Good at picking up intra-abdominal abscess, defining inflammatory masses and confirming diagnosis.
- **Colonoscopy** not usually recommended, especially in the acute setting – greater risk of perforation. Also more challenging to the endoscopist in the presence of many diverticula.

Management

Diverticulitis
Normally conservative with bowel rest.

Intravenous fluids
- Patient is normally **dehydrated**; **cefuroxime and metronidazole** for broad-spectrum and anaerobic cover
- Begin with sips and build up when systemic symptoms start to settle
- **Regular** patient review.

Radiological
Percutaneous drainage of a collection/abscess under CT or ultrasonic guidance.

Surgery

For perforation or non-resolving episode of diverticulitis/abscess formation.

1-2-3 staged procedures

- Diverting colostomy and abscess drainage (first of three)
- Hartmann's procedure (first of two)
- Resection with colonic wash-out and primary anastomosis (one stage).

Lowest operative mortality is with **Hartmann's procedure.**

If a diverticular bleed is life threatening and cannot be localized with angiography, the patient requires a **subtotal colectomy** with **ileostomy** or **total colectomy** with **ileorectal anastomosis**.

56 Gastro-oesophageal reflux disease (GORD) and Barrett's oesophagus

↑ Example viva question

What is the difference between heartburn and GORD?

Heartburn is a lay term for **mild, intermittent reflux** of gastric content into the oesophagus **without tissue injury**. It is relatively common among adults (about **40 per cent**).

GORD implies **oesophagitis** with varying degrees of **erythema, oedema** and **friability** of the **distal oesophageal mucosa**.

EPIDEMIOLOGY

- **7 per cent** of **normal** individuals have GORD
- **5 per cent** of sufferers go on to **surgery**
- **Not** all patients with GORD have a **hiatus hernia** and **vice versa**
- **50 per cent of those aged in their 50s** have a **hiatus hernia; a third** of these suffer with **GORD**.

AETIOLOGY

- **Lower oesophageal sphincter** (LOS) incompetence:
  - normal is pressure of > 5 mmHg over a distance of 1 cm or more
- **Gastric outlet obstruction**: this increases acid reflux
- **50 per cent of GORD** sufferers have an associated **hiatus hernia.**
- **Defective oesophageal action**, e.g. scleroderma, may act as a vicious cycle because reflux can cause oesophageal dysfunction and may therefore predispose to further reflux.

CLINICAL FEATURES

- **Epigastric/retrosternal pain** typically **after meals** or **at night**
- Pain is similar to angina (reflux may be exercise related)
- **Reflux of food** or gastric contents. This is effortless and occurs with bending. Discomfort is relieved by standing or sitting
- **Odynophagia,** especially with hot food/drink
- **Globus** (lump in throat)
- **Pulmonary aspiration**: nocturnal coughing and hoarse voice.

DIAGNOSIS

- **History and examination**: effect of posture and antacids
- **Upper gastrointestinal endoscopy** (70 per cent specificity): shows changes proximal to the squamocolumnar junction
- **Biopsy** (80 per cent specificity): ↑ **eosinophils** + hyperplasia
- **Barium swallow** (60 per cent specificity): can diagnose reflux but frequently **cannot diagnose** oesophagitis, although it can demonstrate **other pathology**
- **Ambulatory 24-hour pH monitoring**: **gold standard** and **90 per cent specific**:
  - antimony probe placed over gastro-oesophageal junction (GOJ) for 24 h
  - diagnosis made if pH < 4 for > 1 per cent of time spent supine or if > 6 per cent of time spent erect
- **Oesophageal + LOS manometry**: used when an oesophageal motility disorder is suspected and before any surgical intervention.

MANAGEMENT

Medical (90 per cent effective)

- **Conservative:** encourage **weight loss** (can be highly effective), avoid large meals before bedtime, **stop smoking**, elevate the head of the bed 4–5 inches (10–15 cm), change diet to avoid foods that are known to induce reflux, e.g. chocolate and coffee, reduce alcohol intake
- **Antacids** for symptomatic relief
- **Metoclopramide:** increases LOS pressure and gastric emptying, but does not relieve symptoms consistently in the absence of acid reduction
- **H_2-receptor blockers**, e.g. ranitidine: 50 per cent of patients show significant healing but only 10 per cent of such patients remained healed at 1 year
- **PPIs**, e.g. omeprazole:
  - **80 per cent** successful in healing severe erosive oesophagitis
  - **70 per cent** remained healed if they continue on this
  - a concern with **prolonged PPI** use is **hypergastrinaemia** secondary to alkalinization of the gastric antrum. Gastrin is known to be trophic to gastric mucosa, which raised the fears of neoplasia, but this has not been borne out by follow-up studies.

INDICATIONS FOR SURGERY

- **Failed medical therapy**: intractable disease, intolerance and allergy to medications, non-compliance and recurrence of symptoms while on medication
- **Complications**: stricture, respiratory symptoms, dental erosions, pre-malignant mucosal changes
- **Patient preference**: cost or lifestyle issues.

GOALS OF SURGERY

- Operations for GORD attempt to prevent reflux by mechanically increasing LOS pressure and, in most procedures, to restore a sufficient length of distal oesophagus to the high-pressure zone of the abdomen
- Hiatus hernia, when present, is simultaneously reduced.

PROCEDURES

- **Nissen fundoplication (NF)**: fundus of stomach is **mobilized** and **wrapped** around the oesophagus. The procedure alters the **angle** of the **GOJ** and **maintains** the **distal oesophagus** within the **abdomen**. There is a **90 per cent** success rate.

- The **Belsey mark IV operation**: accomplishes same anatomical changes as NF but is done via a **thoracotomy**.
- **Hill repair**: this restores the oesophagus to the abdomen by fixing the **fundoplicated OGJ** to the **median arcuate ligament** of the **diaphragm**.
- **Angelchick prosthesis**: this is a **silicone-filled collar** placed around the distal oesophagus within the abdominal cavity. It can increase dysphagia and the prosthesis can **migrate** and cause **erosion.**
- **Roux-en-Y procedure**: for recurrent reflux, but there is associated high morbidity and mortality.

COMPLICATIONS

Oesophageal stricture occurs in **10 per cent** of patients and is treated by **endoscopic dilatation** using balloon dilators or bougies.

Haemorrhage (rare): suspect **Barrett's oesophagus** (see below) or **oesophageal cancer**. Reflux does not cause anaemia so another cause should be sought.

BARRETT'S OESOPHAGUS

This is a **pre-malignant** condition. The relative risk of developing **adenocarcinoma** of the **oesophagus** in patients with Barrett's oesophagus is **50–100 times**.

The **normal surface epithelium** of the oesophagus is mainly **stratified squamous epithelium**. This becomes **columnar lined** at the level of the **GOJ**. If it occurs **more than 3 cm** from the junction this is thought to be **abnormal** and is called a **classic Barrett's oesophagus**.

It is thought to occur via **metaplasia** (transformation of one differentiated cell type into another). The **stimulus** is thought to be **gastro-oesophageal reflux.**

Shorter segments of metaplasia are also currently considered to be **significant**.

Barrett's patients should receive **permanent PPI therapy.**

Treatment of Barrett's oesophagus is **controversial**.

Few surgeons would advocate oesophagectomy for early dysplastic change. The difference between high-grade dysplasia and cancer is sometimes difficult and **severe dysplasia** would warrant **consideration** of **surgery** in the setting of a **multidisciplinary team** (MDT) meeting.

Most surgeons would advocate **regular endoscopic surveillance** once these changes have been identified. If the patient were **frail and elderly** and not fit enough to undergo oesophagectomy, **repeat endoscopy would not be warranted.**

The following are based on the **British Society of Gastroenterology guidelines**.

Patient should undergo **endoscopic surveillance** if:

- The length of Barrett's oesophagus is **> 3 cm**
- **Intestinal metaplasia** is found on histology
- The patient is **fit for surgery** if dysplasia is found and understands the need for surveillance and surgery.

Surveillance endoscopy

Biopsy suspicious areas, then **quadrantic biopsies** every **2 cm** from the tip of the gastric folds to the squamous columnar junction.

Follow-up depends on **histology**.

No dysplasia
Three-yearly upper gastrointestinal (GI) endoscopy: discharge from surveillance if co-morbidity or age rules out surgery.

Low-grade dysplasia
Treat with PPI to reduce inflammation and repeat upper GI endoscopy at **6 months** with quadrantic biopsies every 2 cm.

High-grade dysplasia
Discuss at upper gastrointestinal cancer MDT meeting for surgery.

57 Human immunodeficiency virus and universal precautions in surgery

Possible viva questions related to this topic

→ Who is at increased risk of acquiring HIV infection?
→ What is the mode of transmission of HIV? How can HIV be transmitted from patients to theatre personnel?
→ What is the risk of transmission?
→ What precautions should be taken when operating on a patient who is HIV positive?
→ How would you minimize the risk of transmission?
→ If in the event of exposure to contaminated body fluids or blood what steps would you undertake?
→ What is the rationale for giving prophylactic medication?
→ What surgical conditions are more common in HIV-positive patients?
→ How long is the seroconversion process? What factors increase the risk of seroconversion after a needle-stick injury?
→ What potential problems may arise from operating on HIV-positive individuals?
→ Should patients undergoing surgery be routinely tested for HIV? Justify your answer.

HUMAN IMMUNODEFICIENCY VIRUS

- There are **42 million** HIV-positive people in the world, **65 000** in the **UK**.
- **Retrovirus**.
- **Haematogenous** or **mucomucosal** transmission.
- Transmission to **healthcare workers** by **needle-stick injury** with a hollow needle, contamination of **broken skin** or contaminated fluid splashing into the **eyes** or on to **mucous membranes**.

- **Mechanism**: HIV binds to **CD4 receptors** in lymphocytes, replicates in the nucleus and destroys **T-helper cells, dendritic cells** and **macrophages. T-cell depletion leads** to **immunodeficiency,** including **increased susceptibility** to **opportunistic infections** and **neoplasms.**
- **AIDS-defining illness**:
  - development of **neoplasia** – Kaposi's sarcoma, lymphoma
  - **unusual** or **opportunistic** infection, e.g. *Pneumocystis carinii* pneumonia, aspergillosis, candidiasis
  - probable revision of definition to include HIV-positive people with $\leqslant 200/mm^3$ **T-helper cells (CD-4 count)**
  - **90 per cent 2-year mortality rate**.
- **Seroconversion**: occurs in **85 per cent** of cases within **3 months** of infection. In the other **15 per cent** it may take up to **2 years** to seroconvert. This **seroconversion window** has implications for **blood donation** in that it is possible to donate HIV-infected blood before antibody production has commenced, thereby avoiding detection by antibody screening.
- **Factors** that **increase** the risk of seroconversion:
  - **large inoculum** of infected blood, indicated by a deep injury, visible blood on the device
  - source patient with **terminal** disease
  - **procedures** that entail needles **directly** placed into **blood vessels**.

HIGH-RISK GROUPS FOR HIV INFECTION

- **Homosexual** males
- **Sexually active** adults – incidence of HIV infection is now **higher** in **heterosexual** than in homosexual males (Public Health Laboratory figures)
- **Intravenous drug abusers**
- **People with haemophilia** before October **1985**
- **Children** of **infected mothers**
- Patients from **endemic** areas (**Africa** and **south-east Asia**)

⇡ Key learning points

Most of the questions on HIV can be applied to a **hepatitis B or C viva** question.

Most of the principles for HIV can also be applied to hepatitis except for the pathology.

HIV and hepatitis B and C viruses can **coexist**, so individuals with HIV should be screened for antibodies for hepatitis B and C viruses.

RISK OF TRANSMISSION

Average risk of HIV infection after a **single** percutaneous inoculation is **0.3 per cent.**

Risk is **higher** with **conjunctival** contamination compared with **non-intact skin.**

SURGICAL CONDITIONS IN CARRIERS OF HIV

- **Common acute** or **elective surgical** conditions, e.g. appendicitis, hernia. They can present with **atypical features**, e.g. apyrexia and low WCC. This can make **diagnosis** and **management challenging**. They are **managed** in the **usual way** while taking special precautions (see below).
- **Neoplasia**: HIV carriers have a much higher incidence of cancer.
- Leukaemia and lymphoma.
- **AIDS-related lymphoma** may present in varied **extranodal sites** – perianally, as an intracranial tumour or as an obstructing small bowel tumour.
- **Human papillomavirus infection** causes genital and anal warts. There is an increased risk of developing **anal, cervical** and **vulval** cancers.
- **Epstein–Barr virus** infects **B lymphocytes**. Increased risk of developing **Hodgkin's lymphoma** and **nasopharyngeal carcinoma.**
- **Herpes virus**: associated with Kaposi's sarcoma and multicentric Castleman's disease.
- HIV is a predisposing cause for development of a **fistula *in ano*, anal fissure** and **perianal sepsis.**
- **HIV salivary gland disease** may require superficial parotidectomy to confirm diagnosis.

Postoperatively, HIV-positive patients, particularly in the later stages of the disease, are more prone to developing wound infections after surgery. **Healing** is **compromised** because of their **immunocompromised state** and there is a higher incidence of **anastomotic dehiscence** (see 'Anastomosis and anastomotic leak', Chapter 66, page 270).

PRECAUTIONS TO BE TAKEN

Theatre

- **Routine universal precautions** for **all** patients regardless of HIV or hepatitis status because risk of infection is present in all patients
- Wear a **facemask** with visor or protective eyewear, an **impermeable gown** and **water-resistant footwear**
- Keep cuts and abrasions covered
- **Double glove** – this reduces the contamination risk from glove penetration

- Reduce the **number of people** in **theatre** to a **minimum**:
  - **warn** all **theatre personnel** to this 'category 3' risk and **label all specimens** as such
  - use of a surgical assistant only if strictly necessary
- Maximal use of **disposable items** including drapes; these should be bagged for incineration after the procedure
- **Careful disposal** of **clinical waste** appropriately labelled as hazardous waste
- **Limit use** of **sharps** and use blunt needles where possible
- **Safe handling** of sharps between operators – use of a kidney dish
- **Careful decontamination** of theatre after surgery.

In the event of an exposure

- **Affected area** should be **washed** with copious amounts of **water.**
- Encourage **open wounds** to **bleed.**
- Report incident to **occupational health** for further advice or **A&E** out of hours. Clinicians exposed to communicable viruses should report to the **Communicable Disease Surveillance Centre.**
- **Risk assessment**:
  - **source patient** may provide a sample for testing for hepatitis B or C; with appropriate counselling and consent, the sample can be tested for HIV
  - a sample is also taken from the **affected staff member** to be tested in the event that he or she has any symptoms.
- **Post-exposure prophylaxis** is recommended for significant occupational exposure or high-risk source patient. The rationale is that uptake of HIV and processing of its antigen may take several hours or days, so there is a **window** for **therapeutic intervention** after accidental exposure.
- Should be given within **1 hour** of **exposure.**
- Giving **zidovudine** is associated with an **80 per cent reduction** in the risk of HIV infection.
- **Triple therapy** in the form of **zidovudine, lamivudine** and the protease inhibitor **indinavir** is currently given for **6 months** and may modify the clinical course of the disease.

Should all patients before surgery undergo routine HIV testing?

In the authors' opinion the **answer is no.**

Reasons
- All patients require **formal consent** for an HIV test. This slows down the process of surgery. Some patients may not agree to the test.
- **Added anxiety** for the patient.
- The implications of a positive result would require **appropriate counselling** to both the patient and the rest of family.

- Implications of a **false-positive** (distress to patient) or a **false-negative** result (unduly reassuring to patient).
- **Expense** of testing.
- **Time** to conduct test.
- **Delay** of **treatment**.

HIV AND THE ACUTE ABDOMEN

- **Bacterial enteritis**: atypical mycobacterium, e.g. *Mycobacterium avium-intracellulare*
- **Viral enteritis**: cytomegalovirus (CMV) infection of the colon causing toxic megacolon
- **Pancreatitis**: related to CMV infection
- **GI tract (GIT) haemorrhage**: complication of Kaposi's sarcoma
- **GIT affected by lymphoma**: classically **non-Hodgkin's lymphoma** (NHL).

58 Hyperparathyroidism

Possible viva questions related to this topic

→ How do you classify hyperparathyroidism?
→ What are the clinical manifestations of primary hyperparathyroidism?
→ What is the primary defect in primary hyperparathyroidism?
→ What is the effect on the circulating calcium concentration in primary/secondary/tertiary hyperparathyroidism?

CHARACTERISTICS

- **Prevalence** of 1:1000
- **Most common** in the **fifth** and **sixth decades** of life
- **Females : males** = 3:1
- **Second most common** cause of **hypercalcaemia** after **malignancy**
- Often an **incidental finding**.

CLASSIFICATION

Primary

- **Single adenoma**: 85 per cent
  - **microscopically**: composed predominantly of **chief cells** arrayed in uniform sheets, trabeculae or follicles
- **Multiple adenomas**: 5 per cent
- **Diffuse hyperplasia** of all four glands: 10 per cent
  - **microscopically**: chief cell hyperplasia
- **Parathyroid carcinoma**: < 1 per cent
  - difficult to distinguish from adenomas both grossly and microscopically. Usually involves **one gland** and consists of **grey–white** irregular masses. Can **exceed 10 g** in weight
  - diagnosis of **malignancy** based on the presence of **local invasion, metastases** or both.

Sporadic: 95 per cent cases.

Inherited syndrome: multiple endocrine neoplasia (MEN) types I and IIa.

Secondary

Parathyroid glands' response to **hypocalcaemia** from an underlying cause – usually **chronic renal failure.** Hypocalcaemia is a result of the following.

In the kidneys
• Decreased metabolism of 1,25-dihydroxy-vitamin D
• Decreased renal resorption of calcium.

In the diet
• Decreased vitamin D ingestion.

Physiological
• Decreased exposure to sunlight, and therefore reduced production of **cholecalciferol** in the skin.
• Vitamin D normally inhibits parathyroid hormone (PTH) production, so a decrease in vitamin D causes secondary hyperparathyroidism.

Pregnancy
• Increased demands of calcium can lead to hypocalcaemia.

All glands are enlarged.

Tertiary

Chronic stimulation of all the parathyroid glands by **hypocalcaemia in secondary hyperparathyroidism** eventually renders them **autonomous,** resulting in **hypercalcaemia.** Such hypercalcaemia may manifest for the first time in a patient who has received a **renal transplant,** and then becomes able to metabolize vitamin D normally. Occasionally an **autonomous adenoma** may develop.

DIAGNOSIS

Dependent on the finding of **persistent hypercalcaemia** in the presence of an **inappropriately raised level of serum PTH.**

CLINICAL MANIFESTATIONS OF PRIMARY HYPERPARATHYROIDISM

Symptoms and **signs** of hyperparathyroidism reflect the combined effects of **increased PTH** secretion and subsequent **hypercalcaemia.** Multiple systems are involved.

↑ **Key learning points**

Remember:

'Painful bones, renal stones, abdominal groans and psychic moans'

Bone disease: bone pain, secondary to bone fractures weakened by osteoporosis

Renal disease: **nephrocalcinosis** and **nephrolithiasis** (renal stones) with attendant pain and obstructive uropathy

Gastrointestinal disturbances: abdominal pain, constipation, nausea, anorexia, peptic ulceration, acute pancreatitis and gallstones

CNS alterations: depression, lethargy, and eventually seizures

Neuromuscular abnormalities: weakness and fatigue

Cardiac manifestations: aortic and mitral valve calcifications

Biochemical abnormalities in hyperparathyroidism			
	$[Ca^{2+}]_{serum}$	$[PO_4^{3-}]_{serum}$	$[PTH]_{serum}$
Primary hyperparathyroidism	↑	↓	↑ or →
Secondary hyperparathyroidism	↓ or →	↑ or →	↑
Tertiary hyperparathyroidism	↑	↓	↑

59 Hyperplasia, hypertrophy and atrophy

Possible viva questions related to this topic

→ What do you understand by the terms 'hyperplasia' and 'hypertrophy'? Give examples.
→ Are they mutually exclusive?
→ How are hyperplasia and hypertrophy classified?
→ What is the definition of atrophy? Give examples.
→ What do you understand by the terms 'aplasia', 'atresia' and 'hypoplasia'?
→ What are the differences between necrosis and apoptosis?
→ How is necrosis classified? Give examples.

Related topics		
Topic	Chapter	Page
Carcinogenesis	51	189
Cell cycle	52	194
Wound healing, scarring and reconstruction	83	342

DEFINITIONS

Hypertrophy
This is an **increase** in the **size** of a **tissue** or **organ** because of an **increase** in the **size** of its **cells.**

Hyperplasia
This is an **increase** in the **size** of a **tissue** or **organ** because of an **increase** in the **number** of its **cells.** It can occur only in **cells** that are capable of **DNA synthesis**. Hence **nerve, cardiac** and **skeletal** muscle cells undergo almost only **pure hypertrophy** when stimulated by **hormones** or **increased functional demand.**

Autonomous hyperplasia
This is the increase in the number of cells in an organ or tissue but in the **absence** of a **demonstrable stimulus**, e.g. in **psoriasis** and **Paget's disease** of the **bone.**

Atrophy
This is a **decrease** in the **size** of the **organ** or **tissue**, as a result of a **reduction** in either the **size** or the **number** of **cells** or **both.** The cells have diminished function but are not dead.

Cells exhibit **autophagy** with the **reduction** of **cell organelles** and marked **increase** in the number of **autophagic vacuoles**.

Components that **resist** digestion are converted to **lipofuscin granules**. This makes the organ **brown** ('brown atrophy').

Examples			
	Hyperplasia	**Hypertrophy**	**Atrophy**
Physiological	Hormonal: **Breast** in puberty/pregnancy **Uterus** – pregnancy **Thyroid** in puberty/pregnancy **Bone marrow** at altitude **Pituitary** in pregnancy **Compensatory**: **Liver** after hemi-hepatectomy	**Skeletal** and **cardiac** muscle to exercise **Uterus** – pregnancy	**Thyroglossal duct** **Umbilical vessels** **Thymus** – in early adulthood **Endometrium and breast** – old age
Pathological	Over-stimulation **Thyroid** – Graves' disease **Prostate** – benign prostatic hyperplasia **Adrenals** – Cushing's disease **Endometrium** – excess oestrogen	Over-stimulation **Thyroid** – Graves' disease **Heart muscle** in aortic stenosis and hypertrophic cardiomyopathy **Smooth muscle** in hypertension **Congenital muscular dystrophies**	**Loss of innervation** **Ischaemia** Lack of **nutrition** (adipose) **Disuse** – atrophy of limb **Loss of hormone stimulation** – adrenal atrophy with reduced ACTH secretion, e.g. in hypophysectomy

---

↑ **Key learning points**

Hyperplasia and **hypertrophy** are **NOT mutually exclusive**. They can both occur in:

- Graves' disease
- Adrenal hyperplasia
- Benign prostatic hyperplasia (BPH)

AGENESIS

This is the **complete failure** of an **organ** or **tissue** to **develop** in any way during **fetal development**, e.g. **failure** of development of a **pharyngeal pouch** can result in the **thymus** or **parathyroid glands** not developing.

APLASIA AND HYPOPLASIA

Aplasia

There is **recognizable tissue** that has **failed** to **develop**, e.g. **MacLeod's syndrome**. This is aplasia of a lobe of a lung, or part of a lobe of a child's lung, with consequent emphysema of the contralateral lung as a compensatory mechanism.

Hypoplasia

Failure of an **organ** or **tissue** to attain its **proper size and state of function**, although there is an attempt at this. This follows the **permanent loss** of **precursor cells** in proliferative tissues.

In **hypoplasia** the **development** has **proceeded further** but has not reached normal maturity, i.e. a less severe form of aplasia, e.g. **hypoplasia of the breast or amazia**. This is the absence of a breast with the nipple present. Ninety per cent have absent or hypoplastic pectoral muscles.

Atresia is a form of aplasia but is the **absence** of an **opening**, usually of a **hollow visceral organ** such as the **trachea, bile duct, oesophagus** or **intestine**.

CELL DEATH

Necrosis is the sum of the morphological changes that follow **abnormal death** of **cells** or **tissues** in a **living organism**. **Two processes** cause the basic morphological changes of necrosis:

1. **Denaturation of proteins**
2. **Enzymatic digestion of organelles**.

Classification of necrosis

- **Coagulative** (structured): most tissues, e.g. heart, spleen, kidney and liver. Tissue **architecture maintained** – protein denaturation > digestion.
- **Caseous** (unstructured): tissue architecture is lost, e.g. TB. Gross appearance is of soft, cheesy, friable material. Microscopic appearance is amorphous debris.
- **Colliquative/liquefactive**: CNS and localized bacterial infections (abscesses).

- **Gangrene:**
  - **dry:** mummification of tissue **without** infection
  - **wet: necrosis** where there is **putrefaction** caused by **anaerobic bacteria**.
- Fibrinoid.
- **Fat:**
  - direct trauma: fat necrosis of the breast
  - enzyme digestion: in pancreatitis.

Apoptosis

This is an **energy-dependent** process for **deletion** of **unwanted individual cells** – 'programmed cell death' – to balance mitosis in regulating the size and function of the tissue/organ or to remove unwanted or defective cells with abnormal DNA. Apoptosis may be:

- **Physiological:**
  - thymus degeneration
  - loss of tissue between digits during limb development
  - hormone-dependent involution of tissues, e.g. endometrium and prostate in the adult
- **Pathological:**
  - tumours, e.g. Burkitt's lymphoma
  - graft rejection: damage to cells from viruses, irradiation and T lymphocytes.

↑ Example viva question

What are the differences between necrosis and apoptosis?

	Necrosis	Apoptosis
Energy	Independent	Dependent
Inflammation	Yes	No
Physiological/ pathological	Always pathological	Can be both
Cell membrane	Fragmentation	Integrity maintained
Involves	Usually whole tissue	Single cells
Morphological features	Eosinophilic, glassy and vacuolated cell	Cell shrinkage
	Nuclear changes:	Chromatin condensation and fragmentation
	Pyknosis (small dense nucleus)	Cellular blebbing
	Karyolysis (faint, dissolved nucleus)	Apoptotic bodies
	Karyorrhexis (nucleus broken into many clumps)	Phagocytosis of apoptotic bodies by healthy adjacent cells or macrophages
	Mitochondria swollen Rupture of lysosomes leading to autolysis Dystrophic calcification	
Form of cell death is expressed by	Severity of injury	Specificity of stimulus

60 Malignant melanoma

Possible viva questions related to this topic

→ What is melanin? Describe its role?

→ What is the definition of a melanoma?

→ What are the predisposing factors in the development of malignant melanoma?

→ What are the different subtypes?

→ Can you describe any systems that aid in the diagnosis of a suspicious skin lesion?

→ What are the stages of tumour progression in malignant melanoma?

→ What are surrounding lesions?

→ What are the factors assessed on an excision biopsy?

→ What are the systems used to grade this condition? Which gives the better prognosis and why?

→ What are Clarke's levels and the Breslow thickness?

→ What are the other indicators of prognosis?

→ What preventive aspects can be encouraged?

→ What are the treatment options available?

→ What is the role of adjuvant chemotherapy in the treatment of malignant melanoma?

Melanin is a water-insoluble polymer. It is synthesized from **tyrosine** catalysed by **tyrosinase**. It is found in **melanosomes** in **melanocytes**.

Melanin has **two** roles:

• **Skin pigmentation**
• **Absorption of ultraviolet light** to prevent skin damage.

DEFINITION

Melanoma is a **malignant neoplasm of epithelial melanocytes** primarily arising in the **skin**.

Other sites include the **nasal cavities, retina** and **gastrointestinal mucosa.**

PREDISPOSING FACTORS

Likely to be **multi-factorial** including:

- Excessive **sun exposure**: classically **intermittent high-energy** exposure compared with **continuous low-energy exposure** (for basal and squamous cell carcinoma)
- **Fair complexion** + prominent **freckling** tendency
- Presence of a **changing mole** on the skin
- **Increased number** of commonly acquired and dysplastic moles
- **Family history** of melanoma (2–10 per cent) and dysplastic naevi
- Albinism (lack of tyrosinase) and xeroderma pigmentosa.

More than **50 per cent** of cases are believed to arise anew **without** a pre-existing pigmented lesion.

↑ **Example viva question**

What are the different subtypes of malignant melanoma?

- Superficial spreading melanoma (SSM)
- Lentigo maligna melanoma (LMM)
- Nodular melanoma (NM)
- Acral lentiginous melanoma – more common in dark-skinned individuals
- Amelanocytic melanoma

TUMOUR PROGRESSION

Five stages have been suggested:

1. **Benign** melanocytic naevi
2. Melanocytic naevi with architectural and cytological atypia (**dysplastic naevi**)
3. Primary malignant melanoma, **radial growth** phase
4. Primary malignant melanoma, **vertical growth** phase
5. **Metastatic** malignant melanoma.

Surrounding lesions are **satellite** nodules or **in-transit metastatic** deposits.

↑ **Example viva question**

What systems do you know of that can aid in the diagnosis of a suspicious skin lesion?

MacKie's seven-point checklist
Major (carries 2 points each):
(a) Change in size
(b) Irregularity of pigmentation
(c) Irregularity of outline
(d) Diameter > 6 mm

Minor (carries 1 point each):
(e) Inflammation
(f) Oozing or bleeding
(g) Itch or altered sensation

Needs **further evaluation** in the presence of **one major** or if **scores reach 3**.

American ABCDE system
A – Asymmetry (opposite segments of the lesion are different)
B – Border (irregular representing coastline with bays and promontories, elevation)
C – Colour variation
D – Diameter > 6 mm
E – Examination for other lesions

INFORMATION GAINED FROM AN EXCISIONAL BIOPSY

An excisional biopsy with adequate margins allows:

- Assessment of **tumour depth** (Breslow depth)
- **Anatomical level** of invasion (Clark's level)
- **Ulceration**
- Presence of **mitoses**
- **Lymphatic** and **vascular** involvement
- **Host response** (tumour-infiltrating lymphocytes)
- **Regression**
- **Immunohistochemical staining** for lineage (S-100, homatropine methylbromide 45) or proliferation markers (proliferating cell nuclear antigen, Ki67).

↑ **Example viva question**

What are Clarke's levels and the Breslow thickness?

Clarke's classification (level of invasion)
Level I: lesions involving only the **epidermis** (*in situ* melanoma); not an invasive lesion
Level II: invasion of the **papillary dermis**, but does not reach the papillary–reticular dermal interface
Level III: invasion fills and expands the papillary dermis, but does not penetrate the reticular dermis
Level IV: invasion into the **reticular dermis** but not into the subcutaneous tissue
Level V: invasion through the reticular dermis into the **subcutaneous tissue**

The Breslow (depth) thickness of the lesion
Tumour thickness, as defined by the Breslow depth, is the most **important histological determinant of prognosis** and is measured **vertically in millimetres** from the top of the **granular layer** (or base of superficial ulceration) to the deepest point of tumour involvement. **Increased tumour thickness** confers a higher metastatic potential and a poorer prognosis.

	5-year survival rate (%)
⩽0.75 mm	90
0.76–1.5 mm	80
1.5–4 mm	65
⩾4 mm	35

Breslow gives the **better indication of prognosis**.

In **Clarke's levels**, the thicknesses of the papillary and reticular dermis **vary** around the body: both are thin on the face but thick on the back.

OTHER PROGNOSTIC INDICATORS

- **Male** gender
- **Increasing age**
- **Ulceration**
- **Site**: in order of **poor prognosis**: lower limb, upper limb, trunk, head and neck.

PREVENTION

The preventive aspects are:

- **Adequate clothing**
- **UV-absorbent screens**: UV radiation especially in the wavelength range 320–280 nm is the most carcinogenic
- **Avoiding sunbathing and tanning salons**: UV rays from tanning beds and sunlamps are just as dangerous
- **Avoid sun exposure**, particularly for those patients at risk (albinism, xeroderma pigmentosa)
- Local or systemic **carotenoids** (carotene, retinol, retinoids) prevent malignant transformations; systemic retinoids are more effective
- **Public education**: regular skin check-ups and follow-ups are vital for early detection.

PRINCIPLES OF SURGICAL MANAGEMENT

- Excision margin based on histological confirmation of tumour-free margins:
  - for **melanoma *in situ***: 0.5 cm margin
  - melanoma with Breslow thickness < **2 mm**: 1 cm margin
  - melanoma with Breslow thickness ⩾ **2.0 mm**: 2 cm margin.
- Melanomas near a **vital** structure may require a reduced margin.
- **Aggressive histological features** may warrant a wider margin.
- Sites such as the fingers, toes, sole of the foot and ear need separate surgical consideration.
- **Elective lymph node dissection (ELND)** is defined as the removal of regional lymph nodes draining the site of the primary melanoma in the absence of any clinical evidence of nodal metastases. This is a controversial point. Some studies have shown increased prognosis but other studies have shown no statistical difference.
- **Sentinel lymph node biopsy (SLNB)**: this is based on the premise that the first node draining a lymphatic basin (sentinel lymph node) would be expected to predict the absence or presence of melanoma in that area. One per cent isosulfan blue (Lymphazurin) dye is injected around the cutaneous lesion to allow intraoperative localization of this sentinel lymph node. Alternatively, a radioactive tracer, technetium-99, can also be injected at the lesion site. A gamma probe is used to pinpoint the radiolabelled lymph node, which is then removed for histopathological review. If no melanoma cells are found, no further surgery is done. However, if the node does have involvement, the remainder of the nodes in this area are removed.

- Determination of the status of the **sentinel lymph node** is relevant because:
  - it has been shown to be an important independent prognostic factor, with a positive result predictive of high risk of treatment failure
  - it is a relatively **low-risk procedure** that can help identify high-risk patients who might benefit from additional therapy such as **selective complete lymphadenectomy** or **adjuvant interferon-α-2b**
  - it provides a psychological benefit for the patient whose sentinel lymph node biopsy does not reveal metastases.

ADJUVANT THERAPY: INTERFERON

- May improve the survival of patients with melanoma > **4 mm thick**
- Diminishes the occurrence of metastases
- Prolongs the disease-free survival in patients with melanoma > 1.5 mm.

CHEMOTHERAPY

- Advanced **stage III** (unresectable regional metastases) or **stage IV** (distant metastases).
- **Dacarbazine** remains the most active chemotherapeutic agent for the treatment of advanced melanoma. The response rate is in the range of 10–20 per cent, and patients with metastases in the skin, subcutaneous tissues or lymph nodes respond most frequently.
- **Other combination chemotherapy** and biochemotherapy regimens could achieve higher response rates, but do not appear to lead to durable remission.

BIOLOGICAL THERAPY

Therapy directed towards modulating or inducing the immune system against the melanoma:

- **Interleukin-2 (IL-2)** as a single agent has been utilized in metastatic melanoma. In one study, there was a complete response in 7 per cent of patients, which was durable, with patients remaining disease free for up to 8 years after initiating therapy.
- Another study also showed positive results treating patients with their own tumour-infiltrating lymphocytes and IL-2.
- **Monoclonal antibody therapies** are still experimental and may be of potential use in melanoma.
- **Melanoma vaccines** have been developed to stimulate a specific response against melanoma-associated antigens. Vaccines are currently undergoing clinical trials.

PERFUSION CHEMOTHERAPY

Isolated limb perfusion (ILP)

This involves isolating a limb from the systemic circulation with a tourniquet, using arterial and venous cannulation, and infusing a chemotherapeutic agent by means of a pump oxygenator, and then removing the medication from the limb. It has been developed into the most effective method of treatment for **local recurrent or in-transit metastases of an extremity**. Medications that are used for infusion include melphalan, cisplatin and TNF-α.

Radiation

Radiotherapy is indicated in certain patients with **stage IV disease**, for the purpose of palliation. Specific indications include **brain metastases**, pain associated with bone metastases, and skin and subcutaneous metastases that are superficially located.

61 Portal hypertension

Possible viva questions related to this topic

→ What is portal hypertension?
→ What causes portal hypertension?
→ What is the underlying pathophysiology of this condition?
→ What are the common complications of portal venous hypertension?
→ What are the management options?
→ What is TIPPS?
→ How would you manage an acute oesophageal variceal bleed?

Related topics

Topic	Chapter	Page
Ascites	48	172
Portal vein and portosystemic anastomoses	14	39
Starling forces in the capillaries/oedema	101	401
Starling's law of the heart and cardiovascular equations	102	403

Example viva question

What is portal hypertension?

Portal hypertension is defined as a **portal venous pressure** exceeding 10 mmHg.

PATHOPHYSIOLOGY

Increase in portal pressure is as a result of increased portal blood flow or increased intrahepatic vascular resistance of cirrhosis.

Increased portal blood flow

Patients with **liver cirrhosis** are found to have **systemic** and **splanchnic vasodilatation** as a result of a **decrease** in **vascular tone**. This is accompanied by **hyperkinetic blood flow** in the **splanchnic** and **systemic circulation**.

Patients have **warm, well-perfused extremities, bounding pulses** and **rapid heart rate**. The **increase in blood flow** through the splanchnic organs draining into the portal venous system is a **major contributor** for the **maintenance** and **aggravation** of **portal hypertension**.

Recent evidence has implicated **circulating vasodilators**, e.g. nitric oxide (NO). The recognition of vasodilatation and hyperdynamic circulation has led to the 'forward flow theory', which proposes that increased portal venous inflow plays a central role in the pathogenesis of portal hypertension; this is **independent** of the **increased resistance** in the **portal venous** and **collateral circulation** ('backward flow theory').

Increased intrahepatic vascular resistance of cirrhosis

Previously thought to be the result of **fibrosis, scarring** and **regenerative nodule** formation. However, there is increasing evidence to suggest that this is more of a dynamic process, whereby the **intrahepatic vascular tone** and **resistance** are modulated by **sinusoidal endothelial** cells. **Hepatic stellate** cells located in the **space of Disse** are **contractile** structures that have also been implicated in modifying **intrahepatic vascular resistance**. Along with other extracellular matrix-producing cells, such as **fibroblasts** and **myofibroblasts**, present in the portal tract, they are thought to exert their contractile effects under the influence of mediators such as **NO** and **endothelin** to **increase intrahepatic resistance**.

Combination of both **resistance to portal blood flow** and **increased portal blood flow** are now thought to play a central role in portal hypertension.

PRINCIPAL CAUSES

Pre-hepatic

- Portal vein thrombosis
- Portal vein compression by tumour.

Intrahepatic

- Cirrhosis
- Idiopathic (non-cirrhotic)
- Acute alcoholic hepatitis
- Congenital hepatic fibrosis.

Post-hepatic

- Budd–Chiari syndrome (hepatic vein thrombosis)
- Veno-occlusive disease
- Right heart failure
- Constrictive pericarditis.

COMPLICATIONS

- Haemorrhage from oesophageal varices (most common and dangerous)
- Hepatic encephalopathy
- Ascites
- Hypersplenism
- Rectal varices
- Hepatorenal syndrome (HRS)
- Spontaneous bacterial peritonitis
- Portal hypertensive gastropathy.

MANAGEMENT

Elective

Liver transplantation: established treatment and only cure for chronic progressive liver disease and for complications of portal hypertension. Liver transplantation should be performed before the onset of serious complications, e.g. encephalopathy and hepatorenal syndrome.

Total portosystemic shunts

Non-selective shunts divert all portal blood flow into the systemic circulation and decompress the entire portal system, producing a rapid decompression of varices and relief of portal hypertension.

End-to-side shunt: the portal vein is ligated at the hepatic hilum and transected, and the proximal end is anastomosed to the side of the inferior vena cava.

Main complication: 40 per cent incidence of encephalopathy and exacerbation of underlying liver failure.

Selective shunts: designed for selective variceal decompression without portal diversion, e.g. distal splenorenal (Warren) shunt involves anastomosing the splenic end of the divided splenic vein to the left renal vein end to side. The spleen is left in place and the left gastric vein, umbilical vein and other venous tributaries of the splenic vein are all divided. This effectively excludes the gastrosplenic portal circulation from the rest of the portal circulation. There is reduced hepatic encephalopathy incidence with this method.

The Sugiura procedure

Reserved for patients with recalcitrant haemorrhage or patients who cannot undergo a shunt operation because of portal vein thrombosis. Procedure involves:

- Splenectomy
- Devascularization of the stomach and lower oesophagus

- **Oesophageal transection** with a **circular stapling device** to disrupt flow to the gastro-oesophageal varices.

This is a highly effective method in controlling active bleeding.

Transjugular intrahepatic portosystemic shunting (TIPSS)

This is an alternative to surgical shunting. It **shunts portal blood** across the liver into the **vena cava**.

A **guidewire** introduced through the **jugular vein** is threaded through the liver and forced into an **intrahepatic branch** of the **portal vein**. This **track** is **balloon dilated** and held open with a **metallic stent**, creating a shunt that decompresses the portal system. Use with caution because it can worsen an encephalopathy. Also it is only a **temporary measure** – shunts usually **stenose** or **thrombose** within 1 year (50 per cent).

↑ **Example viva question**

What is the management of acute variceal bleeding?

Effective resuscitation
Patients with massive haemorrhage should be considered for admission to **intensive care**.

Early consideration for transfer to a **specialist liver unit**.

Two large-bore cannulae inserted into antecubital veins.

Obtain **blood** for **grouping, cross-matching, FBC, clotting profile, electrolytes, urea, creatinine, liver biochemistry** and **blood cultures**.

Many patients have some degree of **coagulopathy** and **thrombocytopenia**. These should be corrected with **fresh frozen plasma, vitamin K injection** and **platelet transfusion if platelet count** $< 50\,000/mm^3$.

Upper gastrointestinal endoscopy is essential to establish an accurate diagnosis because 50 per cent patients with documented portal hypertension and varices will have a **non-variceal source of bleeding**. Performed as soon as resuscitation is adequate.

Endoscopic sclerotherapy or **band ligation** for control of active bleeding. This **arrests bleeding** in **80 per cent** of cases as well as **reducing early re-bleeding**.

Pharmacological therapy: used in combination and while waiting for an upper GI endoscopy. Works by causing **splanchnic arterial constriction** and subsequent decrease in pressure and flow in the varices.

Vasopressin (0.4–0.8 U/min IV): efficacious in controlling bleeding and reducing mortality.

Somatostatin (250 µg IV bolus; then 250 µg/h IV) and its synthetic analogue octreotide decrease portal blood flow by **selective splanchnic vasoconstriction** and are free from systemic side effects. Although effective in controlling bleeding it has **no effect on mortality**.

Mechanical balloon tamponade with a **Sengstaken–Blakemore tube**. It consists of a **nasogastric tube** with **two large balloons** at the distal end. Two balloons – one in the **oesophagus** and one in the **cardia** – are blown up to compress the varices. The tube position must be confirmed by radiograph before inflation of the balloons. The distal gastric balloon is inflated with 250 mL of air and then pulled up tight against the gastro-oesophageal junction. If the gastric balloon alone does not control the bleeding the proximal oesophageal balloon is inflated to a pressure that equals portal venous pressure (25 mmHg). The tube is **deflated at 24 h** and if **bleeding** has **stopped** it is removed **48 h** after insertion. If bleeding is not controlled the tube is left inflated for a further 24 h after an interval of 1 h deflation.

Complications of balloon tamponade are **ischaemic necrosis** of the oesophageal mucosa, **oesophageal perforation** and **aspiration pneumonitis**. As a result of these complications, balloon tamponade should be used only as a **temporary measure**.

TIPPS has been shown to be effective in controlling variceal bleeding in more than **90 per cent of patients** who continue to bleed after endoscopic and vasoconstrictor therapy.

62 Thyroid cancer

Possible viva questions related to this topic

→ What are the risk factors for thyroid cancer?
→ How would you investigate a thyroid mass in clinic?
→ What are the principles of management for thyroid cancer?
→ How can thyroid tumours be classified?
→ How is thyroid cancer staged?
→ How does thyroid cancer spread?
→ What percentage of thyroid tumours is secretory?
→ What are the disadvantages of fine-needle aspiration cytology and in which particular type of thyroid tumour is this a problem?
→ If you have performed a hemi-thyroidectomy and the histology comes back as papillary carcinoma, what extra management would you consider for the patient?
→ What are multiple endocrine neoplasia (MEN) syndromes and which specifically are associated with what type of thyroid cancer?

CLINICAL FEATURES

Systemic

• Patients are usually **euthyroid** – unusual to present as thyrotoxicosis. '**Cold**' nodules (no isotope uptake and therefore not secretory) much **more likely** to represent **carcinoma** than 'hot' nodules.
• May present like other goitres in the neck, but often **growing more rapidly**.
• **Dysphagia** may be present but **uncommon** (suggestive of an anaplastic tumour).
• **Odynophagia** is relatively **common** (pain on swallowing).
• **Hoarse voice** is suggestive of **local invasion** of the **recurrent laryngeal nerve** (see 'Thyroid gland and parathyroid glands', Chapter 18, page 49).

↑ **Example viva question**

What are the risk factors for thyroid cancer?

Thyroid cancer is the **most common malignant endocrine tumour**, but represents only about **1 per cent of all malignancies**.

- Every year there are about **900 new cases** and **250 deaths**
- Annual incidence is approximately **2 per 100 000 women** and **1 per 100 000 men**
- Affects those aged **25–65 years**

Risk factors
- **Radiation** administered in **infancy** and childhood for **benign conditions** of the head and neck (e.g. enlarged thymus, acne, or tonsillar or adenoidal enlargement)
- **Radiation exposure** as a consequence of **nuclear fallout**
- History of **goitre**
- **Family history** of thyroid disease (particularly MEN syndromes and papillary carcinomas)
- **Female** gender
- **Asian** race

- Deep **cervical lymphadenopathy**.
- **Most commonly presents as a lump in the neck.**
- **Diarrhoea** in medullary carcinoma.

CLASSIFICATION OF THYROID TUMOURS

If asked to classify thyroid tumours, always remember to **start with benign** and **don't forget** to include **secondaries**.

In terms of **prognosis**, a simpler classification of **well-differentiated** and **poorly differentiated** can be used, although you should know the various types below.

Benign

Adenoma (follicular)
- Relatively **rare**
- Most **functioning** nodules are **adenomas (Plummer's syndrome)**
- Most benign nodules are **part of a multinodular goitre** and are not true benign adenomas.

Malignant

Primary (five main types)
Papillary carcinoma
- **Most common** type of thyroid malignancy
- **60 per cent** of all thyroid cancers
- Most common in **young adults** and children
- **Slow growing** and metastasizes late
- **Good prognosis**
- Can be **multifocal**
- **Histology**: large epithelial cell nuclei – 'orphan Annie'.

Follicular adenocarcinoma
- Most common in young and **middle-aged** adults
- Commonly **associated** with areas where **endemic goitres** are found
- **Worse prognosis** than papillary, although good prognosis if no invasion
- **Haematogenous spread** (lymphatic spread uncommon).

Anaplastic carcinoma
- **Worst prognosis**
- Occurs in **elderly people**
- **Rapid local spread**, often into trachea and oesophagus
- **Early lymphatic spread**
- **Early haematogenous spread** to **lungs**, bone and **brain**.

Medullary carcinoma
- Arises from **parafollicular C cells** of the thyroid and as a result may **secrete calcitonin** as a **tumour marker**
- Can occur at any age
- **Equal sex distribution**
- Associated with other tumours (multiple endocrine neoplasia syndromes **MEN-IIa and -IIb** – see later)
- **Histology**: **amyloid** found between tumour cells.

Lymphoma (very rare)
- Non-Hodgkin's
- Associated with **Hashimoto's thyroiditis**.

Secondary
- **Direct invasion** from adjacent anatomical structures (e.g. oesophagus, larynx)
- **Very rare** site for **blood-borne deposits**.

Example viva question

How would you investigate a thyroid mass in clinic?

Similar to breast lumps, thyroid lumps arguably require a triple assessment of **clinical history and examination, radiological assessment** and **cytological assessment**.

Clinical history and examination
- **Size** and **synchronicity** of the mass
- **Thyroid status** of the patient (bloods should include **calcitonin** to rule out medullary carcinoma as well as **TSH** (thyroid-stimulating hormone) and **thyroid autoantibody** status)
- Evidence of **systemic disease** or local **tumour infiltration** (see above)
- Assessment of any **other similar masses** (?multinodular goitre)
- **Tethered** to underlying structures?
- **Moves up** with **swallowing**?
- Associated **lymphadenopathy** (cervical/subclavian)?
- **Vocal fold** assessment (essential **before surgery**)

Radiological assessment
Ultrasound examination reveals whether the **mass is solitary** and **guides the FNAC**. If not, then the diagnosis is likely to be multinodular goitre and not carcinoma, particularly if the patient is not euthyroid.

Cytological assessment
FNAC is often **ultrasound guided** and gives an **instant cytological diagnosis. It does not reveal histological architecture**, however, and in the case of **follicular carcinoma** is **non-diagnostic** because follicular cells may indicate **follicular adenoma** (benign).

Other investigations
- **Nuclear medicine** examinations can look for a 'hot' nodule, although they are of questionable use above the other clinical tests available
- **MRI** and **CT**: when limits of the goitre cannot be determined, or for fixed tumours or patients with haemoptysis. Note that iodinated material used for CT contrast will reduce subsequent ^{131}I uptake by thyroid tissue and **should be avoided if possible**
- **Chest radiograph**: useful in assessing secondary disease
- **Flow–volume loop**: if **upper airway obstruction** is suspected

STAGING OF THYROID CANCER

TNM definitions for staging

Primary tumour (T)

All categories may be subdivided into (1) solitary tumour or (2) multifocal tumour (the largest determines the classification).

TX: primary tumour **cannot be assessed**
T0: **no evidence** of primary tumour
T1: tumour $=$ **2 cm** and limited to the thyroid
T2: tumour $>$ **2 cm** but $=$ **4 cm** and limited to the thyroid
T3: tumour $>$ **4 cm** and limited to the thyroid, or any tumour with minimal extra-thyroid extension (e.g. extension to strap muscles)
T4a: tumour of **any size** extending **beyond the thyroid capsule** to invade subcutaneous soft tissues, larynx, trachea, oesophagus or **recurrent laryngeal nerve**
T4b: tumour **invades prevertebral fascia** or **encases carotid artery** or **mediastinal vessels**

All anaplastic carcinomas are considered T4 tumours (and therefore have a worse prognosis). The **division** of T4 in this case is **whether or not** the tumour is **resectable**.

T4a: intrathyroidal anaplastic carcinoma – **surgically resectable**
T4b: extrathyroidal anaplastic carcinoma – **surgically unresectable**

Regional lymph nodes (N)

Regional lymph nodes are the central compartment, lateral cervical and upper mediastinal lymph nodes.

NX: regional lymph nodes **cannot be assessed**
N0: **no** regional lymph node **involvement**
N1: regional lymph node involvement
  N1a: metastasis to level VI (pretracheal, paratracheal and prelaryngeal/Delphian lymph nodes)
  N1b: metastasis to unilateral or bilateral cervical or superior mediastinal lymph nodes

Distant metastases (M)

MX: distant metastasis **cannot be assessed**
M0: **no** distant **metastasis**
M1: **distant metastasis**

Although TNM staging is the recommended standard, there are different staging systems based on groups with differing prognoses.

MANAGEMENT

- **Well-differentiated tumours** can be treated by a combination of:
  - ○ **surgery** (usually total or near-total thyroidectomy if tumour > 1 cm)
  - ○ **thyroid suppression** with thyroxine (T_4)
  - ○ ^{131}I (**radio-iodine ablation**)
- All new patients should be seen by a member of the **multidisciplinary team (MDT)**, and the treatment plan discussed
- **Fine-needle aspiration cytology (FNAC)** should be used in the **planning** of surgery (see above)
- Most patients with **tumours > 1 cm** in diameter should undergo **near total** or **total thyroidectomy** with **central node dissection**
- **Serum thyroglobulin (Tg)** should be checked in **all postoperative patients** with **differentiated thyroid cancer**
- Patients will normally start on triiodothyronine (T_3) **20 µg t.d.s. (normal adult dosage)** after the operation (this should be stopped 2 weeks before radioiodine therapy)
- The majority of patients with a **tumour size > 1 cm** in diameter, should have ^{131}I **ablation therapy**
- Always **exclude pregnancy** and **breast-feeding** before administering radioactive iodine
- Patients should be **started on T_4 3 days after** ^{131}I in a **dose sufficient to suppress TSH completely**
- Reassessment with a **post-ablation diagnostic scan** (after stopping T_4 for 4 weeks) is indicated **4–6 months after** ^{131}I ablation, although in low-risk patients measurement of Tg alone may be adequate. If significant uptake of the tracer is detectable, a further ^{131}I therapy dose should be given and a post-treatment scan performed. Following this the patient should restart T_4
- If there is **suspicion of residual disease**, **further scans** should be carried out, usually 6 months later.
- **Recombinant human TSH (rhTSH)** can be used **instead of stopping T_3 or T_4** in appropriate cases as decided by the MDT
  - ○ **external beam radiotherapy** is only **occasionally used**, for patients with T_4 tumours (TNM staging – see above) or **distant metastases**.

↑ **Example viva question**

If you have performed a hemi-thyroidectomy and the histology comes back as papillary carcinoma what extra management would you consider for the patient?

As **papillary carcinoma** can be **multifocal**, and if the patient was young with a life-time follow-up, surgery to **complete the thyroidectomy** may be considered in discussion with the patient.

↑ **Example viva question**

What are MEN syndromes and which specifically is associated with what type of thyroid cancer?

Multiple endocrine neoplasia syndromes
These are a group of **inherited disorders** (autosomal dominant) where affected individuals develop **tumours in two or more endocrine glands** at the same time, making the affected glands overactive. With several endocrine systems being overactive, a diverse range of symptoms is seen.

They are broadly **divided into three.**

MEN type I (Wermer's syndrome)
This is characterized by the coexistence of:

• Parathyroid tumours – 80–95 per cent of cases
• Pancreatic islet cell tumours (including gastrinomas, insulinomas, glucagonomas, VIPomas and PPomas) – 80 per cent of cases (VIP = vasoactive intestinal polypeptide; PP = pancreatic polypeptide)
• Anterior pituitary tumours (prolactin-, growth hormone- and ACTH-secreting tumours and non-functioning tumours) – 50–71 per cent of cases

More rarely tumours of the adrenal cortex, carcinoid tumours (special tumours, often arising in the gut – described in their own section) and lipomas (tumours of fat tissue) may also occur within MEN-I. It is NOT associated with medullary carcinoma of the thyroid.

MEN type II
This is further subdivided into IIa and IIb, both of which include medullary carcinoma of the thyroid:

• IIa *(Sipple's syndrome)*: the most common variant of MEN-II, with:
  ○ medullary carcinoma of the thyroid – almost 100 per cent
  ○ phaeochromocytoma – 50 per cent
  ○ parathyroid tumours – 40–80 per cent
• IIb: this has no parathyroid involvement and is characterized by:
  ○ **medullary carcinoma** of the thyroid – almost 100 per cent
  ○ phaeochromocytoma
  ○ marfanoid habitus
  ○ mucosal neuromas
  ○ medullated corneal nerve fibres
  ○ megacolon

FOLLOW-UP

Clinical follow-up needs to be **life-long** because:
- The disease has a **long natural history**
- **Late recurrences** can occur, and these can be **successfully treated**
- **Cure** and **prolonged survival** are common, even after **tumour recurrence**
- **Monitoring of treatment** (TSH suppression, the consequences of supraphysiological T_4 replacement, treatment of hypocalcaemia)
- **Life-long suppression** of **serum TSH** level below normal (< 0.1 mU/L) is one of the main components of treatment and requires monitoring
- **Late side effects** of ^{131}I **treatment** should be monitored
- **Surveillance** for recurrence of disease is essential and is based on:
  - annual **clinical examination**
  - annual measurement of **serum Tg** and **TSH**
  - diagnostic scanning when indicated (**isotopic imaging** and/or ultrasonography or CT)
- **Support** and **counselling** are necessary, particularly in relation to pregnancy and in **familial medullary carcinoma** and **MEN syndromes**.

63 Tumour markers

Possible viva questions related to this topic

→ What is a tumour marker?
→ How are tumour markers classified?
→ Which tumour markers are characteristically found in testicular tumours?
→ Give examples of enzymes, hormones and oncofetal antigens as tumour markers.
→ What is PSA? How is it used clinically?
→ Can you give some examples of commonly used tumour markers in clinical practice?
→ Name one example of a tumour marker that is used in the surveillance of tumour progression.

↑ Example viva question

What is a tumour marker?

This is a **tumour-derived** or **tumour-associated molecule** found in the **blood** or **body fluids** of a patient **with neoplasia**. It is **directly** related to the **presence** of the neoplasm, **disappears** when the neoplasm is **treated** and **reappears** when the neoplasm recurs.

FEATURES

• **No** tumour marker is **pathognomonic**
• Can **aid** in the **diagnosis**
• May be of value in determining **response** to a treatment

- Most used as a **surveillance tool** to **monitor** for **recurrence** of the neoplasm
- Most are **not stoichiometric** – amount produced is not in direct proportion to the tumour bulk, although there may be some evidence that **carcinoembryonic antigen** (CEA) and **prostate-specific antigen** (PSA) are.

CLASSIFICATION

Classified in terms of **biochemical structure** and **function**:

- Hormones
- Enzymes
- Oncofetal antigens.

Hormones (examples)

Eutopic hormones

These are produced from tumours affecting **endocrine** organs:

- **Pituitary** tumour: produces **ACTH, human growth hormone, prolactin**
- **Adrenal** tumour: produces **cortisol**.

Ectopic hormones

These may be produced **aberrantly** from the tumour, which itself is **not typically** an endocrine organ:

- **Carcinoid** tumours: produce **5-hydroxyindoleacetic acid** (5-HIAA)
- **Oat-cell lung** tumours may produce **ACTH** and **antidiuretic hormone** (ADH)
- **Neuroendocrine** tumours.

Enzymes (examples)

Serine protease associated with **semen**. Normal function is to **liquefy** the **ejaculate** enabling fertilization.

Prostatic acid phosphatase or **PSA**, produced by **normal** and **malignant** prostatic **ductal** and **acinar epithelial** cells.

PSA is **elevated** in most patients with:

- **Prostate carcinoma**
- **Benign prostatic hyperplasia**
- **Prostatitis**
- **After urinary retention**
- **After digital rectal examination** (DRE)
- **Urinary catheterization**

- Used in combination with **DRE**, **transrectal ultrasonography** (TRUS) ± biopsy in the management of prostatic carcinoma for:
  - **diagnosis**
  - **follow-up**
  - **assessment of response to treatment.**

The normal range for the serum PSA assay in men is < **4 ng/mL**, although this varies with **age.**

- **PSA velocity: > 0.75 ng/mL per year** is associated with prostate carcinoma
- Prostatic carcinoma is associated with a **lower free:total (F:T) PSA ratio**.

↑ **Example viva question**

Is PSA a good screening test for prostate carcinoma?

Yes	No
Common disease + major health problem	High number of TRUS biopsies performed
Sensitive	Not specific
Potential for cure if disease picked up early	Poorly defined clinical outcome + best treatment for early disease unknown

---

Placental alkaline phosphatase: carcinoma of the bronchus, pancreas, colon and germ cell neoplasms.

Oncofetal antigens (examples)

α-Fetoprotein (AFP): produced by primary liver tumours and testicular teratomas.

Also raised in **non-neoplastic** conditions:

- Liver cirrhosis
- Chronic hepatitis
- Pregnancy
- Neural tube defects.

CEA: normally produced by **fetal gut, liver** and **pancreas**.

It is elevated in **80 per cent of colorectal cancers**. Twenty per cent of colonic neoplasms are non-expressors of the antigen.

This antigen is of value in estimating **tumour burden** in colorectal cancer and in **detecting recurrences** after surgery

Also **raised** in **carcinoma** of the **pancreas, stomach, ovaries** and **breast** and, less consistently, levels are elevated in **non-neoplastic** conditions, e.g. **alcoholic cirrhosis, hepatitis** and **ulcerative colitis**

Not specific or sensitive enough to be used as a screening tool.

TESTICULAR TUMOUR MARKERS:

Teratoma: β-hCG, CEA, AFP.
Seminoma: placental alkaline phosphatase, sometimes β-hCG.

The measurement of serum levels of **AFP** is used to **monitor** the progress of testicular teratomas. A sample initially taken preoperatively, although **not indicative** of tumour burden, is used as a guide with which the **response to treatment** may be monitored. After orchidectomy, serum levels must be measured frequently until they return to normal. Samples can then be taken less frequently and a rise may indicate tumour recurrence, allowing instigation of further investigations.

OTHER TUMOUR MARKERS USED IN CLINICAL PRACTICE

- **Ca 15-3**: a glycoprotein occasionally elevated in breast carcinoma. **Level** is related to the **stage** of breast cancer.
- **Ca 19-9**: a glycoprotein occasionally elevated in pancreatic and advanced colorectal carcinoma.
- **Thyroglobulin**: elevated in some thyroid cancers.
- **Calcitonin**: raised in medullary thyroid carcinoma (see 'Thyroid cancer', Chapter 62, page 244).
- **Vanillylmandelic acid** (VMA): produced by **phaeochromocytomas** and can be detected in the urine.

PRINCIPLES OF SURGERY

64 Abdominal incisions

Possible viva questions related to this topic

→ What abdominal incisions are you aware of and what are their advantages and disadvantages?
→ What is the ideal abdominal incision?
→ What are the factors to be considered while planning a surgical incision?
→ What are the advantages of transverse abdominal incisions?
→ What are the important principles regarding the closing of the abdominal incision?
→ What is Jenkins' rule?
→ What are the complications of abdominal incisions?
→ What are the differences between Lanz's and McBurney's incisions for appendicectomy?
→ What are the different layers of the anterior abdominal wall that you go through when performing a laparotomy?

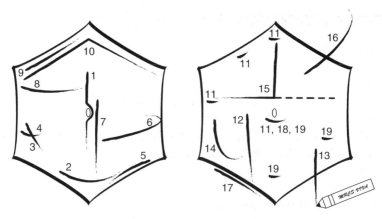

Figure 64.1

Incision	Uses	Notes
1. Midline	Laparotomy	See notes
2. Pfannenstiel's	Pelvic surgery	Gynaecological surgery
3. McBurney's	Caecum/appendix	Allows extension
4. Lanz's	Caecum/appendix	Better cosmesis
5. Inguinal	Inguinal and femoral hernia	
6. Loin	Upper renal tract	Nephrectomy
7. Battle's paramedian	Laparotomy	See notes
8. Transverse	Right colon, biliary	See notes
9. Kocher's subcostal	Open cholecystectomy	Left side for splenectomy
10. Roof top	Hepatobiliary, adrenal	Good access
11. Port sites	Laparoscopic cholecystectomy	
12. Battle's pararectal	Colon, rectum	Now abandoned as a result of damage of nerves on entering rectus
13. McEvedy's (vertical)	Femoral hernia Femoral embolectomy	Can extend to laparotomy Femoral vessels
14. Rutherford–Morrison (hockey stick)	Renal transplantation, difficult appendix	
15. Gable ('Mercedes Benz')	Liver transplantation, hepatobiliary surgery	
16. Thoracoabdominal	Right: liver, portal vein Left: oesophagus, stomach, spleen, aorta	
17. Groin crease	Varicose veins, femoral hernia	
18. Infraumbilical	Umbilical and paraumbilical hernia Laparoscopic camera port	
19. Port sites	Laparoscopic appendicectomy	

PLANNING A SURGICAL INCISION

The following factors are important:

- **Good access** to site of operation
- **Position: over lesion** and **away** from **bony prominences**
- **Adequate size**
- **Safety** with consideration of underlying structures, nerves and blood vessels. Normally made **parallel** to important structures
- **Ease** of access
- **Speed** of access
- **Flexibility** to **extend** the incision if needed
- **Low incidence** of **complications** such as **incisional hernia**
- **Cosmesis:** incisions should be made **parallel** to **Langer's lines** – along natural lines of tension – because they **heal better** and should be made **perpendicular** to skin to avoid undermining, e.g. Pfannenstiel for pelvic surgery
- Presence of **previous scars**
- **Nature** of procedure, e.g. possible stoma
- **Surgeon's preference:** should be **familiar** and **comfortable** with that incision for that operation
- **Shape** of the **abdomen,** e.g. narrow costal angle
- **Age** of the **patient,** e.g. transverse incisions preferred in children.

TRANSVERSE INCISION

Advantages

- Better **cosmesis**
- Less postoperative pain
- Reduced incidence of postoperative **chest infections**
- Preferred incision in **children** to prevent scar puckering with subsequent growth.

Disadvantages

- Division of red muscle involves **more blood loss** and postoperative pain
- Less secure closure than a longitudinal incision – higher incidence of **incisional hernia**
- **Longer** to open and close
- **Cannot** be **extended easily**
- **Limited access** in **adults** to **pelvic** or **subdiaphragmatic** structures.

MIDLINE INCISION

Advantages

- Good access
- **Easy to extend**
- Quick to open and close
- ↓ Blood loss – relatively avascular.

Disadvantages

- **More painful** than transverse incisions because the incision is theoretically **cutting through** more **dermatomes**
- Incision **crosses Langer's lines** and therefore probable **poorer cosmetic** appearance
- May cause **bladder damage** so essential to catheterize patient if performing a laparotomy.

BATTLE'S PARAMEDIAN

- **Muscle cutting** so **increased** postoperative **pain**
- Used less widely today
- Takes **longer** to close
- **Poor cosmetic result**
- Can lead to **infection** in the **rectus sheath**
- **Does not** lend itself to closure by **Jenkins' rule**
- Effective closure without strong sutures and **low incidence** of **incisional hernia** rate – in the olden days used to be closed with catgut!

ABDOMINAL WOUND CLOSURE

- **Mass closure** is the present preferred method as opposed to layered closure, followed in the past.
- The **correct suture** to be used: **Prolene, nylon or PDS (polydioxanone), looped or non-looped**. Other absorbable sutures such as **Vicryl** or **Monocryl** are **not suitable** for closing a laparotomy wound in an adult.
- The **correct size: number 1**; smaller sizes can cut through.
- The **correct length: four times** the length of the wound preferred (Jenkins' rule 1976). It should definitely **not be less** than **twice** the **length**.
- The **correct technique: large bites**, taking care always to incorporate the rectus sheath. The bites should be at **least 1 cm** from the **edge** of the sheath and **1 cm apart**.

- The **correct tightness**: the suture should be just tight enough to oppose the margins together without gaps. It should **not strangulate** the tissues and render them ischaemic.
- The **correct knot technique**: always perform **square knots** and use a **surgeon's knot** (double throw) and **adequate number of knots** for the suture being used.

COMPLICATIONS

Early

- Infection
- Bleeding/haematoma
- Necrosis of margins
- Wound dehiscence.

Late

- Incisional hernia
- Keloid formation or hypertrophic scar with poor cosmesis
- Suture sinus/granuloma
- Chronic pain caused by scar neuropathy.

APPENDICECTOMY SCARS

McBurney's incision was the traditional incision for an appendicectomy. This is sited over McBurney's point, at **right angles** to the line joining the umbilicus and the anterosuperior iliac spine.

Lanz's incision is more **cosmetic**, being more transverse and along the skin crease. It is usually **shorter** than McBurney's incision.

The muscles are split and not cut in both incisions. If the **muscles** are **cut** it is called a **Rutherford–Morrison** incision – rarely used today except for a heterotopic **renal transplantation** or for a **difficult appendicectomy**.

↑ Example viva question

What are the different layers of the anterior abdominal wall that you go through when performing a laparotomy?

From **surface inwards**, the **successive layers** are:

Skin

Superficial fascia (comprising two layers)
- ○ outer adipose layer
- ○ inner fibroelastic layer (Scarpa's fascia)

Musculoaponeurotic layer: comprises:
- ○ rectus abdominis
- ○ external oblique
- ○ internal oblique

Transversalis fascia

Pre-peritoneal adipose layer

Parietal peritoneum

65 Amputation

Possible viva questions related to this topic

→ What are the indications for lower limb amputation?
→ How would you decide the level of amputation?
→ How would you preoperatively assess and manage a patient undergoing amputation?
→ How can you assess the blood supply before deciding on the level of amputation?
→ What types of amputation are there?
→ What are the contraindications to performing a below-knee amputation?
→ What are the complications of performing a below-knee amputation?

Related topics		
Topic	**Chapter**	**Page**
Femoral and brachial embolectomy	31	98

INDICATIONS

- Vascular:
  - complications of **peripheral vascular disease** (85 per cent) – people with diabetes (40 per cent)
  - arteriovenous fistulae
  - thromboangiitis obliterans
- Trauma (10 per cent):
  - burns
  - frostbite
- Malignant tumours (3 per cent), e.g. malignant melanoma
- Infection:
  - osteomyelitis
  - gas gangrene
  - necrotizing fasciitis
- Congenital deformity
- Chronic pain
- 'Useless' limb, usually caused by neurological injury.

> ↑ **Example viva question**
>
> *What are the indications for performing an amputation?*
>
> Indications – **think** *the* **three 'D's**
>
> **Dead**
> - Acute ischaemia
> - Unreconstructable critical ischaemia
>
> **Dangerous**
> - Crush injury
> - Gas gangrene
> - Necrotizing fasciitis
> - Tumour
>
> **Damn nuisance**
> - Useless, insensate limb

CLASSIFICATION

Lower (97 per cent) versus **upper** (3 per cent) limb.

Major (most of limb removed) versus **minor**.

PREOPERATIVE WORK-UP AND ASSESSMENT

Multidisciplinary approach

- Anaesthetic team (patient normally has a high ASA grade with multiple co-morbidities)
- Prosthetic specialist
- Nursing staff
- Physiotherapy
- Occupational therapy
- Psychologist.

Consent

Obtain consent to amputate more proximally than intended.

Assessment of level of amputation

This should include ability of patient to undergo successful rehabilitation:

- Energy expenditure with above-knee prosthesis > below-knee prosthesis
- May limit patients with coexisting ischaemic heart disease (IHD)

- Above-knee or through-knee amputations generally better for wheelchair-bound patients
- Below-knee stump more liable to decubitus ulceration so contraindicated in bedbound individuals, and also those with a fixed flexion contracture > 15°.

Level of amputation

This is influenced by:

- Viability of tissues and degree of tissue loss
- Severity and pattern of vascular disease, including consideration of previous vascular grafts
- Previous orthopaedic prostheses
- Underlying pathology (ensure pathology available)
- Functional requirement
- Comfort
- Cosmetic appearance
- Preserve the knee joint and epiphysis in children.

Assessment of blood supply

Most surgeons rely on **clinical judgement**.

Unproven adjunctive tests include **laser Doppler studies, transcutaneous measurement of oxygenation** and measurement of blood flow in the skin using isotopes.

Bony appraisal is assessed by taking plain radiographs.

Optimization

- Major amputation is **high-risk surgery**
- Patients are normally ASA grade **III/IV**
- Preoperative preparation to minimize perioperative complications would include **DVT** (deep vein thrombosis) **prophylaxis** and **antibiotic prophylaxis**
- Urinary catheter to assess fluid management and allow ease of micturition while bedbound.

↑ **Example viva question**

What are the possible postoperative complications?

Remember early and late.

Early
- Stump haematoma
- Flap necrosis, infection
- Stump trauma from falls
- Wound-related pain

Late
- Neuroma formation
- Osteomyelitis
- Bony erosion
- Ulceration
- Ongoing ischaemia
- Phantom limb pain – good control with a combination of gabapentin and amitriptyline
- Joint contractures

TYPES OF AMPUTATION

- **Toe**: most common; usually through proximal phalanx. Must not be performed through the joint; exposes avascular cartilage and won't heal.
- **Ray**: excision of toe through the metatarsal bone.
- **Transmetatarsal**: divided at mid-shaft level. Indicated for infection or gangrene affecting several toes. Uses a TOTAL plantar flap. Provides excellent function postoperatively.
- **Midfoot**: consider only in patients with correctable or absent ischaemia. Types include **Lisfranc** (disarticulation between metatarsal and tarsal bones) and **Chopart** (disarticulation of the talonavicular and calcaneocuboid joints). Main disadvantage unpredictable healing rates and development of equinus deformity, which limits ambulation.
- **Ankle level** (Syme and Pirogoff): rarely indicated in vascular practice today.
- **Below-knee** (Burgess long posterior flap and skew flap): randomized controlled trial (RCT) comparing two – same healing, revision and successful ambulation rates.
- **Through-knee**, e.g. Gritti–Stokes: useful if orthopaedic metalware in the femur precluded above-knee amputation. Unpredictable healing of skin flaps.
- **Above-knee**.

- **Hip disarticulation and hindquarter**:
  - malignant disease
  - extensive trauma
  - infection or gangrene
  - non-healing high above-knee amputation.

SPECIFIC CONTRAINDICATIONS TO PERFORMING A BELOW-KNEE AMPUTATION

- Specific indication for performing a higher amputation
- Fixed flexion deformity of knee
- Inability to leave a tibial stump of at least 7.5 cm
- Insufficient tissue for adequate healing
- Bedbound patients.

66 Anastomosis and anastomotic leak

Possible viva questions related to this topic

→ What is the definition of an anastomosis?
→ How do bowel and vascular anastomoses differ?
→ What are the reasons for performing an anastomosis?
→ What are the principles of performing an ideal anastomosis?
→ What are the main risk factors for developing an anastomotic leak?
→ What are the signs of an anastomotic bowel leak? When do they typically occur?
→ If an anastomotic bowel leak was found intraoperatively, what are the different options available to the surgeon?
→ What would you do if the patient developed signs of an anastomotic leak a few days after surgery and began to deteriorate?
→ What are the different anastomoses performed in a Whipple's operation?

↑ **Example viva question**

What is the definition of an anastomosis?

Joining of two hollow organs or structures in order to re-establish a lumen through which flow can continue.

AIMS OF AN ANASTOMOSIS

- To **restore** the **continuity** of a hollow organ, e.g. artery or bowel after removing a diseased section of that organ
- To **bypass** an **obstructed segment** of an organ and divert flow through the lumen distally

- To **restore inflow** and **outflow** between a donor organ and the recipient body, e.g. renal and liver transplantations.

BASIC PRINCIPLES OF ANASTOMOSIS

Any anastomosis requires:

- **No tension**
- **A good blood supply**
- **Accurate apposition**
- **Good size approximation** – avoid mismatch between the two ends
- **Accurate suture technique, i.e. no holes or leaks**
- **Good surgical technique:**
  - do **not** perform anastomoses in 'watershed' areas
  - perform **adequate mobilization** of the ends to be joined – avoids tension
  - **invert edges (bowel)** to **discourage leakage** or **evert edges** to **avoid** risk of **lumen narrowing** and **intimal disruption (vascular)**
  - consider use of **preoperative bowel preparation** to **prevent mechanical damage** to the **join** in **bowel anastomosis**
  - **prophylactic antibiotics** – to cover appropriate organisms and **minimize infection**
  - consider the **type** of **suture material**: staples versus suture; absorbable versus non-absorbable or continuous versus interrupted
  - **avoid strangulating** the **tissue** on tying the knots: hand ties advisable
  - **single-layer versus two-layer** in bowel anastomoses – **ischaemia versus leak rate**. Perform technique with which you are familiar.

Bowel anastomosis

- Bowel anastomosis is performed usually using a **3/0 dissolvable monofilament suture**, e.g. PDS with an **atraumatic round-bodied needle**
- This should include the **submucosa** because this is the **strongest** layer
- **Extramucosal inverting** technique advised – discourages faecal or bile leakage
- Bowel can be joined together with either a **continuous** or an **interrupted** suture technique
- Surgical Royal Colleges teach a single-layer, interrupted seromuscular technique of sutures.

Vascular anastomosis

- Between **arteries, veins, prosthetic material** or combination of these
- Invariably performed with a **non-absorbable monofilament suture**, which moves smoothly through the vessel wall, e.g. Prolene

- Vascular anastomoses are performed with a **continuous suture technique** to ensure equal distribution of tension around the **suture line**
- **Use small needles and suture strong enough to hold anastomosis**
- **Prophylactic antibiotics**: to include **staphylococcal cover**
- Requires **gentle handling**: never hold between forceps!
- **Inside-to-outside technique**: prevents displacement and lifting up of atherosclerotic plaques
- A vascular anastomosis aims to achieve **eversion** of the **mucosa** (see above).

ANASTOMOTIC LEAKS

Occurs when there is ischaemia of the two ends of the anastomosis – especially in oesophageal and rectal surgery.

Predisposing factors

Patient factors
- Malnutrition
- Old age
- Malignancy
- Immunosuppression
- Steroids
- Radiotherapy
- Obesity.

Presentation factors
- Peritonitis
- Abscess
- Ileus
- Fistula
- Signs of sepsis.

Intraoperative factors
- Poor surgical technique
- Suture failure
- Stapler malfunction
- Disease process at the level of the anastomosis.

Postoperative factors
- Haematoma formation at the anastomotic line
- Infection.

Signs of an anastomotic bowel leak

Typically occurs around **7–10** days after surgery:

- **Low-grade pyrexia**: usually first sign
- Unexplained **new-onset tachycardia** or **arrhythmia** (usually **atrial fibrillation**)
- Other signs of **sepsis**, including **rise** in **inflammatory markers**
- **Renal impairment**
- **Cardiac** and **respiratory** problems
- Increasing **abdominal pain** and **peritonism**.

Checking for an anastomotic bowel leak (intraoperatively)
Typically performed after a **low rectal anastomosis** (low anterior resection):

- Examine the **anastomotic doughnuts** within the circular surgical stapler carefully, making sure that they are **complete** and of a **good size**
- **Air or fluid test**: using a **syringe** or a **rigid sigmoidoscope** judiciously **per rectally**
- Request a **water-soluble contrast enema** if worried postoperatively. This would demonstrate the site and extent of any leak.

If a leak is found intraoperatively
Options include:

- **Repair** leak with further sutures
- Place a **pelvic drain** near the anastomosis +/−
- Carry out a **defunctioning stoma** to prevent faecal leakage and peritonitis and hence pelvic sepsis. Defunctioning should not be deemed a failure by the surgeon. Not performing one can put the patient at significant risk postoperatively if he or she develops an anastomotic leak. The current trend is to perform a defunctioning loop ileostomy because it has the least morbidity associated with it and is the easier stoma to close at a later date. **Patients** also find it **easier** to manage a **loop ileostomy** compared with a loop colostomy.

Never perform an anastomosis in contaminated surroundings, e.g. perforated diverticular disease leading to faecal peritonitis. The join is likely to break down.

If a **leak** develops **postoperatively** and the patient begins to deteriorate and has not been defunctioned, he or she should be taken back promptly to theatre and an **emergency laparotomy** performed. The surgeon should:

- Drain the resulting collection
- Perform the safe option, which is to take down the anastomosis and bring out both ends as stomas, i.e. defunction the anastomosis
- Perform a full peritoneal lavage

- Place drains as appropriate
- Consider taking the patient to intensive care after discussion with anaesthetic colleagues for ventilation or multisystem support, because the patient is likely to be septic (see 'Sepsis and SIRS', Chapter 121, page 505).

WHIPPLE'S OPERATION

Procedure designed to **resect** the **head of pancreas** for **carcinoma**.

Roux-en-Y anastomosis performed; involves:

- Proximal loop of jejunum divided
- **Distal end** of divided loop anastomosed to stomach **(gastrojejunostomy)**
- **Proximal end** of divided loop anastomosed as an **end-to-side** anastomosis to the jejunum further downstream **(entero-enterostomy)**.

Other anastomoses performed are:

- **Choledochojejunostomy**
- **Pancreaticojejunostomy**.

As part of the operation, a **cholecystectomy** and a **partial duodenectomy** are also performed.

67 Antibiotics in surgery

Possible viva questions related to this topic

→ In what sort of operations should antibiotic prophylaxis be used?
→ What sorts of regimens are used for antibiotic prophylaxis?
→ Through what routes can antibiotics be used in surgery?
→ How should the choice of antibiotic be made?
→ What precautions and practices can be put into place to prevent the transmission of MRSA?
→ Define 'bactericidal' and 'bacteriostatic', giving examples of antibiotics from each class of agent.
→ What are the aims of antibiotic prophylaxis?
→ What is the mechanism of action of bactericidal antibiotics?
→ How do bacteria become resistant to antibiotics and what can surgeons do to help prevent this?
→ What would be the antibiotic of choice for a *Staphylococcus aureus* infection?
→ What are the risks of giving elderly patients second- and third-generation cephalosporins?
→ What are the definitions of narrow- and broad-spectrum antibiotics and when should they be used?

ROUTES, TIMING AND DURATION OF ADMINISTRATION

- **Parenteral** administration
- **Before surgery** to **ensure** effective **tissue levels**
- **Postoperative** antibiotics on their own **do not prevent infection**
- During a **long operation, top-up doses** may be given to maintain tissue levels of the antibiotic
- **Gentamicin** in the **wash** for **colonic on-table lavage**, as well as in **orthopaedic cement**, has proved useful
- **Intrathecal vancomycin** during cerebrospinal fluid (CSF) diversion procedures has been shown to **reduce** the **risk** of **postoperative shunt infection**.

↑ **Example viva question**

What are the aims of antibiotic prophylaxis?

In what sort of operations should antibiotic prophylaxis be used?

Antibiotic **prophylaxis** is intended to **reduce the risk** of **postoperative infection without alteration** of the **normal flora**.

It is **required only** when **wound contamination** is expected (e.g. colorectal surgery) or when **operations** of a **contaminated site** might lead to **bacteraemia** (e.g. incision and drainage of a perianal abscess).

It is **not required** for 'clean' operations except:

- Where a **vascular graft** or **prosthetic implant** (e.g. total hip or knee replacement) is used
- In patients with **pre-existing valvular heart disease** to decrease the risk of **infective endocarditis**
- On an in-patient with **pre-existing source of infection**
- If an infection would have **devastating** or life-altering **consequences** (e.g. all neurosurgical procedures)

↑ **Example viva question**

Define bactericidal and bacteriostatic, giving examples of antibiotics from each class of agent

Bactericidal: an antibiotic capable of **lysing and killing** bacteria (e.g. β-lactams, vancomycin, aminoglycosides)

Bacteriostatic: an antibiotic capable of slowing or **stopping the multiplication** of bacteria. **Final elimination** of pathogens **depends on** host **cellular defence mechanisms** having an effective phagocytotic response (e.g. erythromycin)

MECHANISMS OF ACTION OF ANTIBIOTICS

Inhibition of cell wall synthesis

- Leads to bacterial lysis as a result of defective peptidoglycan molecules in the cell wall
- Examples: β-lactams (e.g. penicillin, ampicillin, cephalosporins), vancomycin, monobactams.

Inhibition of protein synthesis within the bacteria

Inhibition of:

- Transfer RNA (tRNA) via attachment of amino acids (tetracyclines, bacteriostatic agents)
- Nuclear translocation (erythromycin [bacteriostatic at low concentrations], chloramphenicol, fusidic acid [bactericidal at high concentrations])
- Messenger RNA (mRNA) attachment to ribosomes (aminoglycosides – bactericidal)

Inhibition of nucleic acid synthesis

- Decreased mRNA (e.g. rifampicin)
- Decreased RNA replication (e.g. quinolones, suphonamides, metronidazole).

Alteration of call membrane function

- Polymyxin: bactericidal action against Gram-negative bacteria.

BROAD-SPECTRUM VERSUS NARROW-SPECTRUM ANTIBIOTICS

Broad spectrum

- Often **covers wide range** of bacteria
- Useful for prophylaxis
- Tends to **alter normal gut flora** of the patient
- Can lead to complications such as ***Clostridium difficile*** enterocolitis (see below).

Narrow spectrum

- Covers many **fewer types** of bacteria
- Useful for prophylaxis if common infecting organisms are known but, otherwise, **better for use** when **treating** a **known** infective **organism**
- **Less likely** to **alter** the normal **gut flora** of the patient
- **Fewer complications** such as C. *difficile* enterocolitis.

↑ **Example viva question**

What precautions and practices can be put into place to prevent the transmission of MRSA?

- **Handwashing** between patients is the single most important measure that can be taken to curb the incidence of MRSA (meticillin-resistant *S. aureus*) colonization in hospitals
- Many hospitals have instituted **MRSA-only bays** in wards and MRSA **side rooms**
- Before examining a patient with MRSA, **examination gloves** and an **apron** should be worn
- **Stethoscopes** should be disinfected between patients
- MRSA **cases** should be **left for the end of a list** or ensure that a **thorough cleaning** of theatre occurs afterwards
- **Barrier nursing**
- Make it clear to theatre that the patient is MRSA
- The problem of **resistant organisms** has arisen, however, as a result of continued **overuse of antibiotics**, arguably particularly prophylactic antibiotics

A clinician can **minimize this effect** by ensuring **appropriate use** of prophylactic antibiotics (see above) and **compliance** when a patient is prescribed a **full treatment dose** of antibiotics – the patient must **finish the course** to limit the risk of the formation of resistant organisms.

RISKS OF ANTIBIOTICS

One of the most **feared risks** of antibiotic prescription, particularly in elderly people, is that of **C. *difficile*** enterocolitis. This occurs particularly after the intravenous administration of a very broad-spectrum antibiotic such as a second- or third-generation cephalosporin or classically co-amoxiclav (Augmentin). These antibiotics **damage and kill** the **natural protective commensal bacterial flora** of the patient's gut, allowing an **overgrowth of pathogenic bacteria**.

Indeed, some centres will not allow a cephalosporin to be administered to someone aged over 65 unless the infection is very severe (e.g. central nervous system or CNS infection/overwhelming sepsis).

PRESENTATION OF ANTIBIOTIC-ASSOCIATED ENTEROCOLITIS

- Usually occurs in the **first postoperative week**
- Severe **watery diarrhoea** (can be bloody)

- Colonoscopy reveals mucosal inflammation and **pseudomembranes**
- Abdominal distension
- **Shock** secondary to profound fluid loss (see 'Shock', Chapter 122, page 510)
- Treatment is usually a course of **oral metronidazole**, although some strains that are resistant will require **oral vancomycin**
- *C. difficile* toxin positive.

↑ **Example viva question**

What would be the antibiotic of choice for a **S.** *aureus* **infection?**

Vancomycin is an excellent choice for an **MRSA infection**; indeed it is one of a very few antibiotics that would be appropriate, although it is easy to forget that **not all *S. aureus* infections are MRSA!**

For **MSSA** (meticillin-sensitive *S. aureus*) infection, **flucloxacillin is a much better option** because its **tissue penetration** is better. Furthermore, the appropriate use of vancomycin where it is not needed only **increases the chance** of developing further strains of a **vancomycin-resistant MRSA**.

ANTIBIOTIC REGIMENS – EXAMPLES

- **Clean procedures** (e.g. varicose veins) – **no prophylaxis**
- **Abdominal** surgery with **no expected contamination** (e.g. cholecystectomy) requires **single-dose** prophylaxis on **induction only**
- Procedures with a **contaminated field** (e.g. anterior resection, appendicectomy): **dose on induction and two further postoperative doses**
- Wounds **contaminated with skin flora** need prophylaxis against **staphylococcal** infection with **500 mg–1 g flucloxacillin** intravenously
- **Bowel procedures** need **broad-spectrum cover** for Gram-positive, Gram-negative organisms and anaerobes (an example regimen would be co-amoxiclav or a second- or third-generation cephalosporin with **metronidazole (for anaerobic cover)**
- **Biliary tract** operations rarely involve a flora of anaerobes and, in this case, a **cephalosporin** alone would be adequate prophylaxis.
- **Despite being clean, orthopaedic implants** and **heart valve surgery** require **prophylaxis** because **infection** in either case **is disastrous** and potentially **life threatening** (cefuroxime and gentamicin in the case of heart valves and flucloxacillin and gentamicin in the case of orthopaedic implants).

68 Bowel preparation

Possible viva questions related to this topic

→ What is the aim of preoperative bowel preparation?
→ What sorts of bowel preparation regimens are used?
→ How does Picolax work?
→ What are the complications of bowel preparation?
→ When should bowel preparations never be used?
→ What bowel preparations are used for left colon and right colon procedures, respectively?
→ Is there any evidence to suggest that mechanical bowel preparation with polyethyleneglycol reduces the incidence of anastomotic leak postoperatively?

BOWEL PREPARATION REGIMENS

Large bowel surgery or colonoscopy

- **Low residue diet** 3 days before procedure
- **Clear fluids** 2 days before the procedure
- **Bowel preparation sachet × 2, 6 hours apart** (usually **sodium picosulphate** or other purgative) – patient is advised to **continue drinking clear fluids** during this process. If unable to keep up with output, patient may go into **hypovolaemic shock** and bowel preparation for **elderly** people may have to be **in hospital while on intravenous fluids**
- **Phosphate enema** on the morning of surgery
- **Intravenous fluid replacement** is often required on admission.

↑ **Example viva question**

What is the aim of preoperative bowel preparation?

The **aim** of **preoperative** bowel preparation is to **reduce** the **incidence of postoperative sepsis** and other infective complications particularly after large bowel surgery. It attempts to achieve this by **reducing the overall bacterial load** within the gut **before surgery**.

There is **no class I evidence** to support the use the bowel preparation, and indeed a relatively **recent meta-analysis** (see 'Statistics and clinical trials', Chapter 79, page 326) looking at bowel preparation using propylethylene glycol has shown **no benefit** and possibly an **increased risk** of **postoperative anastomotic leak.**

The evidence has, thus far, failed to support the validity of preoperative bowel preparation, although it is still a practice that is **widely used in general surgery**.

There is no doubt that it has a role **pre-colonoscopy** to afford a **much better view** of the whole bowel wall.

Sigmoidoscopy

- **Phosphate enema** on the morning of the procedure or **at home** the previous evening.

Emergency large bowel resections

On-table 'wash out' or **lavage** may be used by some surgeons. This usually involves making a small incision in the bowel wall and inserting a long Foley catheter or similar device through a **caecostomy** or **appendicostomy**, often distal to a soft clamp. Infusion of warm saline with or without gentamicin can be used. Either the fluid is allowed to drain out through the anus or, more commonly, the bowel is divided and fluid escapes distally under controlled conditions (often through a large-bore effluent tube inserted into the bowel) with sterile saline-soaked gauze covering as much of the operative field and wound edges as possible.

Anorectal surgery

- A glycerine suppository is often used preoperatively, although there is no evidence of benefit for this.
- Some colorectal surgeons will perform a rectal wash-out (with Savlon or similar) before making the primary anastomosis in an anterior resection.

Obstructed patients

As a general rule, **preoperative bowel preparation** should **never be used** in the case of an obstructed patient for **fear of perforation**. Some surgeons may choose to use a phosphate or arachus oil enema for left-sided lesions, although there is no evidence in the literature to support this practice.

SODIUM PICOSULPHATE (PICOLAX)

- Diphenylmethane derivative
- Stimulates **myenteric plexus** to **increase the rate of peristalsis** and **decreases transit time**. This decreases the time for large bowel water absorption to take place and results in very watery diarrhoea via two possible mechanisms:
  - **inhibition of the sodium pump** (sodium/potassium adenosine triphosphatase [Na^+/K^+ ATPase]) preventing sodium transport across the gut wall and leading to the accumulation of water and electrolytes in the gut lumen
  - increased production of fluid in the intestine through **cyclic adenosine monophosphate (cAMP)** and prostaglandins, which promote active secretory processes in the intestinal mucosa.

COMPLICATIONS OF BOWEL PREPARATION

Systemic

- **Water and electrolyte imbalance** requiring intravenous fluids (see 'Fluid balance', Chapter 111, page 452)
- **Hypovolaemic shock** (see 'Shock', Chapter 122, page 510)
- **Cardiac arrhythmias** as a result of electrolyte imbalance
- **Death** (reported in elderly people)
- **Cramping pain**
- Nausea and vomiting.

Local

Bowel perforation: large bolus of effluent builds up proximal to a luminal narrowing or obstruction, leading to an increase in intraluminal pressure and subsequent perforation of an oedematous, ischaemic and friable gut wall.

69 Clinical governance

Possible viva questions related to this topic

→ What is the definition of clinical governance?
→ What is audit?
→ What is an audit cycle?
→ What is the difference between audit and research?
→ What is meant by 'closing the audit loop?'

↑ **Example viva question**

What is the definition of clinical governance?

From the original paper on the subject by Scally and Donaldson in the BMJ:

'A framework through which NHS organisations are accountable for continually improving the quality of their services and safeguarding high standards of care by creating an environment in which excellence in clinical care will flourish.'

Clinical governance is a concept, introduced by the government in 1998, to re-structure change within the NHS. It demands a fundamental change in the attitude and culture of the NHS. The main difference under clinical governance is that **a trust**, and ultimately the **chief executive of that trust**, is responsible for creating an environment in which **effective changes** can be made to achieve **high-quality care**, and can be held **accountable** if this is not provided.

For surgeons, clinical governance aims to ensure that:

- There are systems in place to **monitor quality of clinical practice** and that they are **functioning well**
- Clinical practice is **reviewed** and **improved** as a result
- Surgeons continue to meet the **national standards** as issued by the **professional bodies**.

The areas covered by clinical governance are divided into **seven pillars:**

1. **Clinical effectiveness** (the degree to which the organization ensures that 'best practice' is used):
   ○ **evidence-based medicine**
   ○ **NICE (National Institute for Health and Clinical Excellence): this organisation appraises the evidence for and against funding new treatments and produces guidelines for best practice based on the available evidence.**
2. **Risk management** (having systems to monitor and minimize risk to staff, patients and visitors):
   ○ **incident and near-miss reporting**
   ○ **health and safety**
   ○ **complaints.**
3. **Clinical audit** (the systematic critical analysis of the quality of clinical care).
4. **Education and training** (ensuring that support is available to enable staff to be competent at their jobs and to develop their skills to be up to date).
   ○ **continuing professional development (revalidation and appraisal).**
5. **Staffing and staff management** (recruitment and ensuring effective working conditions).
6. **Information use** (systems in place to collect and analyse information on service quality).
7. **Patient experience and public involvement** (ensuring individuals have a say in their own treatment).

RESEARCH

Definition

'The process of trying to find the truth.'

AUDIT

Definition

'A process used by clinicians to improve patient care by assessing clinical practice, comparing against accepted standards and making changes if necessary.'

The audit cycle

- Collect data
- Assess conformity of data to a predetermined standard
- Feedback results
- Update standards if necessary
- Intervene to promote change

- Set standards
- 'Close the loop' and go back to collecting data.

↑ **Example viva question**

What is the difference between audit and research?

Clinical audit is not research, but it does make use of research methodology in order to assess practice.

Although research and clinical audit are two distinct activities with different purposes, they are interrelated in several ways:

- **Research provides a basis** for defining good-quality care for clinical audit purposes
- **Clinical audit** can provide **high-quality data** for **non-experimental evaluative research**
- Research into the effectiveness and cost-effectiveness of clinical audit is needed
- **Research needs to be audited** to ensure that **high-quality work** is performed (refer to www.corec.org.uk for more information on this)

Research	Clinical audit
Aims to **establish best practice**	Aim to see **how close current practice** is to **best practice** and identify ways to bring the two closer together
Designed to be replicated and validated by other groups	Specific to one particular patient group – the **results are not transferable** to other settings
Aims to generate **new evidence**/knowledge	Aim to **improve services**
Usually initiated by **researchers**	Usually initiated by **service providers**
Is **theory** driven	Is **practice** based
Is often a single **one-off** study	Is an **ongoing process** (see the audit cycle)
May involve **randomization** (see 'Statistics and clinical trials', Chapter 79, page 326)	**Never** involves **randomization**
May involve a **placebo**	**Never** involves a **placebo**
May involve a **novel treatment**	**Never** involves a **completely novel treatment**

Benefits of clinical audit

- Identifies and **promotes good practice** and can **lead to improvements** in service delivery and outcomes for users
- Can **provide the information** that you need to show others that your service is effective (and **cost-effective**) and thus ensure its development
- Provides opportunities for **training and education**

- Helps to ensure **better use of resources** and, therefore, increased efficiency
- Can **improve working relationships**, communication and liaison between staff, between staff and service users, and between agencies
- The overall aim of clinical audit is to **improve service user outcomes** by **improving professional practice** and the **general quality of services** delivered.

REVALIDATION AND APPRAISAL

- As part of the government's commitment to delivering the quality agenda, **annual appraisal is being introduced for all doctors** working in the NHS.
- Appraisal for **consultants** was launched in **April 2001**.
- **Work is under way** to roll out schemes for other groups of doctors, including **doctors in training**, public health doctors and locum doctors.
- In effect, **all NHS doctors** (including GPs) will be **discussing their practice** with their **employer** or a **recognized NHS appraiser** on an **annual basis**.
- Part of this appraisal process is a **review of the evidence** used to support the standards set by **good medical practice**.
- During the development of appraisal, the **General Medical Council (GMC)** made proposals to 'revalidate' all registered doctors. This means that **every 5 years** each doctor who wants to remain in practice must **present evidence to the GMC** that he or she is **competent in his or her field** of practice and has **kept up to date** (CME or continuing medical education points are essential to this process).
- The **appraisal system** for NHS doctors is designed to **support** the **process of revalidation**.

70 Day surgery

Possible viva questions related to this topic

→ What is day surgery?
→ What are the criteria for consideration of day surgery?
→ What procedures are suitable for day surgery?
→ What are the advantages and disadvantages of day surgery?
→ What sort of instructions are patients who are undergoing day surgery given?
→ What are the contraindications to day surgery?

↑ Key learning point

Day surgery

Procedures and operations performed on an **elective non-resident** basis but that nevertheless **require facilities** for patient **recovery**.

The government has targeted **75 per cent of all elective surgery** to be performed on a day-case basis by the end of 2006!

CRITERIA FOR CONSIDERATION OF DAY SURGERY

• Patients must be **ASA** (American Society of Anesthesiologists) **grade I or II** (i.e. fit and well)
• Patients must have **body mass index (BMI) < 35**
• **Operations** must be projected to be **less than 1 hour**
• Idea of day surgery must be **acceptable to patient**
• **Pathology** must be **appropriate** (i.e. no massive scrotal hernias, etc.)
• Patient must **live close** to day surgery unit (travel time < 1 hour)
• Patient must have **friend or relative at home** to look after the patient for **24–48 hours** after surgery
• Patient must have a **telephone at home**.

PROCEDURES SUITABLE FOR DAY SURGERY

(These are based on the British Association of Day Surgery 'trolley' of procedures, 1999, of which 50 per cent should be suitable for day-case surgery.)

These procedures need to be **relatively quick** with a **low complication rate**. They can be performed using **local anaesthetic** infiltration or a quick **general anaesthetic** but they must **not involve a spinal or epidural anaesthetic**. Patient should not require strong opioid analgesia postoperatively and **oral analgesics should be sufficient**.

General surgery

- OGD (oesophagogastroduodenoscopy)
- Colonoscopy
- Anal tag removal/haemorrhoidectomy
- Hernia repair (inguinal/femoral/umbilical/paraumbilical/epigastric)
- Varicose vein surgery
- Pilonidal sinus surgery
- Small breast lump excision.

ENT

- Direct pharyngoscopy and laryngoscopy
- Insertion of grommets
- Tonsillectomy.

Orthopaedics

- Arthroscopy (shoulder/knee)
- Trigger finger release
- Dupuytren's contracture surgery
- Digit amputation
- Carpal tunnel release
- Ingrowing toenail surgery.

Ophthalmic surgery

- Cataract surgery
- Strabismus surgery (squint)
- Visual acuity correction surgery (LASIX, radial keratotomy).

Plastic surgery

- 'Bat' ears
- Breast augmentation
- Nipple and areola reconstruction
- Small contracture surgery (z-plasty, etc.).

Gynaecological surgery

- Dilatation and curettage
- Termination of pregnancy
- Laparoscopy and laparoscopic sterilization.

THE DAY SURGERY UNIT

These procedures should ideally be performed in a **dedicated day surgery unit** with its own waiting lists, building, theatres and recovery area on the ground floor. Procedures should be performed by an **experienced consultant** who is **constantly audited** to ensure that **complications remain low**. In some cases an **experienced senior registrar** would be **acceptable**. Patient satisfaction and adequacy of postoperative analgesia should be **regularly audited** as well. A successful unit depends on **day of surgery admission** and **nurse-led discharge** in many cases.

Advantages and disadvantages of day surgery

- **Minimum time** away from home
- **Cost-effectiveness**
- **Less chance** of operation being **cancelled as a result of** emergency work
- Inpatient **beds released**
- Arguably **less** chance of **nosocomial infection**
- Needs **aftercare** at home (friend or relative)
- **Less** opportunity for **training** in 'bread and butter' cases for juniors
- **Inpatient admission** can be required following an **unexpected complication** or inadequate postoperative analgesia

Instructions given to patients

Patients must have **full verbal and printed details** giving a description of the **surgical problem**, and **outline of the surgery** and other possible **alternatives, pre-op instructions, post-op instructions** and advice on when to **return to work** and/or **follow-up** appointment or **suture removal**. A list of possible complications should also be given along with anything that the patient should look out for at home that could indicate a postoperative problem. The process of **informed consent is exactly the same** for day surgery as for any other form of surgery.

Contraindications to day surgery

These can split up into **surgical/anaesthetic** and **social**.

Surgical/anaesthetic
- **Unfit** (ASA III or above)
- Operation **longer than 1 hour**
- Requires **spinal or epidural analgesia**

- Day surgery **unacceptable to patient**
- Patient is **obese** (BMI > 35)
- **Pathology too extensive** to tackle as a day-case procedure.

Social

- **Relative or friend unavailable** to look after them for 24–48 hours
- **No access** to a lift in an upper floor flat or restricted access to a house; lack of appropriate toilet facilities/bathroom
- **Lives too far** from day surgery unit.

71 Diathermy

Possible viva questions related to this topic

→ What are the possible complications with using diathermy in theatre?
→ What different sorts of diathermy do you know?
→ How does diathermy work?
→ What different settings do you know for diathermy and how do they work?
→ Why does diathermy induce very little neuromuscular stimulation?
→ What is the difference between monopolar and bipolar diathermy?
→ What are the problems with using diathermy in patients with pacemakers?

Related topics		
Topic	Chapter	Page
Laparoscopic cholecystectomy and laparoscopy	34	112

Surgical diathermy involves the passage of **high-frequency alternating current between two electrodes** and through tissue. Where the **local current density** is the **highest**, a large amount of **heat is produced** in the tissue, resulting in tissue destruction.

There are two main types: monopolar and bipolar.

Monopolar

Probably the most common sort, using a **high-power generator (400 W)**. A current is generated in the diathermy machine and **passed to a hand-held electrode**. At the **tip** of this electrode, the **current density is very high**, resulting in very high temperatures locally. The **current** then **dissipates** over a large amount of tissue to the patient 'plate' electrode – with a **large surface area** of at least **70 cm²**, ensuring that the **current density at the plate is low**, and thus causing minimal heating.

Bipolar

Here, the current is **passed from one electrode to another** across a small amount of tissue. The two electrodes are usually incorporated into a **pair of forceps** with which the surgeon can **hold and coagulate** tissue. As there is **no need for a plate**, bipolar diathermy requires **much less power (50 W)**. More commonly used in plastic surgery and neurosurgery for very precise coagulation.

DIATHERMY SETTINGS

Cutting

Continuous output from the generator causes an arc to be struck between the active electrode and the tissue in monopolar diathermy. **Temperatures up to 1000°C** are produced and **cellular water is instantly vaporized**, causing tissue disruption without much coagulation. This setting is not available in bipolar diathermy.

Coagulation

Pulsed output from the diathermy generator results in the sealing of blood vessels with the minimum of tissue disruption.

Blend

Many machines have this setting for monopolar diathermy – a continuous output with pulses to help coagulate as well as cut.

CAUSES OF DIATHERMY BURNS

Older earth-referenced machines

These are from **ECG electrodes**, **metal drip stands** or metal components of the **operating table** in contact with the patient's skin. They provide **other earths** for the diathermy machine and, as their **surface area** is relatively **small, current density may be high** and severe burns will result. Modern isolated, as opposed to earth-referenced, machines get around this problem by not needing an earth and using a tight frequency range for the AC current, resulting in less earth current leakage.

Incorrect placement of patient plate (most common cause)

- Needs good contact with **dry, shaved skin** (no kinking because it reduces area)
- **Contact surface** must be at least **70 cm²** (minimal heating)
- Plate must be **away from bony prominences** and tissue with poor blood supply (e.g. scar tissue) – poor heat distribution.

Careless technique

Failure to replace electrode in insulated quiver after use and use of **spirit-based skin preparation** (use of diathermy without allowing sufficient time for the prep to evaporate)

Use of diathermy on large bowel

Methane and hydrogen in large bowel can be **explosive**.

Use of monopolar on appendages (e.g. penis, digits or tissue pedicles)

Current is concentrated along the line of tissue pedicles and can cause **tissue damage far distant** to the site of the electrode. In circumstances such as these where **coagulation** is needed, **bipolar should be used.**

Used close to metallic implants (e.g. hip prostheses)

Current can be **induced** locally around metal implants, causing local heating and tissue damage.

Active electrode not in view in laparoscopy

Diathermy should only be used in laparoscopy when the active electrode is fully in view, along with the tissue that it is about to cut or coagulate. The electrode should **never** be used 'around the corner'.

Metal laparoscopic ports used with plastic insulator cuffs

The use of diathermy in this instance could set up a **capacitance** in the port and local heating at the point where the port meets the skin. Thus laparoscopic ports should always be made up of the appropriate components. Never 'mix and match'.

↑ **Example viva question**

Why does diathermy induce very little neuromuscular stimulation?

To produce profound neurostimulation, alternating current needs to be **below 50 kHz.** The **mains electricity in the UK works at 50 Hz** and a current of only 5–10 mA will cause **painful muscle stimulation**, whereas 80–100 mA across the heart will result in **ventricular fibrillation. Surgical diathermy** involves currents at **400 kHz–10 MHz** and, with these frequencies, **currents of up to 500 mA** may be safely passed through the tissues.

DIATHERMY AND PACEMAKERS

There are two potential problems:

1. **High frequency** of the diathermy may result in **induced currents in the logic circuits of the pacemaker**, resulting in potentially fatal arrhythmias.
2. **Diathermy close to the box** itself may result in currents travelling down the **pacemaker wires**, leading to **myocardial burns.** This could either increase the threshold or at worst cause cardiac arrest.

Thus, for any patients with a pacemaker:

- **Discuss** the case first with a **cardiologist** – type of box, type of pacing, underlying arrhythmia, etc.
- **Avoid diathermy** completely if possible – if not, consider bipolar
- If monopolar must be used, use only for **short bursts** and place the patient's plate so that the **current flows away from the pacemaker system**. If any arrhythmias are noted, stop all diathermy immediately.

72 Drains in surgery

Possible viva questions related to this topic

→ What is the purpose of a surgical drain?
→ What are the complications associated with the use of drains in surgery?
→ What type of drains have you seen or heard about? Give examples.

INDICATIONS

- To **exteriorize actual** (e.g. radiologically placed drain for subphrenic abscess) or potential **collections of fluid** in a wound
- To **minimize dead space**
- To **divert fluid away** from **blockage** or potential blockage, e.g. biliary T-tube and suprapubic urinary catheter and protection of a healing anastomosis
- To **decompress** and allow **air to escape** (chest drain).

TYPES

- **Open**: these would be **non-suction** in nature, e.g. corrugated or Penrose drain
- **Closed**: *suction* versus *non-suction* (under the influence of gravity only)

- **Suction**: *examples* include sump, Redivac, firm multi-holed PVC, for skin flaps
- **Non-suction** (closed): *examples* include Robinson drain, T-tube, urinary (Foley) catheter, chest drain, Blake drain

- **Closed drain systems**: advantage of **reducing** the risk of introducing **infection**

- **Suction drains** provide the advantage of better drainage, but may damage adjacent structures, e.g. bowel, which could precipitate a leak.

COMPLICATIONS

Immediate

- **Air leak** around a chest drain
- **Pain**: chest drain irritates the diaphragm, causing immobility and therefore its potential complications
- **Trauma at insertion and injury to surrounding structures** during drainage or placement, e.g. bowel injury as the result of an improperly placed ascitic drain.

Early

- **Failure to drain adequately** (incorrect placement, too small, blocked lumen)
- **Fracture** of drain
- **Disconnection or removal postoperatively**.

Late

- **Infection:** via the drain track
- **Retraction** of the drain into the wound: surgical removal may be required in this case
- **Herniation**, e.g. bowel at the drain site
- **Fistula** formation
- **Bleeding**: by erosion into a blood vessel – nasogastric tube causing a gastric ulcer
- **Anastomotic leakage**: direct damage to the anastomosis; prevent vascularization of the anastomosis. However, if the anastomosis is not watertight a drain may be useful to prevent the build-up of a collection, which may impede healing of, for example, a urological or biliary anastomosis.

DRAINS USED IN SURGICAL PRACTICE

- **Nasogastric tube**: used to drain stomach air and fluid contents and to prevent aspiration
- **Chest drain**: used to drain the pleural space – this is attached to an underwater seal to prevent backflow from negative intrathoracic pressures
- **Operative wound drain**: used for an anticipated fluid collection in a closed space; this prevents seroma formation, e.g. after an incisional hernia repair
- **Pericardial drain**: used after coronary artery bypass surgery
- **Infected abscess:** cavity drain (intra-abdominal).

73 DVT prophylaxis and coagulation in surgery

Possible viva questions related to this topic

→ What do you understand by Virchow's triad? How does this relate to DVT prophylaxis in the surgical patient?
→ What regimen of DVT prophylaxis would you use for minor/major surgery?
→ What are the risk factors for DVT?
→ What is the definition of a thrombus? How does it differ from a clot?
→ What is the pathophysiology of the process of thrombosis?
→ How does heparin work?
→ What are the indications for intravenous heparin perioperatively?
→ How long before an operation should warfarin be stopped and which patients need perioperative anticoagulation?
→ If a patient's INR (international normalized ratio) is very high and the patient is on warfarin but requires emergency, life-saving surgery such as an abdominal aortic aneurysm repair, how would you reverse the anticoagulation?

↑ **Example viva question**

What is the definition of a thrombus? How does it differ from a clot?

Thrombus: a **solid mass** formed in **flowing blood** from blood constituents

Clot: a semi-solid mass formed in **stationary blood** from blood constituents. It may be formed **after death** or **outside the circulation**

Pulmonary embolus (PE) accounts for **10–25 per cent** of all postoperative **inpatient deaths**. There are three major sources for this embolus:

1. DVT in the deep veins of the leg
2. Thrombosis in the mesenteric veins
3. Atrial fibrillation (AF) resulting in formation of right atrial thrombus (also mural thrombus from myocardial damage).

In addition:

- At least 20 per cent patients with a DVT develop a post-thrombotic limb
- Most calf DVTs are **clinically silent**
- **80 per cent** of calf DVTs **lyse spontaneously** without treatment
- **20 per cent** of calf DVTs **propagate** to the thigh and have **increased risk of PE**.

↑ **Example viva question**

What do you understand by Virchow's triad?

Virchow's triad
The **three factors** that contribute to the **risk of thrombosis**:

1. Damage to the vessel wall and vascular endothelium
2. Alterations in blood flow
3. Alterations in the constituents of the blood

Damage to the vessel wall and vascular endothelium
- **Arterial**: **atherosclerosis** (see 'Atherosclerosis', Chapter 49, page 177)
- **Venous**:
  - **damage to calf veins** by direct **pressure** when in stirrups – therefore **patient positioning** in long operations – **crucial** to **reduce risk** of DVT
  - damage to femoral vein by distortion **during hip replacement surgery**

Alterations in blood flow
- **Stasis and pooling of blood** in leg veins in patients on bedrest postoperatively – **TED (thromboembolic deterrent) stockings** are compression stockings **that limit pooling of blood** in the legs. Dynamic compression of the legs during surgery has been shown to reduce the postoperative **incidence of DVT. Early postoperative mobilization is essential**
- Immobility for long periods (including **air travel**)
- **Stasis in the heart** as a result of AF – if at all possible, **AF should** be cardioverted preoperatively or at the very least **rate controlled**

Alterations in the constituents of the blood
- **Dehydration** (increased viscosity) – **ensure adequate fluid replacement**
- **Thrombocytosis** (infection, asplenia, etc.) – important to **treat all postoperative** infections promptly
- New platelets (increased platelet adhesion after surgery)

Thrombophilia (factor V Leiden, protein C/S deficiency, lupus anticoagulant): **these factors increase the risk of DVT postoperatively.**

RISK FACTORS FOR DVT

- Age
- Previous DVT
- Pregnancy
- Obesity
- **Surgery**
- Varicose veins
- Pelvic disease
- Oral contraceptive pill
- **Malignancy**
- **Immobility**
- Thrombophilias.

CLINICAL FEATURES OF DVT

- Can be asymptomatic
- Warm, erythematous swollen leg
- Calf tenderness and pain
- Rise in skin temperature of leg
- Distended superficial veins
- Low–grade pyrexia at 7–8 days
- **Doppler ultrasonography can be used for diagnosis of distal thrombosis**
- **Venography may be used to diagnose iliac vein thrombosis.**

PATHOPHYSIOLOGY OF THROMBOSIS

- **Platelets stick** to damaged epithelium, releasing various mediators (e.g. platelet-derived growth factor [PDGF])
- **Fibrin** and **leukocytes adhere** to platelets
- **Fibrin network forms** on this layer:
  - clotting cascade (intrinsic system)
  - activation of factor XII by contact with vascular endothelium
  - thrombin catalyses fibrin formation from fibrinogen
- **Second layer of platelets stick** (alternate layers of fibrin network and platelets form pathological **'lines of Zahn'**)
- **Thrombus** eventually **occludes the lumen** of the vein, creating stasis proximally and **promoting proximal propagation** of the thrombus.

RISK STRATIFICATION ACCORDING TO PROCEDURES AND RISK FACTORS

Patients are **risk stratified** into low-, moderate- and high-risk groups according to their **preoperative clinical condition**, **risk factors** and **type of operation**.

Low risk

- Minor surgery (< 30 min) with no other risk factors other than age
- Major surgery (> 30 min), age < 40 years with no other risk factors
- Minor trauma or medical illness.

Moderate risk

- Major general, urological, gynaecological, cardiothoracic, vascular or neurological surgery + age > 40 years or other risk factor
- Major medical illness or malignancy
- Major trauma or major burns
- Minor surgery, trauma or illness in patients with previous DVT, PE or thrombophilia.

High risk

- Fracture or major orthopaedic surgery of pelvis, hip or lower limb
- Major pelvic or abdominal surgery for neoplasia
- Major surgery, trauma or illness in patient with previous DVT, PE or proven thrombophilia (see above)
- Major lower limb amputation.

UNTREATED EPIDEMIOLOGY OF DVT IN RISK GROUPS AND RECOMMENDED REGIMENS

Group	Calf DVT (%)	Proximal DVT (%)	Fatal PE (%)
Low risk	< 10	< 1	0.01
Moderate risk	10–40	1–10	0.1–1
High risk	40–80	10–30	1–10

High risk

- Graduated elastic anti-embolism **stockings** (e.g. Kendal TED)
- **Unfractionated heparin 5000 U s.c. two or three times daily** (there is evidence that heparin given 8-hourly may be more effective than 12-hourly). Start on admission or more than 2 hours before surgery (**not in the case of epidural insertion or removal**) or
  - **low-molecular-weight heparin** or
  - **adjusted-dose warfarin** (INR 2–3) (not commonly used)
- Consider **intermittent pneumatic compression of calves** in theatre.

Moderate risk

- Graduated elastic anti-embolism **stockings** (e.g. Kendal TED) and/or
  - **low-dose unfractionated heparin 5000 U s.c. two or three times daily.** Start on admission or more than 2 hours before surgery (see above) or
  - **low-molecular-weight heparin** (contact hospital pharmacy for available products and dose).

Low risk

- **Early mobilization.**

Heparin

- Commonly used anticoagulant, available in unfractionated or low-molecular-weight (LMW) forms
- Can be given intravenously or subcutaneously
- Acts by inhibition of factor X and binding anti-thrombin III
- Unfractionated heparin also acts significantly on factor II
- LMW heparin more specific to factor X and needs only to be given once daily. It is more expensive than unfractionated heparin
- Intravenous heparin is reversed by intravenous protamine – standard procedure in cardiothoracic surgery.

Warfarin

- **Antagonizes** the action of **vitamin K** in the liver and on the vitamin K-dependent enzymes in the clotting cascade
- **Reduces** prothrombin and **factors VII, IX and X**
- Patients on warfarin are usually converted to some form of heparin perioperatively to minimize bleeding risk and provide as much control as possible to the surgeon.

INDICATIONS FOR INTRAVENOUS HEPARIN

With the advent of LMW heparin, indications for intravenous heparin are shrinking, although it is still used in many centres. It is used where the anticoagulation needs to be **reversed quickly** and cover with anticoagulant is **important up to the last moment** (see below). The decision on whether or not to start intravenous heparin for warfarin anticoagulation cover is based on the reason for the anticoagulation:

- **AF** is **no longer considered** an adequate reason for intravenous heparin, given its difficulties and poor management of APTT (activated partial thromboplastin time) ratios by juniors on the ward.
- Likewise, a **metal aortic valve replacement** is considered by many **no longer to require intravenous heparin cover** because the risk of perioperative thrombosis of the valve is tiny for anything up to 2 weeks after stopping warfarin.
- A **metal mitral valve**, however, has a **higher risk of thrombosis** and should be covered perioperatively with intravenous heparin, bringing the patient in early for the switch to take place on the ward.
- Intravenous heparin is also used in the context of vascular surgery, cardio-thoracic surgery and interventional vascular radiology during procedures or operations.

↑ Example viva question

If a patient's INR is very high and the patient is on warfarin but needs emergency, life-saving surgery such as an abdominal aortic aneurysm repair, how would you reverse the anticoagulation?

Although the use of **intravenous vitamin K** and/or **fresh frozen plasma** is the classic way of reversing a wayward INR, it is **not particularly efficient** or **quick**, often taking several hours to get the INR to a level where an operation would become possible.

Thus, in concert with a haematologist, **activated factor VII and factor IX concentrate** can both be given, which reverses the effect of warfarin **almost instantly**. It is, however, very expensive, carries with it a **small increased risk of ischaemic sequelae**, and should be used only in extremis such as the situation above where any delay could be fatal.

Possible viva questions related to this topic

→ What bone is this (femur) and from which side is it?
→ What is the blood supply to the head of femur?
→ Where does the hip joint capsule attach to the femur?
→ What are the ligaments of the hip joint?
→ What maintains the stability of the hip joint?
→ The sciatic nerve is derived from which nerve roots?
→ What is the surface marking of the sciatic nerve from the pelvis to knee?
→ What are the main branches of the sciatic nerve and what do they supply?
→ How do you classify fractures of the neck of femur and how does this relate to management?
→ What are the possible complications of femoral neck fractures?
→ When is a neck of femur fracture an emergency?
→ Where does a prolapsed intervertebral disc normally occur?
→ What are the signs of an L5–S1 nerve root compression?
→ What does the patient typically present with?

Related topics

Topic	Chapter	Page
Orthopaedic approaches and procedures	38	130

Example viva question

How do you side a femur?

Helpful hints
Proximally: rounded head with a **neck angled 125°** to the femoral shaft. Points **upwards** and **medially**

Distally: two **femoral condyles**. Note prominent **adductor tubercle** proximal to medial condyle. **Lateral condyle more prominent** and acts as a buttress to assist in **preventing lateral dislocation** of the patella

Anterior surface is **smooth** and **convex**. The junction between neck and shaft is marked by the **intertrochanteric line** anteriorly

Posterior surface has the **linea aspera** (prominent ridge). Also note the deep **intercondylar notch** that separates the two condyles

BLOOD SUPPLY TO THE FEMORAL HEAD

Three sources

1. Through **diaphysis**
2. **Retinacular branches** from **medial and lateral femoral circumflex arteries** (trochanteric anastomosis), which pass proximally within joint capsule to anastomose at junction of neck and articular surface
3. Artery in the **ligamentum teres** (**negligible** in **adults** but **essential** in **children**, when the femoral head is separated from the neck by the cartilage of the epiphyseal line).

ANATOMY OF THE HIP JOINT

- Ball-and-socket primary synovial joint
- Ligamentum teres in fovea.

Capsule

The capsule of the hip joint is strong and attached to the **acetabulum** and the **transverse acetabular ligament. Anteriorly**, it extends over the neck of the femur to the **intertrochanteric line. Posteriorly**, it covers the neck only to halfway to the **intertrochanteric crest.**

Reflects back as the retinacular fibres which carry its blood supply.

- **Blood supply**: **trochanteric** (at greater trochanter) and **cruciate** (lesser trochanter) anastomoses
- *Three bursae*: trochanteric, ischial and psoas bursae.

Stabilizing factors of the hip joint

Ligamentous, bony and **muscular** contributions.

Ligaments
Three ligaments support the capsule:

1. **Iliofemoral: triangular ligament of Bigelow** is the **strongest**. Arises from the **anteroinferior iliac spine** and inserts **Y shaped** into the **intertrochanteric line**
2. **Pubofemoral**
3. **Ischiofemoral**: contributes little and is the weakest of the three ligaments.

Bony
Femoral head fits snugly into acetabulum. Deepened by the **acetabular labrum.**

Muscular

The **short gluteal muscles**, e.g. quadratus femoris and piriformis.

Gluteus minimus and **medius** are important stabilizers during weight bearing on one leg; they act to prevent adduction rather than as pure abductors.

The hip joint is **least stable** in the **flexed adducted position**.

NECK OF FEMUR FRACTURES

Broadly divided into **intracaspular** and **extracapsular**.

Intracapsular (subcapital, cervical, basal–cervical)

These tend to **disrupt the blood supply** to the femoral head along the **retinacular fibres** (see above). There is an increased risk of **avascular necrosis** of the head.

Garden classification for intracapsular fractures
This describes the **degree of displacement** at the fracture site:

Type I	Incomplete fracture
Type II	Complete but undisplaced fracture
Type III	Complete fracture with partial displacement
Type IV	Complete fracture with complete displacement

The **degree of displacement** of the fracture dictates surgical management:

- **Undisplaced intracapsular fractures**: internal fixation with two to three cannulated **parallel screws**
- **Displaced intracapsular fractures**: **hemiarthroplasty** in elderly people, e.g. simple unipolar prosthesis – Austin–Moore or Thompson
- **Fit patients aged < 65 years** should be treated by reduction and internal fixation or considered for **bipolar** hemiarthroplasty.

Extracapsular (intertrochanteric, basal, subtrochanteric)

Distal to the insertion of the capsule through an area of well-vascularized bone.

Classification is based on the number of fragments produced by the fracture:

- **Undisplaced (two part)**
- **Displaced (two part)**
- **Three part involving greater trochanter**
- **Three part involving lesser trochanter**
- **Four part**
- **Reverse obliquity**.

Management depends on **site and number of parts** of fracture.

Dynamic hip screw (DHS) for **intertrochanteric** and **basal** fractures.

Subtrochanteric fractures with open reduction internal fixation with **intramedullary hip screw (IMHS)** or **DHS with medialization of the fracture.**

Complications of femoral neck fractures

- **Avascular necrosis**: high risk in displaced fractures caused by disruption of the blood supply; eventually the femoral head collapses, causing pain, loss of function and progressive osteoarthritis
- **Non-union**
- **Osteoarthritis**
- **Systemic**: DVT, PE, chest infection, pressure sores.

↑ **Example viva question**

When is a fractured neck of femur an emergency?

The benefit of preserving the femoral head in younger adults is much greater, so biologically younger patients with displaced intracapsular fractures are rushed into theatre for open reduction and fixation.

There is no evidence for this benefit and a wait of 48 hours will not prejudice outcome of hip fracture surgery.

Prognosis

Neck of femur fractures normally occur in elderly people – a population with extensive co-morbidity.

There is a **50 per cent risk of death** within **6 months** of a neck of femur fracture.

THE SCIATIC NERVE

Formed from the **nerve roots** of **L4, L5** (lumbosacral trunk) and **S1–3** (upper sacral plexus).

Surface anatomy: midpoint between ischial tuberosity and greater trochanter downwards on the posterior thigh to the apex of the popliteal fossa.

Supplies the **posterior compartment** of the thigh.

Main branches

- **Nerves to obturator internus and quadratus femoris**: innervates the short external rotators of the hip joint

- **Common peroneal nerve**: supplies muscles of the anterior (via deep peroneal nerve) and peroneal (via superficial peroneal nerve) compartments of the lower limb. Also supplies sensation to the anterolateral leg and dorsum of foot
- **Tibial nerve**: supplies the muscles of the posterior compartments (superficial and deep) of the leg and sensation to the posterior region of the leg and sole of the foot.

Example viva question

Where does a prolapsed intervertebral disc normally occur?

A tear in the **annulus fibrosus** allows **herniation** of the **nucleus pulposus** and is usually secondary to a **flexion–rotational injury**.

The L4–5 and L5–S1 disc levels are most commonly affected.

Patients usually present with:

- Low back pain
- Pain in the leg in the L5–S1 nerve root distribution
- Limitation of straight-leg raise
- Positive sciatic stretch test

Signs of L5 nerve root compression:

- Decreased sensation in the L5 dermatome
- Weakness of extensor hallucis longus
- Weakness of dorsiflexion of the ankle
- Wasting of extensor digitorum brevis

Signs of S1 nerve root compression:

- Decreased sensation of S1 dermatome
- Weakness of plantarflexion of the ankle
- Weakness of eversion of the subtalar joint
- Absent or diminished ankle jerk

Lumbar 'central disc' prolapse causing **cauda equina syndrome** is rare but is a surgical emergency.

Onset is **sudden**. Pain is felt in the back and radiates down the back of both thighs and legs.

Numbness is in the same distribution, often extending into the soles of the feet and perineum (saddle anaesthesia). Ankles, sphincters of the bowel and bladder are weak or paralysed. There are **absent ankle jerks**. The patient must go for immediate spinal decompression.

---

75 Local anaesthetics

Possible viva questions related to this topic

→ Tell me the action of local anaesthetics.
→ How much anaesthetic is in a 1 per cent solution?
→ What are the different types of local anaesthetics?
→ What are the uses and complications of the various local anaesthetics?
→ How can local anaesthetics be administered?
→ What is the maximum dose of lidocaine 2 per cent that you could give a 70 kg man?
→ Why do local anaesthetics work less well in the presence of infection?
→ How does adrenaline mixed with local anaesthetic act and when should it not be used?
→ What is Marcain Heavy?

Related topics

Topic	Chapter	Page
Action potential	85	353
Anorectal surgery 1: anal fissure and lateral sphincterotomy	23	63
Anorectal surgery 2: fistula *in ano* and pilonidal sinus	24	67
Anorectal surgery 3: injection sclerotherapy and haemorrhoidectomy	25	73
Burr holes and lumbar puncture	26	78
Carotid endarterectomy	27	81
Carpal tunnel decompression	28	87
Circumcision	29	91
Emergency splenectomy	30	94
Femoral and brachial embolectomy	31	98
Femoral hernia repair	32	102
Inguinal hernia repair	33	106
Laparoscopic cholecystectomy and laparoscopy	34	112
Long saphenous varicose vein surgery	35	117
Mastectomy, axillary dissection and breast reconstruction	36	120
Open appendicectomy	37	125
Orthopaedic related approaches and procedures	38	130
Perforated duodenal ulcer and exploratory laparotomy	39	135
Renal transplantation	40	140
Thyroidectomy	41	144
Tracheostomy	42	148

ACTION

Local anaesthetics are all **sodium channel blockers** of some sort. They cause **reversible blockade of motor and sensory nerves** depending on type, concentration and site of administration. They **prevent influx of sodium** in peripheral nerves, thus **inhibiting the propagation of the action potential.**

 Example viva question

How much anaesthetic is in a 1 per cent solution?

1 mL of a 1 per cent solution contains 10 mg of local anaesthetic. Likewise, 1 mL of 2 per cent contains 20 mg.

DIFFERENT TYPES

Ester class

Only cocaine still in frequent use for topical anaesthesia.

Amide class

- Lidocaine (formerly called lignocaine): **short acting**, usually available as 0.5 per cent, 1 per cent and 2 per cent solutions
- Prilocaine: highest therapeutic index, safest **agent for intravenous blockade**.
- Bupivacaine: **longer acting** than lidocaine. Often used in epidurals. Levo-bupivacaine now used extensively for local infiltration to minimize wound pain postoperatively.

Local anaesthetic	Maximum dose (mg/kg) without adrenaline	Maximum dose (mg/kg) with adrenaline	Common uses
Lidocaine	3	5 (infiltration)	Local infiltration Short-acting nerve blocks Epidural top-ups
Bupivacaine (Marcain)	2	3 (do not use adrenaline in spinals or epidurals!)	Local infiltration (either alone or in combination with lidocaine) Epidurals Spinals
Prilocaine	6	6	Regional nerve blocks Bier's block

> ↑ **Key learning point**
>
> *Complications*
>
> Rather than remembering a long list, the complications of local anaesthetics are all related to their **membrane-stabilizing** characteristics. These effects are predominantly on the **CNS** and **cardiovascular system**:
>
> | CNS | Cardiovascular system |
> |-----|------------------------|
> | Fitting | Hypotension |
> | Coma: leading to death (hypoxia) | Cardiac arrhythmias |
> | | Acute cardiovascular collapse |

ROUTES OF ADMINISTRATION

- Local infiltration
- 'Field blocks' and **nerve blocks** (e.g. femoral nerve block for neck of femur fracture analgesia)
- Spinal anaesthesia: 'one-off', medium to short acting
- Epidural anaesthesia: longer acting, indwelling catheter; more problems with potential infection
- Intravenous administration: most often used in a Bier's block for manipulation of a Colles' fracture. Note that resuscitation facilities must be available in case of cuff failure

> ↑ **Example viva question**
>
> *What is the mechanism of hypotension in epidural and spinal anaesthesia and what is the treatment?*
>
> The mechanism is **blockade of the sympathetic outflow** to the vasculature and treatment is **reduction of the epidural rate** if possible, **colloids** to increase blood volume and rarely **vasoconstrictors**, and potential complications.

CALCULATING THE MAXIMUM DOSE

Example

What are the maximum doses, with and without adrenaline (epinephrine), of 2 per cent lidocaine that can be given to a 70 kg man?

- Maximum dose:
  without = 3 mg/kg   with = 5 mg/kg

- For a 70 kg man:
  without $= 3 \times 70 = $ **210 mg**   with $= 5 \times 70 = $ **300 mg**
- As 1 mL of 2 per cent solution contains 20 mg, for a 70 kg man:
  without $= 210/20 = $ **10.5 mL**   with $= 300/20 = $ **15 mL**

LOCAL ANAESTHETICS AND INFECTION

Infection promotes an **acidic** environment in the tissues with a great deal of anaerobic metabolism. **Local anaesthetics penetrate** the cell membrane in an **uncharged form**. In such an **acidic environment** the molecules become **charged** and cannot therefore penetrate the membrane and exert their effect.

Local anaesthetic infiltration can also **spread cellulitis** in the tissues.

LOCAL ANAESTHETICS AND ADRENALINE

Adrenaline is a **vasoconstrictor**; when mixed with local anaesthetics it:

- **Increases the total dose** of anaesthetic possible because it **limits blood flow** though the tissue infiltrated, thus limiting clearance into the plasma.
- Local vasoconstriction can be useful surgically – **blanching of the skin** allows the surgeon to see exactly where the anaesthetic has infiltrated and it provides a **more bloodless surgical field**, particularly in **highly vascular tissue** such as the scalp.
- **It must not be used near end-arteries**, e.g. **digital blocks** and **penile surgery**.

↑ **Example viva question**

What is Marcain Heavy?

This is bupivacaine prepared in a **dextrose solution** to **increase its viscosity** and **weight**. It is used in **spinal anaesthesia** to keep the local anaesthetic localized around the spinal cord for longer.

Care must be taken with its use in this context because **patient positioning** is crucial. If the patient is **too flat**, a high concentration of bupivacaine can gravitate to the high cervical cord and brain stem, causing problems with **respiration** and maintenance of **blood pressure** ('a **total spinal**').

---

76 Operating theatre design and infection control

Possible viva questions related to this topic

→ How would you best design an operating theatre suite?
→ Also what are the features of an operating theatre that promote an aseptic environment?
→ What is the definition of asepsis?
→ What is aseptic technique?
→ What do you understand by the term 'laminar flow'?
→ Describe how you would 'scrub up'.
→ What antiseptics are commonly used to scrub up?
→ Describe clothing used in theatre to minimize infection risk to both surgeon and patient.
→ What patient factors can be involved in reducing risk of postoperative infection?

↑ Key learning point

Operating theatre design neatly leads on to infection control in a viva situation and allows you to show your knowledge of ideal theatre geography and the various mechanisms and procedures designed to control infection risk.

OPERATING THEATRE DESIGN

- **Theatres** should ideally be **situated away** from the ground floor and **main hospital 'traffic' including the main entrance**
- Theatres should be on the **same level as the ITU** (intensive therapy unit) and surgical ward
- There should be a **minimum distance** from the operating theatre to **A&E** and **radiology** (particularly CT, angiography suite and plain radiography)

- **Sterile services** within the unit
- **Anaesthetic rooms adjacent** to theatre
- **Adequate room** for **storage** and **staff recreation**
- **Minimization** of the number of **people** in theatre **reduces** the overall **bacterial load** in the theatre air
- **Theatres** should be **next to each other** to minimize movement of staff and equipment.

INFECTION CONTROL ZONES

- Outer zone: patient reception area
- Clean zone: between reception and theatre; no outside clothing
- Aseptic zone: within the theatre itself
- Dirty zone: disposal areas (sluice) and dirty corridors.

LAMINAR AIR FLOW AND POSITIVE PRESSURE SYSTEMS IN THEATRES

Airborne bacteria are thought to be a source of **postoperative wound infection** and sepsis, now proven in the case of orthopaedic prosthetic joint implants.

Positive pressure ventilation systems use filtered air that **enters via the ceiling** in theatre and **leaves via the door** flaps. There is a **higher pressure** in **clean/ultra-clean areas** and **lower** in **dirty areas**, encouraging the **flow of air** and therefore any potential airborne pathogens from **clean to dirty** areas.

In the case of positive pressure systems, the number of **complete air changes** per hour is a minimum of **20**, but routine checks of bioload are not required.

Laminar flow is an **upgraded version of positive pressure ventilation**, ensuring laminar or **non-turbulent flow of air** at approximately **300 air changes per hour**. The air is recirculated through a HEPA (high efficiency particulate air) filter.

Laminar flow has found particular favour in orthopaedics where the consequences of prosthetic joint infection are disastrous. Laminar flow has been shown to reduce the infection rate in orthopaedic theatres almost as much as getting the surgeons to wear air-tight 'space suits'.

ASEPSIS AND ASEPTIC TECHNIQUE

The term **'asepsis'** refers to methods that **prevent wound contamination** by ensuring that only **sterile objects** and fluids **come into contact**, and also by minimizing the risk of airborne contamination. This should not be confused with **'antisepsis'**, which is the **use of solutions for disinfection** (e.g. alcohol, chlorhexidine, iodine) but **does not** necessarily **imply sterility**.

Thus, when describing an operation, the phrase 'aseptic technique was used at all times' implies that the surgeon maintained strict asepsis towards the wound.

SCRUBBING UP

- **3- to 5-minute scrub at the beginning** of the operating list using sterile, single use sponges or polypropylene bristled brushes
- **Water** should run from '**clean to dirty**' and therefore from fingertips to elbows
- **Hands** should be **dried** using **single-use sterile towels**, again from 'clean to dirty'
- Too much **scrubbing causes skin abrasions** and results in **more bacteria** being brought to the skin surface
- After this, **effective handwashing between cases** should be all that is required.

SKIN ANTISEPTICS

- Chlorhexidine gluconate 4 per cent (**Hibiscrub**): broad spectrum and persists with a cumulative effect
- Povidone–iodine (**Betadine**): used if surgeon is allergic to chlorhexidine. Less prolonged effect than chlorhexidine.

CLOTHING IN THEATRE

- **Gowns**: woven cotton poor at preventing bacterial passage. Disposable, **non-woven PTFE** (polytetrafluoroethylene), **Goretex** or tightly woven **polycottons** are the **ideal.**
- **Masks**: **no evidence** to suggest that in standard abdominal procedures masks decrease the risk of postoperative infection. They continue to be worn to prevent risk of blood-borne viral transmission from the patient to the surgeon. If worn, they should be single use and made of synthetic fibres containing filters of polyester or polypropylene.
- **Eye protection**: as part of 'universal precautions', eye protection should be worn to protect the surgeon from blood-borne viruses.
- **Hair and beards** must be **covered at all times.**
- **Footwear**: **no obvious role** in the spread of infection; need to protect from sharps injury; boots in genitourinary surgery.
- **Gloves**: although improving, **20–30 per cent** of all surgical gloves have **imperceptible holes** in them by the **end of an operation**. Double gloving improves this but at the expense of 'feel' and dexterity. Gloves should be **single use** and **sterilized by irradiation.**

PATIENT FACTORS

- **Short preoperative stay** if possible to prevent nosocomial colonization
- Patient should be **shaved in theatre** and not on the ward because this increases the risk of infection
- **Ward blankets** and **clothing** should be **removed before entering theatre**.

PREPARING THE SKIN

- **Operation site** and surrounding area should be **cleaned** using a sponge or **swab impregnated with detergent**
- **Skin is then prepared** using an alcohol-based solution of chlorhexidine or povidone–iodine. This should **completely dry** for adequate antisepsis. Care with diathermy; alcohol should not be allowed to pool in the umbilicus or under the perineum (see 'Diathermy', Chapter 71, page 291)
- Skin should be prepared **from the cleanest area to the dirtiest area** as with all aspects of aseptic technique. Savlon (cetrimide and chlorhexidine) can be used in perineal or vaginal antisepsis.

77 Screening in surgery

Possible viva questions related to this topic

→ What do you understand by the term 'screening'?
→ What are the desirable features of a screening programme?
→ What characteristics should a screening test have?
→ What do you understand by the terms 'sensitivity' and 'specificity'?
→ What biases are associated with screening?
→ What are the potential advantages and disadvantages of screening for cancer?

↑ Example viva question

What is the definition of screening?

Screening is **population testing** of otherwise well and asymptomatic individuals in order to **identify** a **particular disease** or its pre-morbid state. This can be targeted at the **whole population** (breast cancer screening) or at **certain high-risk groups** (patients with Barrett's oesophagus for oesophageal carcinoma). Screening tests are **not** usually **diagnostic** and further investigations are required to establish the diagnosis.

DESIRABLE FEATURES OF A SCREENING PROGRAMME

Based on the guidelines of the **World Health Organization (WHO)**:

• The disease being screened for should be an **important health problem**
• **Natural history** of the disease must be understood

- There should be a **detectable early stage** to the disease
- **Treatment** at the **early stage** should be of **more benefit** than at a later stage
- There should be a **test available** for **detecting** the **early stage** of the disease. The test should be:
  - **sensitive** (detects most cases, few false negatives)
  - **specific** (few false positives)
  - **replicable**
  - **safe**
  - **acceptable** screening test with a **high compliance rate**
  - **inexpensive**
- **Intervals** for **repeating** the test should have been determined
- There should be **adequate healthcare provision** to manage the **extra clinical workload** brought about by the screening
- **Facilities** for treatment must be available
- **Benefit** of **reduced morbidity** and **mortality** by **detecting** the disease **earlier** in its course by screening.

↑ **Example viva question**

What do you understand by the terms 'sensitivity' and 'specificity'?

Sensitivity: the ability of the test to **detect** all the people who actually have the disease, i.e. **true positives**. A high sensitivity is required so that large numbers of people with the disease are not missed.

Specificity: the ability of the test to **exclude the disease** in those who actually do not have it, i.e. **few false positives**. A high specificity is required so as not to diagnose falsely or worry people who do not actually have the disease.

Biases associated with screening

Selection bias
Health-conscious individuals are likely to take part in screening programmes.

Length–time bias
Increased survival as a result of detection of slow-growing tumours with a better prognosis.

Lead-time bias
Malignant tumours are likely to be picked up at an earlier stage and therefore lead to increased survival time.

Diagnosis bias
This is the inclusion of individuals with pre-invasive conditions that would not have generally progressed to invasive disease.

EXAMPLES OF SCREENING IN SURGERY

Cancer screening

Advantages
- Improved prognosis
- Less radical treatment regimens for early stage of the disease
- Reassurance to patients without pathology.

Disadvantages
- Treatment may not always alter the outcome and therefore patient will suffer morbidity longer as a result of earlier diagnosis
- Screening test may be invasive and have associated complications
- False positives may lead to unnecessary treatment
- False negatives give false reassurance.

There are currently **two national screening programmes** available in the **NHS**.

Breast cancer

- Set up in **1988** following the **Forrest Report**
- All **50- to 70-year-old women** invited for **3-yearly cycle** of screening, although those with a strong family history are screened earlier
- Women aged over 70 no longer receive an invitation but may request screening
- **Mammography** is best screening tool available but detects only **95 per cent** of breast cancers
- **Two views: craniocaudal (CC)** and **oblique views** at each visit.
- Abnormal mammogram initiates patient recall to specialist units for further assessment and treatment
- **25 per cent** of breast cancers are **not palpable** clinically
- NHS breast-screening programme is thought to save at least **300 lives a year** and this is likely to rise to 1250 by 2010, with the continued expansion and uptake of the service. Overall breast cancer screening has been shown to **reduce the mortality rate by about 30 per cent** in women aged over 50. However, there is some debate about the effectiveness of the programme, with some of the decreased mortality attributed to increased health awareness and treatments such as Tamoxifen.

Cervical cancer

- Cervical smear tests begin 3 years after **commencement of sexual activity**
- False-negative rate **10 per cent**
- **Labour intensive**
- Compliance 80 per cent.

Colorectal cancer

Controversial; only in widespread use in the USA.

Main methods for screening are:

- **Digital rectal examination (DRE)**
- **Rigid sigmoidoscopy**
- **Faecal occult blood (FOB)-positive** patients undergo colonoscopy in the USA. There is a low compliance rate and it is a costly exercise
- **Serum tumour markers (CEA)**
- **Flexible sigmoidoscopy**
- **Colonoscopy**
- **Barium enema**.

Better to screen for **high-risk individuals** for developing colorectal cancer, e.g.

- Long-standing ulcerative colitis
- Familial adenomatous polyposis coli
- Peutz–Jeghers syndrome
- Ureterosigmoidostomy
- Strong family history of colorectal cancer.

Abdominal aortic aneurysm

Not yet in place as a national screening programme but should be.

The **Multicentre Aneurysm Screening Study (MASS)** showed reduced mortality from screening men over the age of 65 by a single abdominal ultrasound for abdominal aortic aneurysms. Shown also to be cost-effective and give a better quality of life. There was a high acceptance rate (80 per cent) in this study.

Prostate cancer

There is currently no national programme for screening for prostate cancer. There is no definitive treatment available and there is the debate of using **prostate-specific antigen** (PSA) as a screening tool (see 'Tumour markers', Chapter 63, page 252).

Stomach cancer

This is effectively performed in **Japan** with **endoscopic surveillance**.

Neonatal screening

In the form of **postnatal checks**, e.g. congenital dislocation of the hip, imperforate anus and sexual abnormalities.

78 Skin grafting and flap reconstruction

Possible viva questions related to this topic

→ What is a skin graft?
→ What are the differences between a split- and a full-thickness skin graft?
→ When would you use a skin graft?
→ From where would you harvest a skin graft?
→ Describe how you would harvest a split-skin graft.
→ Why do skin grafts fail?
→ What tissues do skin grafts not take on?
→ What is a flap?
→ How does a flap differ from a graft?
→ What are the principles of flap surgery?
→ How would you classify flaps?
→ How is the viability of a flap assessed?
→ What measures can be undertaken in the event of vascular compromise?
→ How is the donor site managed?
→ What complications need to be discussed with the patient before surgery?

Related topics

↑ Key learning points

Definitions

A **skin graft** is a piece of skin transferred **without a blood supply** from a donor site to reconstruct a defect

A **flap** is a volume of tissue transferred from a donor site to reconstruct a defect while maintaining its **own blood supply**

A **flap is dependent** on its **own blood supply**. A **graft** is entirely **dependent** on a vascular bed at the **recipient site** to establish a **new blood supply**

A **pedicle** is the attachment of a **flap** through which it receives its **blood supply**

SKIN GRAFTS

Types of skin grafts

Skin grafts can be split thickness, full thickness, dermal or composite; they can also be autografts, allografts or xenografts.

- Split thickness: epidermis and a thin layer of dermis
- Full thickness: epidermis and entire dermis
- Dermal: dermis only
- Composite: skin and an underlying structure (e.g. skin + cartilage from the ear).

Full thickness vs split thickness	
Graft type	**Advantages of each type**
Split thickness	• More likely to 'take' – can survive longer by imbibition
	• Less donor site scarring
	• Suitable for larger grafts
	• Can be meshed to cover a larger area
Full thickness	• Better skin colour match
	• Less contour defect
	• More durable
	• Less contracture of graft bed
	• Adnexal structures are maintained (hair follicles, sweat glands)

Stages of graft take

- **Adherence**: a fibrin bond is formed between the graft and the bed.
- **Imbibition**: intracellular proteoglycans within the graft break down into smaller, more osmotically active subunits. **Interstitial fluid is absorbed**, providing nutrition to the graft, but causing graft swelling.
- **Re-vascularization**: ingrowth of vascular tissue into the graft differentiates into afferent and efferent vessels, linking with graft vessels and restoring circulation. Thicker grafts take longer to re-vascularize.
- **Maturation**: regeneration of appendages (hair follicles and sweat glands). Re-innervation from graft edges.

Failure to take

Acute graft failure can occur as a result of the patient, the graft bed or the graft. Although many factors can affect graft take, the three main causes for failure are indicated in bold below:

- **Shearing forces between graft and bed** (disrupts re-vascularization)
- **Graft separated from bed** by seroma or haematoma
- **Infection** (especially beta-haemolytic streptococci)

- Unsuitable or avascular graft bed (poorly perfused tissues, exposed tendon, cartilage, bone)
- Poor healing
- Poor graft handling
- Graft laid incorrectly.

Skin grafting technique

Graft type	Common donor sites
Split-thickness skin graft	• Thigh • Abdomen • Buttock • Back • Palm
Full-thickness skin graft	• Groin crease • Base of neck • Pre-auricular • Post-auricular • Upper arm • Upper eyelid

Split-thickness skin grafts are harvested with a **dermatome**, slicing a predetermined thickness of skin from the donor site. This can be either a hand-held guarded knife (e.g. **Watson knife**) or an air-powered dermatome (e.g. **Zimmer air dermatome**). During graft harvest, the donor site is thoroughly **lubricated** with paraffin. An assistant ensures that the site is **flat** by supporting the surrounding tissues and stretching the area with a flat edge (e.g. a wooden board). The graft is harvested with the dermatome and laid onto a flat board, and covered with a saline-soaked swab until ready for use. The graft can be **fenestrated**, reducing the risk of fluid accumulating under the graft, or **meshed**, allowing the graft to cover a **larger area**. Common mesh sizes are **1:1.5** and **1:3**.

Full-thickness grafts are **excised** with a scalpel as an ellipse of skin, which is **closed directly**. Any beads of **subcutaneous fat** are **excised** from the underside of the graft and it is stored in a saline-soaked swab until ready for use. Full-thickness grafts can also be **fenestrated**.

To minimize the chances of graft failure, **haemostasis** is achieved at the recipient site to avoid development of a haematoma under the graft. The graft is laid onto the bed, **dermal (shiny) side down**, and secured with a **pressure dressing**, reducing shearing between the graft and the bed, and further reducing the likelihood of haematoma or seroma under the graft.

Complications of skin grafts

- Partial or total graft failure
- Infection
- Bleeding
- Donor site pain and morbidity
- Need for further surgery.

FLAPS

Classification

Flaps can be classified in terms of the type of tissue transferred, the nature of the vascular patterns of the tissues and the proximity to the defect requiring reconstruction.

Type of tissue
- Skin
- Fascia
- Fasciocutaneous
- Muscle
- Myocutaneous
- Bone/Osseocutaneous/Osseomyocutaneous
- Visceral (e.g. colon, small intestine, omentum)
- Innervated muscle flaps.

Vascular patterns
- Random pattern
- Axial pattern.

Random pattern flaps have no dominant blood supply. They rely on many unnamed small vessels to provide a blood supply via the base of the flap. This limits the length:breadth ratio to 1:1. Axial pattern flaps rely on a blood supply from a single vessel or a group of recognized vessels, allowing flaps to be raised that are as long as the vascular territory of their axial vessels.

Proximity to defect
- Local
- Distant
- Free.

A local flap is immediately adjacent to the defect and is transposed, advanced or rotated into place. A distant flap remains attached to the body at the pedicle and can be moved over a greater distance. A free flap is completely detached from the body and regains a blood supply by microsurgical anastomosis of the vessels within the pedicle to recipient vessels near the defect.

Flap failure and monitoring

Clinical evaluation is the best method of flap assessment:

- Flap **colour** (relative to skin adjacent to the **donor site**)
- **Capillary refill** time
- Skin **turgor**
- Skin **temperature**
- Bleeding after a **pinprick** or **scratch** test (avoid the pedicle)
- Hand-held **Doppler** ultrasonography
- Pulse oximetry
- Adhesive skin temperature probes.

Insufficient arterial supply – clinical signs

- **Pallor**
- Skin **coolness**
- **Slow** capillary refill > 2 seconds
- Slow or **absent bleeding** on pinprick test
- No palpable pulse.

Insufficient venous outflow – clinical signs

- Blue to purple **dusky** hue
- **Brisk** capillary refill < 1 second
- Brisk **dark blood** on pinprick test
- **Tense**, swollen flap.

Factors leading to vascular compromise

- Tight dressings: **loosen** any tight **dressings**
- Tight sutures: **release** alternate/all **sutures** as necessary
- Pressure on the flap or pedicle from positioning: **reposition the patient** away from the flap
- **Haematoma** impeding vascular in-/outflow: immediately **release sutures** and return to theatre to **evacuate the haematoma**
- **Vasoconstriction:** avoid:
  - dehydration – **urine output** < 1 mL/kg per h
  - cold – ensure room is **warmed**
  - nicotine
  - caffeine
  - pain – adequate **analgesia**
- Kinking of, or clot within, the flap pedicle: urgent **return to theatre** and consider the use of local thrombolysis, dextran, heparin or aspirin.

Urgent re-exploration is **essential** if these fail to provide a **rapid** improvement.

Complications of flap surgery

- Partial or total flap failure
- Infection
- Bleeding and blood transfusion
- Anticoagulation requirements
- Donor site morbidity
- Need for re-exploration
- Reoperation for flap adjustment
- Anaesthetic complications of major surgery, including death.

79 Statistics and clinical trials

Possible viva questions related to this topic

→ What types of clinical trial do you know?
→ What is meant by the power of a trial?
→ Define type I and type II statistical error.
→ What is meant by the sensitivity and specificity of a clinical test?
→ Which type of clinical trial has the most statistical power and why?
→ What is an odds ratio?
→ What is a 95 per cent confidence interval?
→ What is the difference between parametric and non-parametric statistics?
→ What is a meta-analysis and what is its purpose?

CLINICAL TRIAL TYPES

Clinical trials can be **prospective** or **retrospective** with the **latter** having a **higher statistical power** than the former.

Observational cohort study

• Usually retrospective but can be prospective
• Observational investigation where a group of individuals with a specific disease or characteristic are followed over a period of time to detect complications or new events
• Comparisons may be made with a control group
• No interventions are normally applied to the participants.

Case–control study

• Usually retrospective but can be prospective
• Observational investigation in which characteristics of people with a condition (cases) are compared with a selection of the population without the disease (controls).

Cross-sectional study

• Usually retrospective
• A survey of the frequency of a disease or risk factor in a defined population at a given time

- Used to assess prevalence
- Cannot evaluate statistical hypotheses but can suggest statistical associations and generate hypotheses.

Controlled trial

- Intervention under investigation is applied to one set of individuals
- Outcome compared with a similar group (the control group) not receiving that particular treatment
- In drug trials the control group usually has a placebo, eliminating placebo effect in the intervention group.

Randomized trial

- Participants are placed in a particular arm of the investigation in a random way, rather than via the conscious choice of the investigator or participant
- Eliminates selection bias
- Ensures that confounding factors are spread evenly throughout the trial groups.

Blinded (or masked) trial

- Either investigators or patient is unaware of treatment group to which the participant has been assigned
- Eliminates assessment bias.

Double-blinded (double-masked) trial

- Both investigators and patient are unaware of treatment group to which the patient has been assigned
- Eliminates both assessor and patient bias.

↑ **Example viva question**

Which type of clinical trial has the most statistical power and why?

A **double-blind randomized placebo-controlled trial** has the most statistical power by eliminating as much bias as possible and spreading confounding factors evenly between the different trial arms. It ensures that statistical samples come from truly random dataset, allowing the use of more powerful statistics that make assumptions about randomization and population distributions (see later).

STATISTICAL POWER AND *P* VALUES

Statistical power is defined as the **ability of a study** to demonstrate **an association or causal relationship** between **two variables**, given that an **association actually exists**. For example: **90 per cent power** in a clinical trial means that the study has a **90 per cent chance** of ending up with a *p* **value** < 0.05 in a **statistical test** if there really is an important difference (e.g. 30 per cent versus 15 per cent mortality rate) between treatment groups.

The *p* values

The probability (ranging from 0 to 1) that the results observed in a study (or more extreme results) could have occurred by chance.

Convention dictates that we take a *p* **value** < 0.05 to indicate statistical significance. It is worth bearing in mind that this could still mean that there is a **1 in 20 chance** that a 'statistically significant' result could have **occurred by chance!**

The meta-analysis

Although not strictly a clinical trial, this is a study that attempts systematically to merge the results from many clinical trials that are trying to answer the same clinical question, in an attempt to **increase the statistical power** through an increase in the overall number of cases.

STATISTICAL ERROR

Broadly statistical error can be divided into two: type I and type II errors.

Type I error

A true null hypothesis is incorrectly rejected (i.e. although there is no difference between two groups, chance has shown there to be a statistical difference and the null hypothesis is incorrectly rejected).

Type II error

Rejection of the alternative hypothesis when it is true (i.e. although there is a difference between two groups, it is determined that there is no difference).

The 95 per cent confidence intervals

This quantifies the **uncertainty in measurement** of a value. A 95 per cent confidence interval (CI) gives a range in which there is a 95 per cent confidence that the unknown value will lie within that range. Usually expressed as 95 per cent CI in clinical journals and gives much more information than a simple *p* value. Many high-impact factor journals now insist on the quotation of 95 per cent CIs.

↑ Example viva question

What is meant by the sensitivity and specificity of a clinical test?

Sensitivity: the sensitivity of a test is the **proportion of people with the disease** who have a **positive test result** (the higher the sensitivity, the greater the detection rate and the lower the false-negative rate)

Specificity: the specificity of the test is the **proportion of people without the disease** who have a **negative test** (the higher the specificity, the lower will be the false-positive rate)

Predictive value
- The **positive** predictive value of a test is the **probability of a patient with a positive test** actually **having a disease**
- The **negative** predictive value is the **probability of a patient with a negative test not having** the **disease**

A confidence interval that **includes 0** implies that the treatment effect is **not statistically significant**.

Odds ratios in clinical trials

The ratio of the odds of having the target disorder in the experimental group relative to the odds in favour of having the target disorder in the control group.

An odds ratio is calculated by dividing the odds in the treated or exposed group by the odds in the control group.

Parametric and non-parametric statistics

For **parametric statistics** to be valid, they make an assumption that the groups being compared are **randomly sampled** and **conform to a normal distribution**. Typical examples of parametric statistics are Student t-tests and χ^2 (chi-squared) tests.

For **non-parametric statistics** to be valid, they make an assumption that the groups being compared are **randomly sampled,** but they make **no assumptions** about the distributions that they follow. Non-parametric statistics are **not as statistically powerful** as parametric statistics but are useful in circumstances where populations **do not conform** to the **normal distribution**.

80 Stomas

Possible viva questions related to this topic

→ What are the indications for forming a stoma?
→ What are the uses of a stoma?
→ How would you classify them further?
→ How would you prepare a patient who is going for surgery that will involve formation of a stoma?
→ What are the principles of siting a stoma?
→ What are the potential complications of a stoma?
→ What are the differences between an ileostomy and a colostomy?
→ Why are ileotomies fashioned with a spout?
→ How would you rehabilitate a patient following creation of a stoma?
→ What is a mucous fistula?

DEFINITION

A stoma is an **artificial opening** brought up on to the **body surface**.

INDICATIONS

- **Decompression**, e.g. caecostomy
- **Exteriorization/drainage**:
  - perforated or contaminated bowel, e.g. distal abscesses/fistula
  - permanent stoma, e.g. abdominal perineal excision of rectum (APER)
- **Enteral feeding**, e.g. percutaneous endoscopic gastrostomy (PEG) after gastrointestinal (GI) surgery, in CNS disease or in coma
- **Faecal stream diversion**:
  - protect a distal anastomosis: previously contaminated bowel; technical considerations – low anterior resection or ileorectal anastomosis
  - urinary diversion after a cystectomy

- **Diversion**, e.g. pharyngostomy or oesophagostomy: to divert solids and liquids in order to protect the bronchial tree in neonates with oesophageal atresia or tracheo-oesophageal fistula
- **Lavage**: appendicostomy for large bowel washout.

CLASSIFICATION

Temporary

PEG tube, pharyngostomy, oesophagostomy, caecostomy, loop ileostomy or transverse colostomy.

Permanent

End-colostomy after an abdominoperineal resection (APER), or end-ileostomy after a panproctocolectomy.

PREOPERATIVE PREPARATION

- Psychosocial and physical preparation
- Informed consent with risk and benefits explained
- Use of a clinical nurse specialist in stoma care – who would also mark the site.

STOMA SITE

Generally:

- 5 cm away from umbilicus (not for PEG)
- Away from scars or skin creases
- Away from bony prominences or waistline of clothes
- Site that is easily accessible to the patient – not under a large fold of fat!
- Stoma must be within the rectus abdominis, otherwise parastomal herniation will occur and obstruction and pain will ensue (not for PEG)
- Need to consider patient's mobility and eyesight.

COMPLICATIONS

- **General** versus **specific**
- **Technical** versus **general** versus **practical**
- **Immediate** (< 24 hours), **early** (< 1 month) or **late** (> 1 month).

General

This is related to the underlying disease:

- **Stoma diarrhoea**: water and electrolyte imbalance, hypokalaemia
- **Nutritional disorders**: vitamin B deficiency, chronic microcytic/normochromic anaemia

- **Stones**: both gallstones and renal stones are more common after an ileostomy
- **Psychosexual**
- **Residual disease**, e.g. Crohn's disease and parastomal fistula, metastases.

Specific

- Ischaemia and gangrene
- Haemorrhage
- Retraction
- Prolapse/intussusception
- Parastomal hernia
- Stenosis – leads to constipation
- Skin excoriation.

PRACTICAL PROBLEMS:

- **Odour**: advice on hygiene, diet and deodorant sprays
- **Flatus**: improved with diet and special filters
- **Skin problems**
- **Leakage**: especially transverse loop colostomies.

↑ **Example viva question**

What are the differences between an ileostomy and a colostomy?

	Ileostomy	Colostomy
Site	Right iliac fossa (RIF)	Left iliac fossa (LIF)
Surface	Spout (prevents irritation of underlying skin)	No spout Flush with skin
Contents	Watery – small bowel	Faeculent
Effluent	Continuous	Intermittent
Permanent	Panproctocolectomy	APER
Temporary	Loop ileostomy after low anterior resection	Hartmann's procedure

---

MUCOUS FISTULA

Used in similar circumstances to Hartmann's procedure but, instead of dropping the rectal stump back into the abdomen, it is brought out as a **separate** stoma, which being an **efferent limb** produces only **mucus**. This makes the distal limb more accessible when the bowel is later rejoined. Also performed in **inflammatory bowel surgery** because of fear of **rectal stump blow-out**.

REHABILITATION

- **Diet** should be **normal**
- Bag should be changed once or twice a day (needs to be emptied more frequently if urine or watery small bowel contents)
- **Ileotomies** should have a **base plate** under the bag changed every 5 days and the bag changed daily
- **Psychological** and **psychosexual** support.

81 Surgical sutures and needles

Possible viva questions related to this topic

→ What criteria would the ideal suture fulfil?
→ How do the characteristics of a suture material affect its behaviour?
→ What are the characteristics of natural versus synthetic suture materials?
→ What are the differences between monofilament and multifilament sutures?
→ How would you classify sutures? Give examples of commonly used sutures.
→ Name some examples of absorbable and non-absorbable sutures. Describe some features of one of each.
→ What suture-related factors may lead to wound dehiscence?
→ When might you use clips instead of sutures?
→ Describe the type of needles in common surgical use and their characteristics.
→ What are the various parts of a needle called?

CRITERIA OF AN IDEAL SUTURE

- Ease of handling
- Ease of knotting
- Knot securely without fraying
- Minimal tissue reaction
- Maintain tensile strength until it has served its purpose
- Provides effective duration of wound support appropriate to the tissue and operation in question
- Narrow diameter to minimize tissue damage and scarring
- Unfavourable suture surface for bacterial colonization
- Inexpensive
- Easily sterilized
- Not electrolytic, carcinogenic or allogeneic and does not demonstrate capillary action.

Related topics

CLASSIFICATION

- Source: **natural** or **synthetic**
- Filament type: **braided** versus **monofilament**
- Absorbability.

Natural sutures

- Handle well and relatively inexpensive
- Unpredictable absorption
- Can incite tissue reaction and fibrosis
- Absorbed by enzymatic action. They can trap bacteria and set up a localized infection because they are not monofilament. This can lead to wound sinus formation.

Synthetic sutures

- Inert; absorbed by hydrolysis
- Predictable absorption and strength
- More difficult to handle.

Braided sutures

- Easier to handle and to perform knot tying
- Can create friction, more difficult to pass through tissue than monofilament, so therefore more likely to incite more tissue reaction
- Infection can sit within the braids.

Monofilament sutures

- Glides more smoothly through the tissues and incites less tissue reaction
- More difficult to knot and handle than braided materials.

↑ Example viva question

Give examples

Suture	Type	Description
Polyglactin (Vicryl)	Synthetic Braided Absorbable	Gives wound support for 30 days. Vicryl Rapide more rapidly degraded with wound support for 10 days
Polydioxanone (PDS)	Synthetic Monofilament Absorbable	Slowly hydrolysed (180 days). Good tensile strength for 56 days. Alternative to nylon for abdominal closure
Catgut	Natural Absorbable	Rapidly hydrolysed 7–10 days wound support. Rarely used today
Silk	Natural Braided Non-absorbable	Evokes marked tissue reaction. Encourages formation of suture sinuses and abscesses. Avoid in vascular anastomoses and skin closure
Polypropylene (Prolene)	Synthetic Monofilament Non-absorbable	Slides well – good for vascular anastomoses, memory (difficult to handle and knot)
Nylon (Ethilon)	Synthetic Monofilament Non-absorbable	Loses 10–20 per cent tensile strength per year. Similar characteristics to Prolene but less memory

FACTORS INVOLVING THE SUTURE THAT CAN LEAD TO WOUND DEHISCENCE

- Weak suture material or inappropriate choice
- Damage to suture by a surgical instrument
- Diathermy damage to the suture
- Poor surgical technique in knotting
- Wound under high tension that can lead to necrosis.

USE OF STAPLES

Staples confer **only speed** of application in wound closure. They are useful when rapid wound closure is desirable or when the **wound is large** and suture closure would be laborious. Also, if there is a **high chance** of **infection**, it may be easier to remove staples rather than sutures to open up the wound.

TYPES OF SUTURE NEEDLES

Various parts are:

- Point
- Body
- Swage – for attachment to the suture.

Characteristics

Type of needle governed by the **procedure, tissue, access, gauge of the suture** and **surgeon's preference**. The **body** of the needle can be:

- **Straight:** used to suture skin wounds which are easily accessible; used by hand.
- **Curved:** ranging from 0.5 to 0.75 of the circumference; usually manipulated with needle holder.
- **Rounded**: separates but does not cut tissue; this creates a watertight suture line.
- **J-shaped**: used to approximate two tissues that are typically difficult to access within a surgical wound, e.g. closure of umbilical port site after laparoscopy.

- **Round-bodied needle**: this causes minimal tissue trauma so it is suitable for fragile or delicate tissue, e.g. bowel anastomosis.
- **Conventional cutting needle**: triangular in cross-section with the cutting edge on the concave side of the needle.

- **Reverse cutting needle**: for tough tissue; triangular cross-section with the cutting edge on the convex side of the needle. This strengthens the needle and, with the sharp edge on the outside of the curvature, protects tissue on the inside.
- **Atraumatic or blunt needle**: used for friable tissue, e.g. liver, spleen, kidney, minimizing tissue trauma. This reduces the chance of an operative needle-stick injury.
- **Taper cut needle**: provides effective initial tissue penetration.

82 Tourniquets

Possible viva questions related to this topic

→ When would you use a tourniquet in surgery?
→ What are the contraindications for using a tourniquet?
→ What are the potential problems associated with tourniquet use? How would you avoid them?
→ What are the complications of tourniquet use?
→ What size of tourniquet should you use and to what pressure should the tourniquet be inflated?
→ For how long should you leave a tourniquet on?
→ Describe the procedure for application and removal of a tourniquet. Will you ignore your anaesthetist when removing the tourniquet?

Related topics		
Topic	**Chapter**	**Page**
Carpal tunnel decompression	28	87
Compartment syndrome	108	433
Long saphenous varicose vein surgery	35	117

INDICATIONS FOR TOURNIQUET USE IN SURGERY

• To produce an effective **bloodless surgical field**; this facilitates the surgical procedure and allows demonstration of important structures, e.g. median nerve during carpal tunnel decompression
• To allow **effective regional anaesthesia**, e.g. during a Bier's block, which requires a double tourniquet
• To provide **temporary haemostasis** in the face of catastrophic and uncontrollable blood loss when local pressure has failed
• **Tourniquet test**: to look for **venous incompetence** in the lower limb.

CONTRAINDICATIONS

All are **relative** contraindications:

• Crush injury
• Peripheral vascular disease

- Pro-thrombotic states
- Sickle cell disease and trait
- Also generally avoid in elderly patients.

TOURNIQUET SIZE AND INFLATION PRESSURES

The size of tourniquet can be estimated by the **cuff width** approximating the **diameter** of the **limb plus 20 per cent.**

A **lower pressure** is required to occlude the arterial circulation when using a **wider** tourniquet.

There is **no consensus** regarding what pressure the tourniquet should be inflated to, but ideally **as low a pressure** as will provide arterial and venous occlusion. A common recommendation is:

- **Upper limb**: 50 mmHg above normal systolic blood pressure
- **Lower limb**: 100 mmHg above normal systolic blood pressure.

SAFE TOURNIQUET ISCHAEMIC TIMES

There is no consensus on this subject either.

This needs to be considered **in relation** to the patient's other **co-morbidities** and problems. A long ischaemic time will not be safe for patients with known relative ischaemia or injury.

Correct answer is as **short as possible!**

Ideally **90 minutes** should not be exceeded.

Ischaemia time should not exceed **120 minutes** without a **20-minute reperfusion time.**

PRECAUTIONS WHEN USING A TOURNIQUET

- See above
- **Neurovascular status** should be documented before tourniquet application and after removal
- Check **monitor** and **cuff** before applying to patient
- A **well-covered area** of the limb should be chosen – **avoid joints** for tourniquet application; also avoid encroachment on surgical field
- The limb should be **well padded** with wool
- The tourniquet should have a width of at **least half** the **limb circumference**
- **Limb exsanguination** should be performed ideally with an **Esmarch bandage** or **rubber Rhys–Davies exsanguinator**. This process can also be done by **limb**

elevation for **2 minutes**. **Avoid** expressive exsanguination in the presence of **tumour, infection** or known **DVT**

- Note **time of inflation** and the **surgeon** should be **informed** every **30 minutes** of ischaemic time; note the time of deflation.

Always request the **anaesthetist's** permission to **deflate** and **remove** the tourniquet. During prolonged ischaemia, products of **anaerobic metabolism** accumulate in the limb and are effectively excluded from the general circulation. When the tourniquet is released, there is not only a release of an **acidotic blood load** but also a general **decrease** in **cardiac afterload**. In a patient with a **limited cardiac reserve** and function this can **precipitate cardiac arrhythmias** and **ischaemia**.

COMPLICATIONS

Immediate

- **Post-deflation bleeding**: tourniquet deflation and meticulous haemostasis before wound closure is one way of dealing with postoperative bleeding and haematoma formation
- **Cardiovascular collapse** post-deflation: caused by afterload or reperfusion injury
- **Muscle damage**: rhabdomyolysis
- **Skin necrosis**
- **Arterial damage**: vascular endothelial injury and thrombosis (rare).

Early

- **Venous congestion**: caused by inadequate pressure
- **Pressure neuropathy**: not caused by ischaemia
- **Pulmonary embolism** (rare).

Late

- **Post-tourniquet palsy**.

83 Wound healing, scarring and reconstruction

Possible viva questions related to this topic

→ How do wounds heal?
→ What factors influence the quality of a scar?
→ What are hypertrophic scars?
→ What is the difference between a hypertrophic and a keloid scar?
→ What is the reconstructive ladder?
→ How would you determine which reconstructive technique to consider?

NORMAL WOUND HEALING

There are **three phases** of normal wound healing.

Inflammatory phase (days 0–4)

- **Injury** causes local **bleeding**
- **Haemorrhage** is limited by **vasoconstriction**, mediated by adrenaline, thromboxane A_2 and prostaglandin 2α
- **Collagen**, exposed by the injury and subsequent retraction of endothelial cells, activates the **clotting cascade** and allows platelets to attach, forming a **platelet plug**
- Platelets release platelet-derived growth factor (PDGF), fibronectin, fibrinogen and von Willebrand's factor, **stabilizing the wound** through **clot formation**
- **Capillary vasodilatation** occurs as a result of release of histamine, bradykinin, prostaglandins and nitric oxide, allowing **inflammatory cells** to reach the wound site
- **Neutrophils** scavenge for debris, **débriding the wound**, and help to **kill bacteria** by oxidative burst mechanisms and opsonization; the neutrophil peak occurs at **24 hours** after injury

- **Monocytes** enter the wound and become **macrophages**, which secrete numerous enzymes and cytokines, including collagenases and elastases, to break down injured tissues; and PDGF, macrophage-derived growth factors, interleukins, tumour necrosis factor (TNF) and transforming growth factor β (TGF-β) to **stimulate proliferation of fibroblasts, endothelial and smooth muscle cells**
- **Lymphocytes** also enter the wound at day 3 and have a role in **cellular immunity and antibody production**.

Proliferative phase (days 4–21)

- **Angiogenesis**, stimulated by TNF-α, is the migration of endothelial cells to form **new capillaries** within the wound bed
- **Type III collagen** is laid down by **fibroblasts**, attracted and activated by TGF-β and PDGF. **Total collagen** content **increases until day 21**
- The combination of **collagen deposition** and **angiogenesis** forms **granulation tissue**
- **Epithelialization** occurs by one of two mechanisms, depending on whether the **basement membrane** has been breached. If the basement membrane is **intact**, epithelial cells migrate upwards in the normal pattern, resulting in epithelialization in **2–3 days**. In a deeper wound, a **single layer** of epithelial cells **advances** from the **wound edges** to cover the wound, which then stratifies when cover is complete. **Adnexal structures** such as hair follicles and sweat glands can also provide a source of cells for epithelialization.

Remodelling phase (days 21–360)

- During remodelling, collagen is **reorganized**; collagenases continue to break down existing collagen while **fibroblasts** and **myofibroblasts** continue to synthesize new collagen along lines of tension
- **Type III** collagen is replaced with **type I** collagen
- Water is removed from the scar, allowing collagen to **cross-link**
- Wound **vascularity decreases**
- Collagen cross-linkage allows **increased scar strength**, scar **contracture** and a decreased scar thickness.

WOUND STRENGTH

Wounds have **little strength** during the **inflammatory** and **proliferative** phases of wound healing. As **remodelling** occurs, wounds rapidly **gain strength**. At **6 weeks**, the wound is at **50 per cent** of its final strength. **Maximum strength**, which is only **75 per cent** of the pre-injury tissue strength, is achieved between **6 and 12 months** after the injury.

ABNORMAL SCARRING

Hypertrophic scars

- Raised, red, thickened scar
- **Limited** to the **boundaries** of the original scar
- Occurs **soon** after injury
- Related to wound tension and prolonged inflammatory phase of healing
- Common in wounds on the **anterior chest** and over **shoulders**
- **Spontaneous regression** over years.

Keloid scars

- Raised, red, thickened scar
- **Extends beyond** the original scar **boundary**
- Occurs **months after injury**
- **No regression**
- More common in **dark skin** colour
- Significant **familial** tendency
- **Autoimmune** phenomenon
- Worsens in **pregnancy**, resolves after menopause
- Worsened by **surgery**.

FACTORS INFLUENCING SCARRING

Patient factors

- Age: **infants** and **elderly people** scar well
- Skin type: **Celtic** skin types are more likely to form **hypertrophic** scars; **dark-skinned** patients are more likely to form **keloid** scars
- Anatomical region: anterior midline, **chest** and **shoulders** scar poorly
- Concurrent morbidity: **nutritional state, diabetes,** wound **infection**
- Local tissue: **oedema,** previous **radiotherapy, vascular insufficiency.**

Surgical factors

- **Atraumatic** skin handling
- **Eversion** of wound edges: inversion places keratinised epidermis (dead material) between healing surfaces
- **Tension-free** skin closure
- Clean, **healthy** wound **edges**
- Scar **orientation**: parallel to lines of relaxed skin tension
- Suture **tension**: over-tightening leads to pressure necrosis; under-tensioning can lead to wound gaping and widening of scar

- Scar length: **skin ellipse length** should be at least **four times the width** to minimize tension and avoid dog-ears
- Suture type: non-absorbable **synthetic sutures** cause least inflammation
- Timing of **suture removal**:
  - 7 days or less leaves no stitch marks
  - 14 days or more leaves stitch marks
  - between these times depends on skin type and wound location.

THE RECONSTRUCTIVE LADDER

Closing wounds and repairing defects are fundamental surgical skills. There are **many techniques** available for reconstruction and the **reconstructive ladder** is a useful **systematic approach** to the process of reconstructing a defect. As the ladder is descended, surgery becomes more complex and **risk to the patient increases**. This approach of considering **simple techniques before complex techniques**, allows defects to be reconstructed with the least risk to patients (see 'Skin grafting and flap reconstruction', Chapter 78, page 320):

- Allow to heal
- Primary closure
- Delayed primary closure
- Tissue expansion
- Split-thickness skin graft
- Full-thickness skin graft
- Local flap (a flap raised immediately next to the defect)
- Distant flap (a flap raised some distance from the defect, maintaining a vascular supply through a pedicle)
- Free flap (a flap completely detached from the body and re-anastomosed to vessels close to the defect).

APPLIED SURGICAL PHYSIOLOGY

84 Acid–base balance

Related Topics		
Topic	**Chapter**	**Page**
Respiratory failure and respiratory function tests	119	495
Altitude	86	356
Functions of the kidney I–IV	92–95	376–383
Criteria for admission to ITU and HDU	109	439

Key definitions

An **acidosis (or acidaemia)** is an excess of H^+ ions in the blood (buffered or otherwise).

An **alkalosis (alkalaemia)** is a deficiency of H^+ ions in the blood (buffered or otherwise).

Normal range of pH is 7.35–7.45.

Base excess (normal value 0) measures how far removed bicarbonate is from its normal value.

A **buffer** is a weak acid, the presence of which prevents large fluctuations in the concentration of H^+. This text deals mainly with the **bicarbonate/carbonic acid** system, but, in the urine, **phosphate** buffers H^+ ions.

Buffering in the blood

A small proportion of H^+ is buffered by **haemoglobin** and the **plasma proteins**, but the majority is buffered by the **bicarbonate/carbonic acid** system.

$$H_2O + CO_2 \rightleftharpoons H_2CO_3 \rightleftharpoons H^+ + HCO_3^-$$

CO_2 acts as an **acid**, because it pushes the equilibrium to the right and produces more H^+.

HCO_3^- acts as a **base**, because it pushes the equilibrium to the left and eliminates H^+.

The equilibrium between bicarbonate and carbonic acid and the H^+ concentration is referred to by the Henderson–Hasselbalch equilibrium:

$$pH = pK + \log[HCO_3^-]/[H_2CO_3]$$

where K = dissociation coefficient of carbonic acid.

The **kidney** is responsible for HCO_3^- homoeostasis (see 'Functions of the kidney II', Chapter 93, page 377) and the **lungs** control CO_2, enabling the pH to be tightly controlled (discussed below).

Diagnosing blood gases: an algorithm

Step 1: what is the pH?

If < 7.35, it is an **acidosis**.

If > 7.45, it is an **alkalosis**.

Step 2: what is the cause of this?

Acidoses
- If $P_{CO_2} > 5.3\,kPa$, **respiratory acidosis** (high P_{CO_2}; retained CO_2, which is an acid)
- If $HCO_3^- < 24\,mmol/L$, **metabolic acidosis** (high H^+, low HCO_3^-) (see above; equilibrium pushed to left)

Alkaloses
- If $P_{CO_2} < 4.8\,kPa$, **respiratory alkalosis** (low P_{CO_2}, CO_2 being lost)
- If $HCO_3^- > 28$, **metabolic alkalosis** (low H^+, therefore high HCO_3^-) (equilibrium to right).

Can use **base excess** quickly to diagnose **metabolic** alkalosis or acidosis in the clinical setting (negative in acidosis, positive in alkalosis).

Note that the base excess is positive in a respiratory acidosis by the Henderson–Hasselbalch equation. It refers to the amount of acid that should be added to the solution to make it neutral.

Step 3: compensation?

This is more difficult. Respiratory causes are always compensated for by metabolic change and metabolic causes are always compensated for by respiratory change.

In vivo, **respiratory compensation** is **fast** (breathe faster to eliminate CO_2 [acid] or slower to retain it) and **metabolic compensation** is **slow** (kidney buffers and excretes or retains HCO_3^- [base]).

Compensated respiratory acidosis
HCO_3^- rises to try to correct high PCO_2.

Compensated metabolic acidosis
PCO_2 drops to try to correct high H^+.

Compensated metabolic alkalosis
PCO_2 rises to try to correct high HCO_3^-.

Compensated respiratory alkalosis
HCO_3^- drops (eliminated by kidney) to try to correct low CO_2 (acid) and hence low H^+.

Separate to acid–base analysis, but relevant to blood gases, is the assessment of the patient's **oxygenation**, which involves looking only at the PO_2 and PCO_2.

If the PO_2 is **< 8 kPa**, the patient has respiratory failure.

Assuming respiratory failure, if the PCO_2 is < 6.7 kPa, this is called type 1 respiratory failure; if it is above this figure it is called type 2 respiratory failure.

Of course, these figures depend on the concentration of inspired oxygen – FIO_2 – in ventilated patients. The difference between the PO_2 in the alveoli and arteries is referred to as the alveolar–arterial or A–a **gradient**. As a guide, it should be no more than 10, so the expected PAO_2 can be calculated by subtracting 10 from the FIO_2.

If the FIO_2 is 50 kPa, the PAO_2 should be no less than 40 kPa (see 'Intubation and ventilation', Chapter 114, page 470).

CAUSES

Respiratory acidosis

Any cause of **hypoventilation** – cardiac arrest, COPD, pneumonia, asthma.

Metabolic acidosis (see 'Anion gap' below)

- Body **produces too much acid** – lactic acid – as a result of anaerobic respiration; many forms of illness cause shock and hypoxia (e.g. severe sepsis). Important surgical causes include pancreatitis (as a result of shock), ischaemic bowel (shock) and crush injury
- **Diabetic ketoacidosis** (this is why these patients hyperventilate – they are trying to compensate)
- Body **cannot get rid of acid** – renal failure

- **Poisoning** with acid (e.g. aspirin)
- **Loss of bicarbonate** (e.g. diarrhoea).

Respiratory alkalosis

Increased respiration (e.g. hyperventilation, PE).

Metabolic alkalosis

Loss of H^+ (e.g. vomiting).

↑ **Example viva question**

What are the harmful effects of acidosis?

- Suboptimal enzyme action
- Depressed myocardial contractility/arrhythmias
- Decreased oxygen-carrying ability of haemoglobin
- Decreased response to vasopressor agents
- Hyperkalaemia and impaired potassium excretion
- Hyperventilation and exhaustion

ANION GAP

The anion gap is a calculation used to detect an **unmeasured concentration of anion** (acid) in the blood.

It helps in the differential diagnosis of causes of a **metabolic acidosis**.

The number of anions and cations in the blood should be equal.

The main anions and cations (Na^+, K^+, HCO_3^-, Cl^-) are measured when calculating the anion gap. So:

$$([Na^+] + [K^+]) - ([Cl^-] + [HCO_3^-]) = [\text{Unmeasured anions}] - [\text{Unmeasured cations}]$$

Normal range is 10–18 mmol/L because there are more unmeasured anions than cations.

If the anion gap is increased, an unmeasured anion is present in the blood in increased quantities.

Causes of **metabolic acidosis** with an **increased anion gap** include lactic acidosis, ketoacidosis and salicylate poisoning.

Examples of causes of a **metabolic acidosis** with a **normal anion gap** include diarrhoea and renal tubular acidosis.

85 Action potential

Possible viva questions related to this topic

→ Describe how an action potential is created and propagated?
→ Why is there a resting membrane potential and how is it maintained?
→ Define action potential.
→ What drugs affect the action potential?
→ What types of nerve do you know and how fast do they conduct?
→ What is the 'all or nothing' principle?
→ What is meant by the terms 'threshold' and 'summation'?
→ What is the difference between skeletal and cardiac action potentials?
→ What drugs affect the action potential and how do they work?

Example viva question

What is the resting membrane potential and how is it generated and maintained?

High **sodium** levels **outside** the cell (extracellular fluid) and high **potassium inside** the cell.

This chemical gradient is maintained by the action of **Na⁺/K⁺ ATPase**.

Both sets of ions try to cross the membrane and flow down their concentration gradient, but this is limited by the formation of an electrical gradient that occurs because they take their charge with them. This potential (for each ion) is called the **Nernst potential.** It is also limited by the fact that the cell membrane is impermeable to proteins, which are also charged.

The overall resting potential is $-70\,mV$ in nerve (see Fig. 85.1).

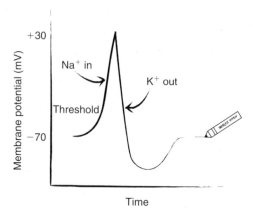

Figure 85.1

DEFINITION

An action potential is a **rapid change** in the **membrane potential** caused by **influx of positive ions**, followed by a **return to resting membrane potential** caused by **efflux of positive ions**; this leads to the generation of an **electrical impulse that** enables signalling to occur in excitable tissue (nerve and muscle).

THE ACTION POTENTIAL

The initiating event for an action potential is **depolarization** of the membrane. The membrane must be depolarized beyond a set **threshold for this to occur.**

In sensory nerves this is caused by activation by **stimulus transducers** (e.g. pressure sensors, pain transduced by blind nerve endings). It can also by initiated by potentials at **synapses**, or experimentally by applying a potential to the nerve directly.

Voltage-gated sodium channels open locally in response to this.

Sodium flows down its concentration gradient at this point, **depolarizing** the membrane to about +40 mV (see Fig. 85.1, left).

The depolarization causes **voltage-gated potassium channels** in the membrane to open. Potassium flows down its concentration gradient and the membrane repolarizes.

The potential **propagates** along the nerve as depolarization causes more and more sodium channels to open.

The sodium channels **close** and become **refractory,** i.e. they cannot open for a time period of 1 ms. This prevents the action potential from propagating backwards.

The changes in membrane potential are illustrated in Fig. 85.1 for a peripheral nerve (left) and cardiac muscle (right). This diagram is often asked for in vivas.

↑ **Example viva question**

What is summation, *and the* 'all or nothing' *principle?*

As described above, the initiating event for an action potential is a stimulus that depolarizes the membrane. **Summation** describes the process whereby depolarizing stimuli can be **added together** (although the depolarizing effect of this stimulus will be reduced), resulting in the generation of an action potential if the threshold is reached.

The all or nothing principle refers to the **action potential** itself. Once the threshold is reached, as described above, a positive feedback loop occurs whereby **all** of the sodium and then the potassium channels in the area of membrane excited become activated. An action potential must necessarily involve all of the channels so it is an all or nothing phenomenon; there are no weak or half-strength action potentials (in contrast to the depolarizing potential responsible for their generation).

SALTATORY CONDUCTION

Some axons are coated with **myelin**, which does not conduct the impulse. There are small interruptions to the myelin, called the **nodes of Ranvier.**

Conduction occurs only at these points and the current 'jumps' from node to node, speeding up propagation. This process is called **saltatory conduction**, and explains why, in **myelinated** fibres, such as in **motor** and **large sensory** neurons, the speed of conduction is greater.

In smaller unmyelinated fibres, such as **pain fibres**, the speed of conduction is slower.

Axon diameter also affects the speed of conduction, with large diameters being faster.

DRUGS

The action potential is abolished by sodium channel blockers – this is how local anaesthetics work (see 'Local anaesthetics', Chapter 75, page 308 and 'Neuromuscular junction' Chapter 98, page 391).

86 Altitude

Possible viva questions related to this topic

→ What are the physiological changes that take place at altitude?

Related topics

Topic	Chapter	Page
Acid–base balance	84	349
Oxygen transport	99	394
Control of respiration	91	373
Cerebrospinal fluid and the blood–brain barrier	90	369

The topic is a good test of applied physiology and understanding across a variety of topics.

PHYSIOLOGY AT ALTITUDE: THE PROBLEM

At altitude, the partial pressure of oxygen decreases, as does atmospheric pressure. This leads to a number of physiological changes and resultant compensations. The primary problem here is **chronic hypoxia** which leads to a drop in arterial P_{O_2}.

PHYSIOLOGICAL CHANGES

Altitude leads to a decrease in the arterial P_{O_2}.

Immediate changes

Respiratory and acid–base

Peripheral chemoreceptor detects a drop in P_{O_2} which leads to a **reflex tachypnoea** and **increase in depth of respiration** (see 'Control of respiration, Chapter 91, page 373).

This, however, results in a **respiratory alkalosis** and its associated features (tingling fingers, etc.). It also results in hypocapnia, which reduces the drive of the central chemoreceptor (not desirable). This is compensated for in the short term by **removal of bicarbonate ions** by the choroid plexus from the CSF.

Alkalosis has an adverse effect on oxygen delivery, because alkalosis shifts the oxygen–haemoglobin dissociation curve to the **left**, thus making it more difficult for the haemoglobin to give up oxygen at the tissues at a given P_{O_2} (see 'Oxygen transport' Chapter 99, page 394).

Reduced humidity can lead to a dry cough.

Cardiovascular

Reflex tachycardia and **cardiac output** increase initially, via stimulation of the peripheral chemoreceptors by hypoxia, to increase oxygen delivery to the tissues. This settles with acclimatization.

Cerebral blood flow increases to increase delivery of oxygen to the brain.

Slow changes

Respiratory and acid–base

The alkalosis created by the tachypnoea is **compensated for in the kidney** by increased **excretion of HCO_3^- ions**, a slow metabolic compensation.

Increased production of **2,3-diphosphoglycerate (DPG)** compensates for the left shift of the O_2–haemoglobin dissociation curve and facilitates release of oxygen to the tissues (see Fig. 99.1).

The chronic hypoxia leads to increased production of **erythropoietin** by the kidney, which causes increased haemoglobin synthesis. This improves oxygen carriage, and individuals chronically exposed to altitude become chronically polycythaemic (see also 'Oxygen transport', Chapter 99, page 394).

There is a **blunted response to hypoxia** as the individual acclimatizes and the alkalosis improves over time. There may also be an increase in the alveolar size and a decrease in the thickness of the alveolar membranes, leading to more efficient gas transfer.

Cardiovascular

Chronic hypoxia leads to **pulmonary vasoconstriction** and hypertension, and this can lead to **pulmonary oedema**.

The alkalosis leads to **cerebral vasoconstriction**; intracranial pressure increases, which can lead to **cerebral oedema**.

Blood **viscosity increases** at altitude.

Other medical problems

- Thrombosis
- Retinopathy
- Immunosuppression.

87 Blood pressure control

Possible viva questions related to this topic

→ What is blood pressure?

→ How is blood pressure measured?

→ What factors determine arterial blood pressure?

→ What are the homoeostatic mechanisms that control blood pressure?

→ What are the causes of hypertension?

→ Tell me what homoeostatic mechanisms maintain blood pressure in the face of acute haemorrhage?

→ Why do anaesthetists worry about blood pressure?

↑ **Key learning points**

Some definitions

Arterial blood pressure: the systemic arterial pressure

Systolic blood pressure: maximum arterial pressure during cardiac systole

Diastolic blood pressure: minimum pressure during diastole

Pulse pressure: systolic minus diastolic value

Mean arterial pressure: diastolic pressure plus one-third pulse pressure

MEASUREMENT OF BLOOD PRESSURE

Manual versus invasive (via an arterial line).

Manual blood pressure is derived by listening to **Korotkoff's sounds** (five different sounds as the cuff is released).

Five phases

1. At systolic pressure the sound appears
2. Sounds become muffled
3. Reappears
4. Becomes softer
5. Disappears (diastolic blood pressure).

Invasive blood pressure monitoring gives a second-to-second indication of patients' blood pressure, which is an advantage over serial manual readings (see 'CVP lines and invasive monitoring', Chapter 110, page 443).

IMPORTANT RELATIONSHIPS

$$BP = CO \times SVR \text{ (Ohm's law)} \tag{1}$$

$$CO = SV \times HR \tag{2}$$

where BP is blood pressure, CO is cardiac output, HR is heart rate, SVR is systemic vascular resistance, and SV is stroke volume.

↑ **Key learning point**

Start a viva by writing these equations out on the paper provided and use them to explain the physiology in a structured fashion

Cardiac output and **systemic vascular resistance** both have a direct bearing on **blood pressure**. These two contributors can be explained separately in the context of the question asked.

Cardiac output can be further broken down by the second equation.

Systemic vascular resistance is predominantly affected by the diameter of the arterioles – the resistance vessels, with a calibre that can be quickly controlled neurally or hormonally.

NEURAL HOMOEOSTATIC PATHWAYS

Blood pressure is monitored by **baroreceptors** (pressure receptors) in the aortic arch and carotid sinus. Sensory information is carried to the brain via **afferent glosso-pharyngeal** and **vagal** fibres. Integration takes place in the **midbrain**.

Efferent sympathetic fibres to the heart and arterioles make necessary alterations: if BP is **high**, afferent firing **increases** and **efferent** sympathetic activity reflexly **decreases**. This leads to **vasodilatation** and **decrease** in **heart rate** and **force of contraction**.

Arteriolar dilatation leads to a **decrease in TPR** (total peripheral resistance) and hence a **decrease in blood pressure** (Eqn 1).

A **decrease in stroke volume** and **heart rate** lead to a **decrease in blood pressure** (Eqns 2 and 1).

ENDOCRINE MECHANISMS

The blood vessels and heart, the main contributors to blood pressure, are also under endocrine control.

Adrenaline (epinephrine) is released if there is a sustained decrease in mean arterial pressure. This acts on α_1-receptors in the arterioles and veins to increase TPR (Eqn 1) and also on β_1-receptors in the heart to increase the rate and force of contraction (Eqns 2 and 1).

Loss of blood volume will lead to renal **renin** secretion, which ultimately leads to **angiotensin II** secretion. This has a direct vasoconstrictor effect (Eqn 1) and leads to **aldosterone** secretion, which causes sodium and fluid retention by the kidney. This indirectly increases cardiac output (Eqn 2).

↑ Example viva question

Tell me what homoeostatic mechanisms maintain blood pressure in the face of acute haemorrhage?

Use the two equations above.

Baroreceptor pressure falls, leading to reflex increase in vasomotor and cardiac sympathetic tone.

This leads to increased adrenaline secretion.

Renin is secreted by the kidney in response to decreased perfusion.

CAUSES

In hypertension, the set point for the above homoeostatic mechanisms is altered.

- 90 per cent essential (no cause found)
- Other endocrine causes: phaeochromocytoma, aldosteronoma, Cushing's disease, acromegaly
- Chronic renal failure.

88 Calcium homoeostasis

Possible viva questions related to this topic

→ How is calcium homoeostasis maintained?
→ What are the different types of hyperparathyroidism?
→ What are the causes of hypercalcaemia?
→ How is a corrected calcium calculated and why would you do it?
→ How do hyper- and hypocalcaemia present?
→ How are hyper- and hypocalcaemia treated?
→ What are the functions of calcium?
→ What are the effects of pH on calcium metabolism?

KEY FACTS

- Over **99 per cent** of total body calcium is **stored in bone** as hydroxyapatite; only 1 per cent is free
- Of this free calcium, **40 per cent is bound to serum albumin** and 60 per cent is free. It is only the unbound free calcium that is physiologically important
- **Acidosis increases** the amount of ionized calcium in the blood by dissolving mineralized bone; the osteoclasts dissolve bone by this mechanism
- The **functions of calcium** include:
  - **muscle contraction**
  - cardiac action potential propagation
  - constituent of bone and teeth
  - enzymatic cofactor
  - blood clotting
- Its intracellular release from stores (sarcoplasmic reticulum) is often responsible for initiating cellular function, because physiologically there is very little intracellular calcium
- It is also an intracellular second messenger.

> ### ↑ Example viva question
>
> #### *How do you correct the serum calcium?*
>
> The normal serum **calcium** level is **2.2–2.6 mmol/L**. A normal **albumin** is **40 mmol/L**. If the albumin level drops, the amount of free calcium rises and, as this is the active calcium, an adjustment needs to be made under these circumstances. For **every 5 the albumin drops below 40 mmol/L, the calcium level should be increased by 0.1 mmol/L.**
>
> This is important in **hypoalbuminaemia** in, for example, postoperative undernourished patients in whom the uncorrected calcium may not seem high.

CALCIUM HOMOEOSTASIS – HORMONES

Three hormones are responsible for keeping the serum calcium at this level within the blood: parathyroid hormone (PTH), 1,25-dihydroxycholecalciferol (1,25-DHCC), a metabolite of vitamin D, and calcitonin.

Parathyroid hormone

This hormone is the most important in the metabolism of calcium. It is a **peptide** hormone, produced by the **parathyroid glands**. It is secreted in response to a **decrease in serum calcium,** and high levels of serum calcium decrease its secretion (a **negative feedback** loop; see Fig. 88.1).

It acts on **osteoclasts** that have PTH receptors, to **increase resorption of bone** and release calcium into the blood. It also acts to **increase** the **production of 1,25-DHCC** by the kidney, and increases secretion of **phosphate** by the kidney.

1,25-DHCC

This is a metabolite of **vitamin D**, which is obtained from the diet or action of UV light on the skin. It is metabolized first in the **liver** to 25-hydroxycholecalciferol and then in the kidney to produce the active hormone.

Its synthesis is **potentiated by PTH**, in the proximal tubule of the nephron. It causes increased resorption of calcium from the **gut** (see Fig. 88.1).

Calcitonin

Not thought to be an important hormone physiologically. It is secreted by the **medullary (parafollicular) cells of the thyroid**.

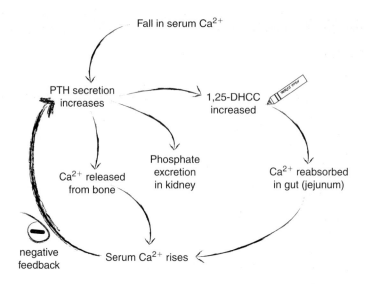

Figure 88.1

It causes a **decrease in serum calcium** by **inhibiting osteoclast** function. It is secreted abnormally in the **medullary carcinoma of the thyroid**, for which it is a **tumour marker**.

HYPERCALCAEMIA

Clinical features

'Stones, bones, abdominal groans, psychic moans.'

- Renal stones
- Bone pain
- Abdominal pain (gallstones and pancreatitis)
- Psychosis.

Causes include (mechanism in brackets) the following:

Common (80 per cent of all causes)
- Primary and tertiary hyperparathyroidism (see below)
- Malignancy (bone destruction).

Rarer
- Sarcoidosis (excess vitamin D)
- Myeloma (bone destruction)
- Thiazide diuretics
- Iatrogenic (excess administration of vitamin D)
- Milk alkali syndrome.

HYPOCALCAEMIA

Clinical features

- Paraesthesia
- Trousseau's sign (twitching of facial muscles on tapping facial nerve) and Chvostek's sign (carpopedal spasm)
- Convulsions
- Tetany
- Rickets (may be a chronic association).

Causes include (mechanism in brackets):

- Parathyroidectomy (loss of PTH secretion)
- Thyroidectomy (transient, damage to parathyroids)
- Chronic renal failure (calcium loss)
- Massive blood transfusion (chelation of Ca^{2+})
- Vitamin D deficiency
- Pancreatitis.

HYPERPARATHYROIDISM

Primary

Caused by parathyroid adenomas and excessive PTH secretion.

Secondary

Caused by renal failure. PTH levels are high but calcium is being lost faster so levels are low or normal.

Tertiary

Occurs in longstanding renal failure. The parathyroids become autonomous and hyperplastic and behave like adenomas, secreting PTH autonomously. Calcium levels become high again despite renal loss of calcium. Treatment is by **parathyroidectomy**

TREATMENT OF HYPERCALCAEMIA AND HYPOCALCAEMIA

Hypercalcaemia is an emergency, because it can cause **arrhythmias**. It is treated in the short term by vigorous fluid resuscitation and administration of pamidronate, which lowers the calcium levels. The cause should be sought and treated where possible.

Hypocalcaemia can be treated by administration of calcium or calcium-raising preparations such as **Calcichew** (vitamin D derivative) and **calcium gluconate**.

89 Cardiac action potential

Related Topics		
Topic	**Chapter**	**Page**
Action potential	85	353
Neuromuscular junction	98	391
Calcium homoeostasis	88	362

- The **heart muscle has an intrinsic ability to beat**.
- The heart acts as a **functional syncytium**, so that depolarization of a pacemaker will rapidly lead to depolarization and contraction of the entire heart.
- All parts of the conducting apparatus are capable of pacing.
- The **sinoatrial node** does so because its intrinsic rate is **fastest**.
- In the absence of a pacemaker, other parts of the conducting system take over (with a slower rate), e.g. in either complete AV block or ventricular escape, the ventricles depolarize at a slower rate, which is why the patient's heart continues to beat in the absence of an atrial pacemaker, but a bradycardia is present.
- In some arrhythmias, there is abnormal pacemaker function, e.g. in atrial fibrillation (AF) there are multiple pacemakers that lead to fibrillation.
- The physiological resting heart rate is 90/min, which is **slowed** physiologically by **increasing vagal tone**.

⬆ **Example viva question**

Tell me how a transplanted heart functions

(A common MRCS question to make you think about the physiology.)

It has intrinsic rhythmicity, it is autonomically denervated, so there are no direct effects of noradrenaline or acetylcholine (sympathetic and parasympathetic neurotransmitters) but circulating hormones do (adrenaline – see below) affect heart rate.

⬆ **Example viva question**

Draw the cardiac action potential for me. How does it differ from a somatic action potential? Label the ion fluxes.

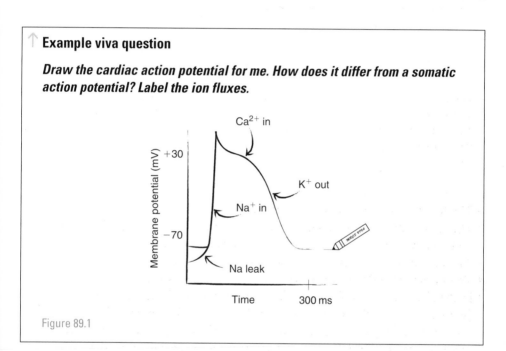

Figure 89.1

The cardiac action potential necessarily differs from that in somatic nerve or muscle.

- There is a constant sodium leak into the cell:
  - this causes a gradual **increase** in the **resting membrane potential**; cardiac myocytes derive their intrinsic rhythmicity from the presence of this sodium leak, which is not present in other excitable cells
  - when the membrane potential reaches threshold, **voltage-gated sodium channels open**, resulting in **rapid depolarization** as sodium flows down its concentration gradient into the cell
- There is now an **influx of calcium**, which **lengthens the cardiac action potential**. This period is the equivalent of the refractory period in somatic nerve.

 Key learning point

The influx of calcium **prevents tetany**, which occurs physiologically in skeletal muscle but is obviously undesirable in cardiac muscle.

- Eventually, **voltage-gated potassium channels open** and potassium flows out of the cell down a concentration gradient, **repolarizing the cell membrane**.

Key learning points

Drugs that affect the cardiac action potential – mechanism of action

- Adrenaline: this **increases the rate of sodium leak, decreases the time between action potentials** and hence increases heart rate
- Acetylcholine: this **decreases the rate of sodium leak**, which has the opposite effect to adrenaline, and hence **slows down the heart rate**
- Calcium channel blockers: these shorten the plateau phase of the action potential and hence decrease the force of contraction of cardiac muscle.

Sodium channel blockers and calcium channel blockers can act as antiarrhythmics by decreasing the excitability of the cell membrane. They do not affect the sodium depolarization, but prevent, for example, premature beats because many of the channels are still blocked.

Example viva question

Don't forget, $CO = SV \times HR$ and the physiology of the cardiac action potential can be used in discussions relating to Starling's law and relationships with respect to heart rate. (see 'Starling's law of the heart and cardiovascular equations', Chapter 102, page 403, and 'Inotropes', Chapter 113, page 466).

---

90 Cerebrospinal fluid and the blood–brain barrier

Possible viva questions related to this topic

→ What are the functions of the CSF?
→ Where is CSF produced?
→ Where does CSF flow and how is it resorbed?
→ What does normal CSF contain? How do its constituents change in meningitis and subarachnoid haemorrhage?
→ How would you perform a lumbar puncture?
→ How does epidural and spinal anaesthesia work?
→ What is hydrocephalus? How is it classified?

Related Topics

Topic	Chapter	Page
Control of respiration	91	373
Local anaesthetics	75	308

CSF FLUX

Cerebrospinal fluid (CSF) is produced by the **choroid plexus** of the lateral, third and fourth ventricles. It flows from the lateral ventricles to the **third ventricle**, and then via the cerebral aqueduct into the **fourth ventricle.**

After this it flows into the **subarachnoid space** via the two foramina of **Luschka** (lateral) and the single foramen of **Magendie** (midline). The fourth ventricle is diamond shaped and its floor consists of **pons and rostral brain stem**, and the roof includes the **cerebellar peduncles**. The caudal part of the roof contains an opening into the cerebromedullary cistern and then into the subarachnoid space; this is the foramen of Magendie. There are two lateral openings in the roof into the pontine cistern and then into subarachnoid space (the foramina of Luschka). The **basal cisterns** (two described above) are dilated areas, here containing CSF.

CSF is reabsorbed by **arachnoid villi/granulations** of the **venous sinuses**, passively under CSF pressure. Normal CSF pressure is **120–180 mmH$_2$O.**

There are **140 mL** present in the adult, although **four times** this amount is produced and resorbed each day.

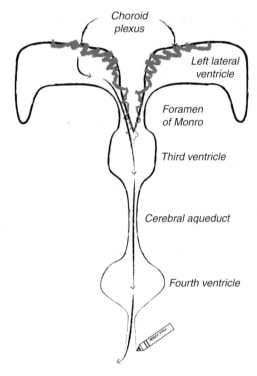

Figure 90.1   Schematic anteroposterior view illustrating the ventricular system and CSF flux.

CONTENTS OF THE CSF

Normal CSF is crystal clear and contains:

- Water
- Protein: 0.15–0.45 g/L
- Glucose: 0.45–0.7 g/L
- Small numbers of white cells (leukocytes, neutrophils and monocytes)
  < 5 white cells/mm^3.

FUNCTION OF THE CSF

It acts as a **shock absorber** for the brain, bathing it in fluid. This is important, because the brain is in the skull, which is fixed and hard.

It **reduces the effective weight** of the brain. It provides a route for **excretion of waste products** from the brain.

It delivers glucose to the brain, and is important in its homoeostasis (e.g. 'Acid–base balance', Chapter 84, page 349, and 'Control of respiration', Chapter 91, page 373).

ABNORMALITIES OF THE CSF

In meningitis

CSF samples are **turbid** in bacterial meningitis. The CSF contains several neutrophil polymorphs and depleted glucose levels.

In subarachnoid haemorrhage there is **xanthochromia** (CSF looks yellow when spun down in the lab).

Spinal and epidural anaesthesia

In spinal anaesthesia, a needle is passed into the subarachnoid space, below the level at which the spinal cord ends (L1–2). The local anaesthetic is delivered directly to the subarachnoid space where all the nerve roots are anaesthetized for a short time.

In epidural anaesthesia, the local anaesthetic is delivered to the epidural space, where it remains for longer periods of time. This is why epidural block lasts for longer.

Hydrocephalus

This is an increase in CSF volume, usually resulting from impairment of absorption of CSF. It is divided into obstructive and communicating:

Obstructive	Communicating
Caused by a **obstruction within the ventricular system**	Obstruction **outside the ventricular system**
Tumours (primary, secondary), colloid cysts	Subarachnoid haemorrhage (involvement of arachnoid granulations)
Aqueductal stenosis (post-infective, post-haemorrhage or congenital)	
Aqueductal haematoma	Excessive CSF production
Abscess	High CSF protein content
Dandy–Walker syndrome (atresia of foramen of Luschka or Magendie)	

Note that **normal pressure hydrocephalus** (NPH) relates to the triad of dementia, gait ataxia and incontinence, despite a 'normal' CSF pressure. It may be idiopathic, or arise insidiously after a subarachnoid haemorrhage or meningitis. In actual fact, studies show that NPH is usually associated with abnormal peaks of pressure that oscillate throughout the day.

Diagnosed on computed tomography (CT) – dilated ventricular system.

Treated with ventriculoperitoneal shunting, third ventriculostomy ± treatment of the cause (e.g. resection of an obstructing posterior fossa tumour).

↑ **Example viva question**

How is raised intracranial pressure measured?

- **Clinical assessment**: headache, nausea and vomiting, papilloedema on fundoscopy
- **Lumbar puncture**: although the CSF pressure can be measured during this procedure, this is not routinely used because diagnostic lumbar puncture is contraindicated in raised intracranial pressure (ICP) (see 'Head injury and intracranial pressure', Chapter 112, page 459)
- **Ventricular catheter**: a catheter is inserted into the anterior horn of the lateral ventricle via a frontal burr hole to measure pressure directly. A pressure > 20 mmHg is moderately elevated and > 40mm Hg is severely elevated. It is used postoperatively and during treatment aimed at reducing the ICP, where the CSF can be aspirated to reduce the overall ICP (see 'Head injury and intracranial pressure', Chapter 112, page 459)

THE BLOOD–BRAIN BARRIER

The blood–brain barrier selectively controls the **entry of substances into the extracellular fluid of the CNS** and the rate of their entry. This limits access of toxins but also of immune mechanisms.

The blood–brain barrier is located in the smallest capillaries supplying the brain and consists of tight junctions and transport mechanisms. **Fat-soluble drugs** (e.g. diamorphine) cross quickly, and **glucose** and **anaesthetic agents** can also cross.

Hydrogen ions do not usually cross and this has implications for control of respiration and acid–base balance (see 'Acid–base balance', Chapter 84, page 349).

The blood–brain barrier is absent in a number of areas:

- **Median eminence** of the hypothalamus where hypothalamic neurons release hormones that act on the anterior pituitary into the portal system of capillaries.
- **Posterior pituitary**, where ADH- (antidiuretic hormone) and oxytocin-secreting neurons secrete directly into the blood (see 'Pituitary', Chapter 100, page 397).
- **Circumventricular organs** adjacent to the third and fourth ventricles. This area is adjacent to the chemotrigger zone.

The blood–brain barrier may be compromised in severely raised ICP and is often disrupted in the context of aggressive intra-axial tumours.

91 Control of respiration

Possible viva questions related to this topic

→ What types of respiratory failure do you know?
→ Why is pure oxygen contraindicated in patients with COPD (chronic obstructive pulmonary disease)?
→ What are the roles of central and peripheral chemoreceptors in controlling respiration?
→ Tell me about how breathing is controlled?
→ What is the interrelationship of PaO_2, $PaCO_2$ and respiratory rate/minute volume? Can you draw a graph?
→ What are the main sensors that maintain respiratory homoeostasis and what is their relative importance?
→ What is the importance of the pH of CSF in control of respiration?

SET-UP AND TERMINOLOGY

Homoeostasis is achieved by feedback systems that keep PO_2 and PCO_2 within tight limits.

Sensors monitor levels and provide input to the respiratory centre if too low or high.

The **respiratory centres** control normal involuntary respiration. It can be overridden voluntarily. They are in the brain stem (pons and medulla).

The **effectors** are the respiratory muscles that act to bring about change. The respiratory centres control these effectors. They consist of **diaphragm, intercostals** and, where a greater respiratory effort is required, **accessory muscles** (abdominal, serratus anterior, scalenus anterior, sternocleidomastoid, etc.).

RESPIRATORY CENTRES

These consist of the **medullary** respiratory, apneustic and pneumotaxic centres. Their relationships are complex: they involuntarily produce a rhythmic respiratory cycle.

They can be overridden voluntarily by the cortex, when we breathe voluntarily.

SENSORS

Peripheral chemoreceptors

- The less important of the two sets of sensors
- They are situated in the **carotid body** and the **aortic arch** and receive a high blood flow
- They primarily **sense the P_{O_2}** and if this is low they increase afferent firing to the respiratory centre, which reflexly beings about an increase in respiratory rate and depth, and hence a return to normal P_{O_2}
- They are also, to a much lesser degree, **sensitive to pH**. This underpins the increase in respiratory rate and depth seen in respiratory compensation of metabolic acidosis (see 'Acid–base balance', Chapter 84, page 349).

Central chemoreceptors

- These are the most important sensors, and are situated on the **ventral surface of the medulla**; they lie within the blood–brain barrier
- CO_2 readily crosses the blood–brain barrier where it undergoes the conversion
  $H_2O + CO_2 \rightleftharpoons H_2CO_3 \rightleftharpoons H^+ + HCO_3^-$.
  H^+ does not cross the blood–brain barrier, so **changes in H^+ in the CSF equate to a rise in P_{CO_2}**
- They are sensitive to the **level of H^+**, hence, indirectly, to CO_2 in the CSF
- Therefore a rise in central H^+ (CO_2) brings about a reflex increase in respiratory rate and depth to reduce the P_{CO_2}
- If the P_{CO_2} remains chronically high the central chemoreceptors reset their set point for the 'correct' P_{CO_2} at a higher level.

↑ **Example viva question**

Why is pure oxygen contraindicated in patients with COPD?

In COPD, the **central chemoreceptors** are chronically exposed to **high levels of CO_2** as a result of poor gas exchange in the lungs. Hence, the **set point for P_{CO_2} increases** for the central chemoreceptors, and they no longer respond to small changes in P_{CO_2}.

These patients therefore purely **rely on hypoxia** to stimulate the **peripheral chemoreceptors**, which in turn stimulates the respiratory centres to increase the drive to breathe.

If 100 per cent oxygen is given, there is no hypoxia to stimulate the peripheral chemoreceptors and, because the central chemoreceptors also no longer respond to a build-up of CO_2 (as H^+), the patient has no drive to breathe.

Note that, in practice, however, it is more dangerous to leave the patient in life-threatening hypoxia than to administer oxygen!

Effect of P_{aCO_2} and P_{aO_2} on minute volume and respiratory rate

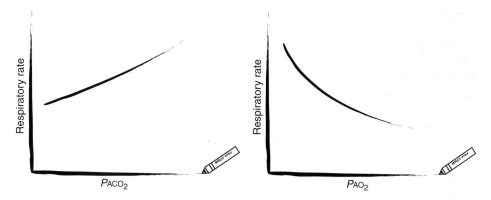

Figure 91.1

Figure 91.1 illustrates the relationship.

On a minute-to-minute basis, the P_{aCO_2} is proportional to the respiratory rate. This is brought about by the central chemoreceptors.

The P_{aO_2} brings about an increase in respiratory rate and minute volume only at quite low values (6.5 kPa), this being effected by the peripheral chemoreceptors. **See 'Altitude, Chapter 86, page 356 for another illustration of how it works.**

92 Functions of the kidney I

Possible viva questions related to this topic

→ What are the functions of the kidney?
→ What hormones does the kidney secrete?
→ What happens in renal failure?
→ How does the kidney act in electrolyte homoeostasis? (How does the kidney handle Na^+, K^+ and H^+ ions?)
→ How does the kidney conserve water?
→ How does the loop of Henle work? Draw a diagram to illustrate.

Example viva question

What are the functions of the kidney?

A common question in vivas and each function can lead into a separate viva as can be seen by the numerous related topics. The key is dividing this up into categories and having these ready, with an explanation of each. The key functions are:

• Fluid balance and electrolyte homoeostasis (see Chapter 93, page 377)
• Acid–base balance (see Chapter 84, page 349)
• Nitrogen excretion, excretion of toxins and drugs (see Chapter 95, page 383)
• Endocrine functions (renin–angiotensin system, erythropoietin, ADH system, calcium metabolism) (see Chapter 94, page 381).

93 Functions of the kidney II: fluid and electrolyte balance in the kidney and loop of Henle

This is the kidney's key function.

ELECTROLYTE BALANCE

Anatomy of the nephron (Fig. 93.1)

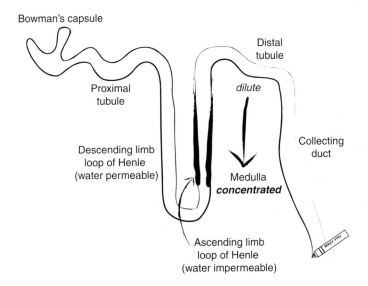

Figure 93.1

The blood is filtered at high pressure in the **glomerulus**; the large proteins and cells remain in the blood and water, and solutes pass into the **Bowman's capsule** and the nephron; **170–180 L** of plasma are filtered a day.

Several solutes are actively reabsorbed in the proximal tubule, including **sodium, glucose, calcium, phosphate** and **chloride**. **Water** is also reabsorbed, as are amino acids.

The renal medulla contains a **gradient** of sodium, which is most concentrated at the centre and more dilute at the periphery. More sodium is pumped out actively at the thick ascending limb of the loop of Henle to maintain the **sodium gradient** (see below).

THE LOOP OF HENLE

Figure 93.2 explains how the **sodium gradient** is generated. The thin **descending limb** of the loop of Henle is **permeable** to **water** and the thick ascending limb is **not**.

Sodium is pumped actively from the tubular fluid in the **ascending limb** of the loop of Henle to the interstitium (at the centre of the loop in Fig. 93.2). Fluid moves from left to right through the loop. The sequence of events is as follows (Fig. 93.2):

1. All concentrations are equal
2. Sodium is pumped out of the thick ascending limb
3. The increased concentration of sodium in the interstitium equilibrates with the fluid in the descending limb
4. Fluid moves around the loop of Henle
5. Again, fluid is pumped from the thick ascending limb into the interstitium
6. The fluid concentrations equilibrate as before
7. The fluid moves once again.

A **gradient** has started to form. This is maintained by the sodium pumps and the constant delivery of the sodium to the loop of Henle.

The fluid leaving the loop of Henle is very **hypotonic** because sodium has been pumped away from it. Water is later reabsorbed through **water channels** (see below) in the collecting system.

This sodium gradient, together with the **countercurrent multiplier** arrangement of the loop of Henle and the blood supply, allows the urine to be concentrated, because **water follows sodium**, the main anion in the blood. As the fluid filtered by the Bowman's capsule enters the loop of Henle and progresses through the permeable descending limb, water enters the more concentrated interstitium by osmosis.

Sodium and chloride are reabsorbed here.

⬆ **Example viva question**

How do loop and thiazide diuretics work?

As water follows sodium, blocking of the sodium channels in the proximal tubule, loop of Henle or distal tubule causes a diuresis (sodium not reabsorbed, so excreted with water); this is the basis of the action of different types of **diuretic**.

In the loop of Henle, blocking of the sodium channels dissipates the sodium gradient and the kidney cannot concentrate urine (loop diuretics such as frusemide).

In the proximal tubule, if sodium reabsorption is blocked (thiazide diuretics such as bendrofluazide) more water and sodium are excreted.

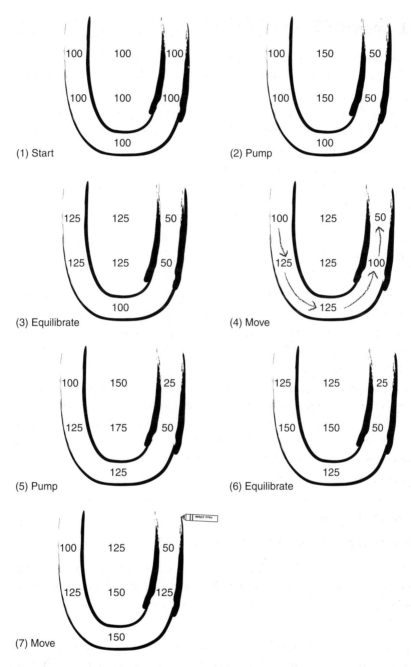

Figure 93.2

DISTAL TUBULE

In the distal tubule, **potassium is excreted** under the control of **aldosterone,** in exchange for sodium.

In the collecting duct, water is reabsorbed via **water channels**, the synthesis of which is mediated by **ADH**. Some urea is passively reabsorbed, but the main contents of the urine here are urea, sodium and water. These movements are summarized in Fig. 93.3.

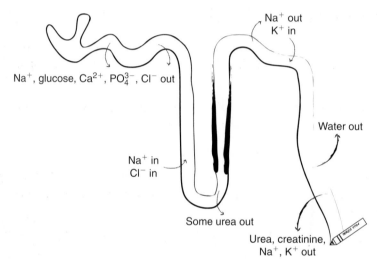

Figure 93.3

94 Functions of the kidney III: endocrine functions of the kidney

Fluid balance is controlled by two main endocrine mechanisms:

1. The **ADH system** controls the tonicity of the blood.
2. The **renin–angiotensin–aldosterone** system controls the blood volume.

ADH SYSTEM: TONICITY OF THE BLOOD

The tonicity of the blood is sensed by cells in the lamina terminalis of the hypothalamus and the magnocellular ADH-secreting neurons of the hypothalamo-neurohypophyseal system (see 'Pituitary', Chapter 100, page 397).

If the blood becomes **hypertonic** (dehydration), these neurons become excited. This causes the release of ADH from the posterior pituitary.

The site of action of ADH is the **collecting duct** of the nephron.

ADH causes the epithelial cells of the collecting duct to increase synthesis of **water channels**, which results in increased **water reabsorption** and production of a concentrated urine.

The sodium gradient (see 'Function of the kidney II, Chapter 93, page 377) is necessary for this system to function.

THE RENIN–ANGIOTENSIN–ALDOSTERONE SYSTEM

This homoeostatic mechanism is mainly concerned with the regulation of **blood volume**. This system will override the ADH system if there are conflicting interests (i.e. low blood volume but dilute blood, as in haemorrhage).

Blood volume is sensed by blood pressure in the afferent arteriole of the **juxtaglomerular apparatus**. A drop stimulates the production of the enzyme **renin**, which converts circulating **angiotensinogen to angiotensin I**, which is in turn converted to **angiotensin II** by **angiotensin-converting enzyme** in the lung.

Angiotensin II has a potent **vasoconstrictor** effect, which raises the blood pressure in the face of hypovolaemia. It also causes increased secretion of **aldosterone** from the adrenal cortex (zona glomerulosa).

Aldosterone causes sodium (and hence water) retention by the distal tubule of the nephron, to **increase blood volume**. Its other function is potassium excretion.

This system **overrides the ADH system**, e.g. if renal perfusion is low, but the blood is hypotonic. This makes sense because, in shock, it is more important to maintain blood volume than to get rid of water from hypotonic blood (if the two coexist).

Erythropoietin is the other hormone that is secreted by the kidney. It causes proliferation of erythrocytes in chronic hypoxia.

The kidney also metabolizes **vitamin D derivatives**, in the metabolism of calcium (see 'Calcium homoeostasis', Chapter 88, page 362).

95 Functions of the kidney IV: other functions

ACID–BASE BALANCE

The kidney is important in **compensating for acidosis or alkalosis** produced by lung disease (respiratory acidosis/alkalosis) – this is called metabolic compensation (see 'Acid–base balance', Chapter 84, page 349 for a more detailed discussion.)

The kidney achieves this by a complex system of **buffers**, which result in the excretion of H^+ or HCO_3^-. This is a **slow** process that occurs over days.

The pH of the urine must not fall below 4.5, and this is also achieved by the buffering system (see also 'Acid–base balance, Chapter 84, page 349).

EXCRETION OF NITROGEN, TOXINS AND DRUGS

Urea and creatinine are excreted by the kidney, because most of these small waste products of nitrogenous metabolism are not reabsorbed by the nephron. Many drugs are excreted by the kidney.

There are two main routes of excretion:

1. Some drugs are **filtered and not reabsorbed** by the kidney. If such drugs are highly polar, they can be trapped in the tubule (e.g. **digoxin**).
2. Drugs can also be **actively secreted** by the transporter systems in the **proximal tubule** (examples include **penicillins, morphine** and **salicylate**).

96 Functions of the liver

Possible viva questions related to this topic

→ What are the functions of the liver?
→ Tell me about liver function tests (LFTs)?
→ Tell me about what happens in starvation?
→ How are drugs metabolized here? What drugs interact with the metabolism of warfarin and how?

Related Topics

Topic	Chapter	Page
Liver	10	28
Portal vein and portosystemic anastomoses	14	39
Biliary tree and gallbladder	5	17

Example viva question

What are the functions of the liver?

A common question. The key is dividing this up into categories and having these ready, with an explanation of each. The key functions are:

• Production of bile
• Protein, fat and carbohydrate metabolism
• Storage of glycogen and vitamins (A, D, E, K, B_{12})
• Detoxification of drugs, hormones and toxins
• Reticuloendothelial and haematopoietic (fetus) functions

PRODUCTION OF BILE

Bile is secreted by the **hepatocytes** and ducts add to its fluid content. About 1 L of bile is produced per day.

It contains **bile salts** (cholate and chenodeoxycholate) and HCO_3^-, as well as the breakdown products of red cell metabolism such as **conjugated bilirubin.** These are responsible for the **digestion (emulsification) of lipids**, which form **micelles** that facilitate their absorption (mainly in the **jejunum**).

Bile produced by the liver flows into the **gallbladder** when not required (not down the common bile duct because the **sphincter of Oddi** is closed).

When a fat-rich meal enters the duodenum, the **gallbladder contracts** and the **sphincter of Oddi relaxes** to allow bile to reach the duodenum.

Most of the bile salts are reabsorbed in the **terminal ileum** where they are returned via the portal circulation to the liver and recycled. This is called the **enterohepatic circulation** and the bile salts are recycled six to eight times a day. Some bile salts are lost in the faeces.

METABOLISM

Protein metabolism

The liver is responsible for **gluconeogenesis** ('new glucose formation'), the **synthesis of glucose** from other small molecules, such as amino acids. Muscle is broken down in starvation to amino acids and transported to the liver for gluconeogenesis.

Protein is broken down in the liver to form nitrogenous waste products such as **urea** via the urea cycle.

The liver is responsible for the **synthesis** of all **non-essential amino acids**. It is also responsible for the **synthesis of proteins**, such as albumin, clotting factors and complement proteins. For this reason, measurement of plasma **albumin** and **clotting** (international normalized ratio or INR) constitute useful LFTs to look at **synthetic function**; albumin decreases and clotting time increases if synthetic function is deranged.

Fat metabolism

The liver is responsible for synthesis of transport proteins for fatty acids, and in starvation it synthesizes **ketone bodies.**

Very-low-density lipoprotein (VLDL) is a lipoprotein synthesized by the liver. Its function is to transport fatty acids from the **liver** to the **peripheral tissues** for storage. VLDLs are synthesized from **chylomicron remnants** after absorption by the small bowel.

Fatty acids are cleaved to produce **acetyl-CoA** for the production of ATP.

In starvation, the brain requires glucose to function but can also metabolize **ketone bodies** for energy. The liver can produce ketone bodies from fatty acids (which cannot be used to produce glucose).

Carbohydrate metabolism

This occurs during **gluconeogenesis** (see above). In 'times of plenty', **glucose** is converted into **glycogen**, for storage, a process termed 'glycogenesis'. The breakdown of **glycogen** to **glucose** takes place in the liver in early starvation (fasting), and is called **glycogenolysis**.

STORAGE

The liver stores **glycogen**, **vitamins A, D, E, K and B$_{12}$, iron** and **copper**.

Glycogen is a quick source of glucose in starvation as outlined above. It will last as long as an overnight fast although other mechanisms are brought into play.

DETOXIFICATION

Peptide hormones (e.g. insulin) and **steroid hormones** (e.g. testosterone) are degraded in the liver. The cytochrome P450 system is involved in their metabolism, which includes increasing water solubility.

Drugs that increase or decrease the activity of the cytochrome P450 system may have an effect on other drugs being administered concomitantly; this is a major source of ADRs, and is particularly significant where the drugs being used have a narrow therapeutic window.

↑ **Example viva question**

What drugs interact with warfarin and how?

Erythromycin inhibits the cytochrome P450 system and **phenytoin** increases it, so warfarin, which is metabolized via this system, would have its effects potentiated if administered together with erythromycin, and reduced if administered with phenytoin. More details of such drugs are available in the *BNF*.

RETICULOENDOTHELIAL AND FETAL

The liver has an erythropoietic function in the embryo. The Kupffer cells in the sinusoids are responsible for removal of bacteria in the portal blood.

↑ **Example viva question**

What is the role of the liver in starvation?

Early starvation: glycogenolysis and gluconeogenesis (muscle breakdown to form amino acids).

Late starvation: breakdown of fatty acids.

Formation of ketone bodies, for use by the brain. **Ketosis** occurs when the liver's glycogen reserves are used up and the liver metabolizes fat to produce ketones. These are used as an energy source by respiring tissues, sparing glucose for the brain, which relies on a proportion of glucose for metabolism but can also use ketone bodies.

97 Functions of the stomach

Possible viva questions related to this topic

→ What are the functions of the stomach?
→ How is acid production controlled?
→ What does the stomach secrete?
→ What are the effects of gastrectomy?

Related Topics		
Topic	Chapter	Page
Stomach	17	46

Example viva question

What are the functions of the stomach?

The key is dividing this up into categories and having these ready, with an explanation of each. The key functions are:
• **Reservoir** for food, **mixing** of food with gastric secretions to form chyme
• Endocrine function: secretion of **gastrin**
• Exocrine functions:
  ○ production of **acid** – digestion of food and immune function
  ○ enzyme production (**pepsin**) for protein digestion, **intrinsic factor** and **mucus**

RESERVOIR AND MIXING FUNCTIONS

The stomach has highly distensible smooth muscle walls, which relax on the arrival of a meal. Its volume can increase to **1.5 L** without an increase in pressure.

The stomach undergoes **peristaltic waves**, which expel only a small amount of chyme into the duodenum with each wave. These waves, generated by inherent electrical activity in the smooth muscle of the stomach, combined with hormonal influences, help to mix the stomach's contents and produce **chyme**.

ENDOCRINE FUNCTION

The stomach produces a hormone called **gastrin (G cells of the antral mucosa)**.

This hormone is released in response to the **cephalic phase** controlling acid secretion in the stomach.

Gastrin acts to **increase the secretion of acid** by the parietal cells in the stomach. It also causes histamine release, which potentiates the release of acid.

H_2-receptor blockers such as ranitidine and cimetidine reduce gastric acidity by blocking this mechanism.

EXOCRINE FUNCTIONS

Acid secretion

- Two litres of HCl secreted per day
- Converts **pepsinogen** to **pepsin**, the active protease
- Converts ferric (Fe^{3+}) **iron** to ferrous (Fe^{2+}) for jejunal absorption
- Creates an acid environment in duodenum to facilitate **iron** and **calcium** absorption
- Acid also provides **innate immunity** to infection.

There are three phases of **control of acid secretion**.

Cephalic phase
- Initiated by **sight and smell of food**
- Vagally mediated increase in acid production
- Stimulates gastrin secretion.

Gastric phase
- Food present in the stomach causes chemical and mechanical stimulation
- This causes further gastrin release, and reflexly (via vagal afferents and efferents) increases acid secretion.

Intestinal phase
Duodenal distension and presence of degradation products bring about a reflex **decrease in acid secretion**. Hormones released that mediate this include secretin, gastric inhibitory peptide (GIP) and cholecystokinin (CCK).

The goblet cells in the stomach produce **mucus**, which lines the gastric mucosa and prevents the formation of ulcers secondary to the acidity.

INTRINSIC FACTOR

This is produced by the parietal cells. It binds to **vitamin B$_{12}$** in the stomach and is necessary for its absorption in the **terminal ileum**.

Loss of the parietal cells and intrinsic factor by autoantibodies (pernicious anaemia) or gastrectomy causes a lack of vitamin B$_{12}$, an essential **co-factor for red cell production**. This leads to megaloblastic anaemia.

Resection of the terminal ileum in, for example, Crohn's disease has a similar effect.

↑ **Example viva question**

Based on your knowledge of the functions of the stomach, what are the effects of a total gastrectomy?

- **Early dumping syndrome**: food of high osmolarity, not mixed in the stomach, causes rapid fluid shift and oligaemia. This causes fainting and sweating from hypovolaemia
- **Late dumping syndrome**: caused by rebound hypoglycaemia, or high insulin levels experienced after a high carbohydrate load is presented and absorbed by the duodenum. Similar symptoms to above
- **Pernicious anaemia** (see above) and iron deficiency anaemia (see below)
- **Early satiety**: loss of reservoir function
- **Bilious vomiting**: loss of pyloric sphincter
- **Hypocalcaemia and iron deficiency**: hypochlorhydia (reduced HCl secretion) interferes with the absorption of Ca^{2+} and iron
- **Gastric stump carcinoma**: cancers occur at the gastrojejunal anastomosis 20 years or so after surgery. This may be a result of chronic irritation of gastric mucosa by duodenal secretions
- **Gallstones:** caused by decreased gallbladder motility post-vagotomy

---

98 Neuromuscular junction

SEQUENCE OF EVENTS AT THE NMJ

The NMJ is the junction of an **α motor nerve** (somatic) terminal with the **motor end-plate** (e.g. phrenic nerve on diaphragm).

The sequence of events at the neuromuscular junction is as follows:

- **The action potential arrives at a motor nerve terminal**
- This nerve terminal is **depolarized**
- **Calcium** enters the cell via voltage-gated calcium channels
- **Acetylcholine**-containing vesicles are mobilized on interaction with calcium and **exocytosis** occurs; the acetylcholine is released into the NMJ
- Acetylcholine interacts with its **receptor** at the muscle end-plate, inducing an **excitatory post-synaptic potential** (EPSP); it is broken down by **acetylcholinesterase** in the nerve cleft
- The summation of EPSPs beyond threshold for the muscle induces an **action potential** in muscle
- **Excitation–contraction coupling** occurs as the action potential is propagated along muscle and causes release of calcium from the **sarcoplasmic reticulum** within the muscle cell; Ca^{2+} causes muscle contraction.

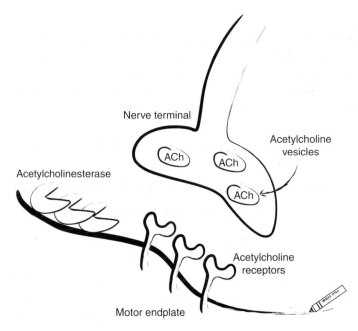

Figure 98.1   Diagrammatic representation of the neuromuscular junction.

DRUGS

Muscle relaxants

Suxamethonium

Short-acting muscle relaxant (lasts 5 minutes). Acts by **mimicking acetylcholine** but it is hydrolysed much more slowly than acetylcholine, so a **depolarizing block** occurs as the muscle becomes refractory. The depolarization is the reason that this drug causes **twitching** in patients. Its action cannot be reversed. It does not compete with acetylcholine for the receptor.

Vecuronium and atracurium

Derivatives of curare from the poison arrow frog. They are **long-acting muscle relaxants** and act by antagonizing the action of acetylcholine (competitively) through action on its receptor. They **do not produce depolarizing block** so they **can be reversed**.

Muscle relaxants aid the surgeon and the anaesthetist in **control of the airway** and **muscle tone** of the patient, allowing the inspection of the abdominal contents and the **closure of a laparotomy without undue tension**, and also allowing the abdominal contents to fall back into the wound.

Neostigmine

An **acetylcholinesterase inhibitor**, neostigmine is applied when reversal of long-acting block is desired. The resulting increased acetylcholine competes with these agents for the receptor, relieving the block. It causes prolonged (4-hour) **gut contraction** and **bradycardia** (acetylcholine excess) so **atropine** (muscarinic blocker, parasympathetic effect) is given in combination with it.

↑ **Example viva question**

What is the molecular basis of myasthenia gravis and how is it diagnosed?

Antibody-mediated **destruction of acetylcholine receptors.**

This results in **weakness** and **fatiguability** of skeletal muscle (e.g. fatiguable ptosis of eyelid clinically on prolonged upward gaze).

Edrophonium (Tensilon) is a **short-acting acetylcholinesterase inhibitor**, and its administration briefly reverses the weakness, by increasing the amount of available acetylcholine in the neuromuscular junction. This is used as a diagnostic tool.

Thymectomy can be curative.

---

99 Oxygen transport

Related Topics

Topic	Chapter	Page
Acid–base balance	84	349
Starling's law of the heart and cardiovascular equations	102	403
Intubation and ventilation	114	470

HAEMOGLOBIN: THE MOLECULE

- Each molecule consists of **four** subunits (two α, two β), bound to a central Fe^{2+} ion
- Each subunit consists of a molecular group called **haem,** and a polypeptide chain called **globin**
- Oxygen binds reversibly to haemoglobin; 97 per cent of oxygen in the blood is carried this way, the remainder being dissolved
- Each subunit binds **one** oxygen molecule (each molecule binds four oxygen molecules)
- Once one oxygen molecule has bound to the haemoglobin molecule, this **increases the affinity of the other sites for oxygen** via a change in conformation of the haemoglobin structure
- Haemoglobin also carries **carbon dioxide**, by combining reversibly with it to form **carbaminohaemoglobin**, although the majority of CO_2 combines with H_2O to form H^+ and HCO_3^- (see 'Acid–base balance', Chapter 84, page 349); a small proportion is dissolved
- Haemoglobin may also combine reversibly with H^+ **ions** and buffer them
- It combines irreversibly with carbon monoxide to form **carboxyhaemoglobin**, which is then no longer of any use for oxygen transport

- **Carbon monoxide** has a much higher affinity for haemoglobin than oxygen; this is why carbon monoxide is so toxic
- **Fetal haemoglobin** has a higher affinity for oxygen than adult Hb, because the globin chains are different (has two δ rather than β subunits)
- Point mutations can occur, resulting in abnormal types of haemoglobin such as HbS (sickle cell).

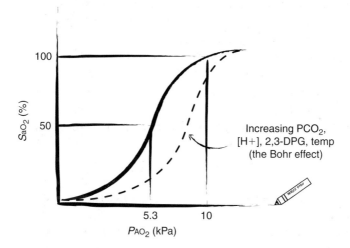

Figure 99.1

The relationship between arterial Po_2 (the partial pressure of oxygen in the blood) and oxygen saturation (percentage of haemoglobin molecules carrying oxygen) is a **sigmoid-shaped** curve (Fig. 99.1).

The steep part of the curve corresponds to the fact that binding subsequent O_2 molecules becomes easier after binding the first one and enables easy oxygenation for small increases in Po_2 as described above.

It also enables the haemoglobin to be released at low partial pressures of oxygen (as in the tissues).

CHANGES IN AFFINITY FOR OXYGEN

The curve is shifted to the right in conditions that decrease its affinity for oxygen (it takes a higher Po_2 to produce the same saturation) – dotted curve on Fig. 99.1.

Such conditions include:

- Increasing **CO_2 concentration**
- Increasing **DPG concentration**
- Increasing **acidity**
- Increasing **temperature**.

↑ **Example viva question**

What factors shift the curve to the right?

This list may be difficult to remember under pressure. The way to remember it is to remember that in the tissues, where the oxygen is to be offloaded, the affinity of haemoglobin for oxygen needs to be reduced. So an increased temperature (respiring tissue), acidity (lactic acidosis), CO_2 concentration (produced by the tissues) and DPG (also produced by the tissues) would all be expected to produce such a change.

Note that the fetal haemoglobin curve lies to the left of the adult curve because its affinity for oxygen is higher as it takes oxygen away from maternal blood.

↑ **Example viva question**

What factors determine oxygen delivery to the tissues?

This is determined by the oxygen delivery equation:

$$Do_2 \propto [Hb] \times Sao_2 \times CO \times 1.34$$

1.34 = no. of millilitres of O_2 carried by 1 g Hb
Do_2 = oxygen delivery
CO = cardiac output

This is a useful equation to write in an exam, when faced with a hypoxic patient to manage.

Improving any of the constituents of the equation will improve the patient.

Cardiac output in surgical patient can often be improved by giving intravenous fluid (see Starling's law of the heart and cardiovascular equations' Chapter 102, page 403).

Oxygen saturation can be improved by putting the patient on high-flow oxygen (see 'Control of respiration', Chapter 91, page 373).

The concentration of Hb may be improved by transfusion (remember that the oxygen-carrying capacity of stored blood is limited).

---

100 Pituitary

Possible viva questions related to this topic

→ How is the pituitary functionally and anatomically divided?
→ What hormones does the pituitary secrete?
→ How is pituitary secretion controlled?
→ What is Sheehan's syndrome?
→ What are the physiological effects of hypophysectomy? What hormone replacements are necessary?
→ How does the pituitary gland develop?
→ Describe the pituitary portal system.

PITUITARY ANATOMY

The pituitary is divided, functionally and anatomically, into **anterior** and **posterior.** The anterior part is also called the **adenohypophysis**, derived embryologically from Rathke's pouch – pharyngeal epithelium. The posterior part or **neurohypophysis** is derived from hypothalamic tissue.

The pituitary stalk is called the **infundibulum.** It lies in the **pituitary fossa** and is inferior to the **hypothalamus**.

The posterior pituitary consists of nerve terminals. The cell bodies of these nerves are in the **paraventricular** and **supraoptic** nuclei of the hypothalamus, and this is where the hormones are synthesized before release.

The anterior pituitary cells themselves synthesize hormones, which are under the control of releasing hormones synthesized by the hypothalamus and released into the portal system of capillaries (see 'Portal vein and portosystemic anastomoses', Chapter 14, page 39).

The **optic chiasm** lies immediately anterior to the infundibulum. Tumours of the pituitary affect the central fibres within the chiasma, producing a **bitemporal hemianopia**.

HORMONE SECRETION

Anterior pituitary				
Hormone	**Site of action**	**Action**	**Controlling influence**	**Pathologies**
Growth hormone (GH)	Liver Peripheral tissues	Hyperglycaemia Secretion of insulin growth factor I (IGF-I), which stimulates growth of unfused bone Several anabolic metabolic functions	GHRH secreted by the hypothalamus is excitatory and somatostatin is inhibitory	Acromegaly (epiphyses fused) Gigantism Dwarfism
Thyroid-stimulating hormone (TSH)	Thyroid gland	Promotes secretion of thyroxine (T_4) and triiodothyronine (T_3) by the thyroid, and increases their synthesis	Thyroid-releasing hormone (TRH) secreted by hypothalamus T_3 and T_4 feed back negatively on the pituitary	Hyper- and hypothyroidism
Prolactin	Breast	Promotes breast development and milk production	Dopamine produced by the hypothalamus has an inhibitory effect	Prolactinoma
Adreno-corticotrophic hormone (ACTH)	Adrenal cortex (zona fasciculata)	Promotes secretion of cortisol	CRH (corticotrophin-releasing hormone) and negative feed-back by cortisol	Cushing's disease, Addison's disease
Follicle-stimulating hormone (FSH) and luteinizing hormone (LH)	Gonads	Promotes secretion of oestrogen and progesterone in the female, in a cyclical fashion (menstrual cycle) and testosterone in the male	Gonadotrophin-releasing hormone (GnRH) by the hypothalamus and complex feedback mechanisms by their target hormones	

Posterior pituitary				
Hormone	**Site of action**	**Action**	**Controlling influence**	**Pathology**
Vasopressin (antidiuretic hormone or ADH)	Collecting duct of the nephron	Water retention	Its release is increased by increased tonicity of blood (dehydration), which is sensed by the lamina terminalis and the neurons themselves	Syndrome of inappropriate ADH secretion (SIADH), diabetes insipidus
Oxytocin	Uterus Collecting duct of the nephron	Initiation of parturition/ uterine contraction	Neural inputs from stretch receptors in uterus	
	Smooth muscle cells in breast	Milk secretion Water retention	Neural inputs from suckling child (breast) – milk ejection reflex	

IMPORTANT PATHOLOGIES

This section is not exhaustive.

Hypopituitarism

Causes

Hypophysectomy, pituitary adenoma, irradiation, Sheehan's syndrome – pituitary infarction following postpartum haemorrhage. Symptoms related to lack of hormones:

- Gonadotrophin: amenorrhoea, osteoporosis, loss of libido
- Corticosteroid: tiredness, postural hypotension, weight loss, hyponatraemia
- Androgen: impotence, loss of muscle and hair.
- Thyroid: constipation, weight gain, (hypothyroidism).

Diagnosis

Hormone levels (paired T_4/TSH; Synacthen test).

Treatment

Hormone replacement – hydrocortisone, T_4, testosterone/oestrogen and GH.

Pituitary tumours

Almost always benign adenomas; 35 per cent secrete prolactin, 20 per cent GH, 30 per cent non-functioning.

- Signs/symptoms: bitemporal hemianopia, hypopituitarism (above), headache
- Diagnosis: hormone tests and magnetic resonance imaging

- Treatment: dopamine agonists may shrink tumour; hypophysectomy (trans-sphenoidal versus open); radiotherapy (usually for remnants or if unfit for surgery).

Cushing's syndrome

Called Cushing's disease if secondary (pituitary ACTH hypersecretion).

Can be caused by adrenal cortical tumours (cortisol secreting) or ectopic ACTH secretion (e.g. small-cell lung cancer), or iatrogenic (steroids).

- Signs/symptoms: glucocorticoid excess: weight gain with truncal obesity, muscle weakness, depression, thin skin and bruising, hyperglycaemia
- Diagnosis: dexamethasone suppression test (to diagnose Cushing's syndrome); CT/magnetic resonance imaging (MRI) of adrenals/pituitary (localization) and chest radiograph; inferior petrosal sinus sampling
- Treatment: adrenalectomy for tumours; hypophysectomy for pituitary lesions.

Acromegaly

Caused by hypersecretion of GH from a pituitary tumour.

- Signs/symptoms: as for pituitary tumour (above), proximal myopathy, carpal tunnel syndrome, overgrowth of bones (prognathism, prominent supraorbital ridges, large spade-shaped hands)
- Diagnosis:
  - clinical to an extent, review past photographs as well as physical examination
  - oral glucose tolerance test
  - CT/MRI of pituitary
- Treatment: hypophysectomy ± radiotherapy.

101 Starling forces in the capillaries/oedema

Related topics		
Topic	**Chapter**	**Page**
Mastectomy, axillary dissections and breast reconstruction	36	120
Acute inflammation	45	161

STARLING FORCES IN THE CAPILLARIES

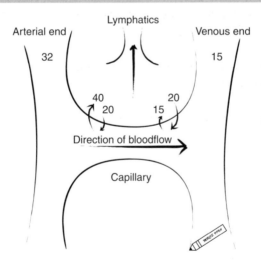

Figure 101.1

Figure 101.1 can be drawn in any viva question asking to explain the Starling forces in the capillaries or mechanism for formation of oedema. Explanation of Fig. 101.1:

- Blood flows from the arterial end, through the capillary, to the venous end
- The **hydrostatic pressure** (generated by the pressure from the left ventricle) at the arterial end is obviously higher

- At the arterial end of the capillary (1), which is leaky to fluid, the **hydrostatic pressure exceeds** the **colloid oncotic pressure** (this is the osmotic pull of the large molecules in the blood, pulling any fluid pushed into the interstitial space by hydrostatic pressure back into the capillary). Net movement of water here is out of the capillary into the interstitial space
- At the venous end of the capillary (2), the **colloid oncotic** pressure now **exceeds** the **hydrostatic pressure** and water is pulled back into the capillary. Hence the Starling 'filtration–reabsorption' forces.

Any excess fluid in the interstitial space goes into the lymphatic system and is returned to the circulation.

OEDEMA

The various causes of oedema can be explained using Fig. 101.1.

Increased *leakiness of capillaries*
- Occurs in burns, sepsis or acute respiratory disease syndrome (ARDS).

Increased *hydrostatic pressure* at the *venous end*
- This leads to increased hydrostatic pressure throughout the capillary and more net movement of fluid into the interstitial space
- Occurs in DVT, venous hypertension (which often accompanies varicose veins and ulcers), pelvic venous compression (by tumour), liver cirrhosis, renal cell carcinoma infiltration and right-sided heart failure.

Decreased *colloid oncotic pressure*
- Basically any cause of hypoalbuminaemia
- Liver failure (lack of synthesis), increased loss: nephrotic syndrome, protein-losing enteropathies, poor nutrition, etc.

Failure of *lymphatic system* to drain = *lymphoedema*
- Primary lymphoedema (unknown aetiology)
- Secondary lymphoedema: damage of the lymphatic system caused by surgery (especially breast), radiotherapy or carcinoma.

Note that hypertension at the arterial end, according to this model, might be expected to generate oedema, but does not.

102 Starling's law of the heart and cardiovascular equations

Possible viva questions related to this topic

→ What is the effect on blood pressure of losing a litre of blood? What mechanisms compensate?

→ What are the immediate cardiovascular effects of cross-clamping the aorta in an aneurysm repair?

→ What are the cardiovascular effects of amputating the right leg?

→ What are the cardiovascular effects of standing up from a lying position?

→ Why would an anaesthetist be worried about a patient in heart block?

→ What are the cardiovascular effects of a Valsalva manoeuvre?

↑ Key learning point

This section will come up in some guise in almost every physiology and critical care viva, and can be applied to all of the above questions. This topic will provide a methodical approach to tackling such questions.

IMPORTANT RESTING VALUES

Stroke volume (SV): the amount of blood ejected by the left ventricle in one cardiac cycle (70 mL).

Cardiac output (CO): the amount of blood ejected by the heart in 1 minute. If resting heart rate is also taken at 70: 70 × 70 = 4900, which is near enough 5000 or 5 L.

IMPORTANT RELATIONSHIPS

$$BP = CO \times SVR \text{ (Ohm's law)} \tag{1}$$

$$CO = SV \times HR \tag{2}$$

where SVR is systemic vascular resistance, HR heart rate and BP blood pressure.

↑ **Key learning point**

On any question related to this topic, start by writing these equations out on the paper provided and use them to explain the physiology and responses (see examples below).

DETERMINANTS OF CARDIAC OUTPUT

Cardiac output is determined by three determinants: **preload, contractility** and **afterload** on the heart.

Preload is determined by **Starling's law of the heart** (see below).

Contractility is affected by disease, which affects the heart muscle or mechanics; pathologies such as myocardial infarction, cardiomyopathy and pericardial effusion will affect this. **Sympathetic activity** also increases contractility.

Afterload is determined by increased **blood pressure** or SVR or such pathologies as aortic stenosis.

STARLING'S LAW OF THE HEART

Definition

The relationship between left ventricular end-diastolic volume (LVEDV) and stroke volume (SV) in the heart, as shown in Fig. 102.1, which illustrates the relationship between **LVEDV** and **SV**.

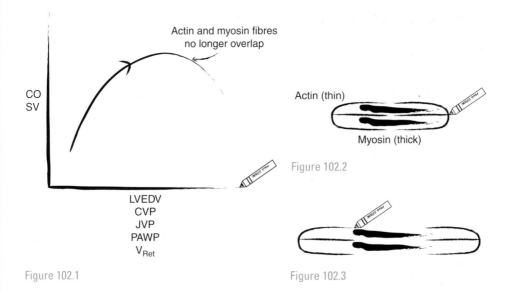

Figure 102.1

Figure 102.2

Figure 102.3

At low values of LVEDV, the **amount ejected** by the heart (SV) is **proportional** to the degree that the actin and myosin fibres are stretched by the blood returning to the heart. (Figure 102.2 shows one sarcomere: the myosin fibres are thick and the actin is thin).

> ↑ **Key learning point**
>
> Actin rhymes with thin

At the point at which the interdigitating fibres of actin and myosin in cardiac muscle **no longer overlap** (Fig. 102.3, see arrow in Fig. 102.1), increasing LVEDV no longer causes an increase in SV. This is because there are no longer strong **cross-bridges** between the actin and myosin.

CO is **SV in a unit time** and the two are proportional, the **relationship between CO and LVEDV** produces a **similar graph**.

Similarly, **central venous pressure (CVP)** and jugular venous pressure **(JVP)** are measures of, and proportional to, **LVEDV**, as is pulmonary artery wedge pressure **(PAWP)**, so any of these could be placed on the x axis (as above). The importance of this will become clear in the discussion below.

Figure 102.4 illustrates the effects of certain treatments on this curve, a commonly asked MRCS viva question.

Intravenous fluid will increase the venous return, or JVP or CVP, so will move you along Starling's curve (see arrow).

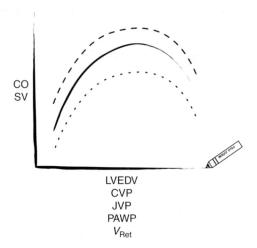

Figure 102.4

Inotropes increase the **contractility** of the heart. Giving an inotrope (or sympathetic activation), or **decreasing the afterload** by giving a **vasodilator** such as **GTN**, will move the patient to a **higher curve** (dashed line in Fig. 102.4), because the same preload will now result in more blood ejected (or a higher stroke volume).

β Blockers or treatments that **antagonize the sympathetic nervous system** will move the patient to a **lower Starling's curve** (dotted line in Fig. 102.4) for the opposite reason.

↑ **Example viva question**

What are the cardiovascular effects of cross-clamping the aorta in AAA repair?

1. CO = SV × HR
2. BP = CO × SVR

TPR increases markedly, pushing up blood pressure (2)
To compensate, there is a reflex **bradycardia** to reduce **CO** and hence **BP** (1)

Example viva question

What happens to your capillaries when you stand up/perform a Valsalva manoeuvre?

1. $CO = SV \times HR$
2. $BP = CO \times SVR$
3. Draw Starling's curve

Standing up leads to pooling of blood, and a decrease in **venous return**

This leads to a decrease in **SV** and hence **CO** (Starling's curve)

This leads to a decrease in **BP** (2)

This drop in **BP** is sensed by the **baroreceptors** (see 'Blood pressure control', Chapter 87, page 358) and there is a reflex **constriction of the capillaries** and **arterioles** to maintain **BP** as the **CO** component of Eqn (2) has dropped. There is also a **reflex tachycardia** (1), and an **increase** in **contractility** caused by sympathetic activation of the heart.

A Valsalva manoeuvre (forced expiration against a closed glottis) causes increased intrathoracic pressure and hence a **decrease in venous return** as above.

Example viva question

Why would an anaesthetist be worried about a patient with heart block?

1. $CO = SV \times HR$
2. $BP = CO \times SVR$
3. Draw Starling's curve

This question needs lateral thinking.

Induction agents cause vasodilatation and a decrease in **SVR** (2)

This causes the **BP** to drop (2)

To maintain reflexly the BP the **SV and HR** need to increase (1), but the **heart block prevents a reflex tachycardia.**

See also 'Blood pressure control' Chapter 87, page 358 for discussion of the effects of haemorrhage.

103 Swallowing and oesophageal physiology

Possible viva questions related to this topic

→ What is the sequence of events in swallowing?
→ What sphincteric mechanisms are there in the lower oesophagus and how is reflux normally prevented?
→ How is reflux investigated?

SWALLOWING

Oral phase

- Food is chewed and a bolus is formed, which is pushed to the posterior pharynx by the **tongue**
- Here, afferent impulses in cranial nerves IX and X are transmitted to the **swallowing centre** (medulla), which reflexly triggers swallowing via efferent impulses in cranial nerves IX and X
- **Respiration** is also reflexly **inhibited**.

Pharyngeal phase

- The **soft palate is pulled upward** and **palatopharyngeus** helps to close the nasopharynx and prevent reflux
- The **true vocal folds** are apposed and the **larynx elevates**. The bolus pushes against the **epiglottis** to close the entrance to the respiratory tract and prevent aspiration
- **Upper oesophageal sphincter (cricopharyngeus muscle)** relaxes
- The **constrictor muscles** (superior, middle, inferior) sequentially contract and force the bolus down into the oesophagus.

Oesophageal phase

- Bolus is propelled along the oesophagus by a **primary peristaltic wave** behind the bolus

CRITICAL CARE

104 Acute pancreatitis

Possible viva questions related to this topic

→ What is pancreatitis?
→ What are the clinical features of pancreatitis?
→ What are the possible causes of pancreatitis?
→ How would you manage pancreatitis?
→ What are the complications of pancreatitis?
→ What scoring systems do you know of for pancreatitis and what use are they?
→ How useful is serum amylase in the diagnosis of acute pancreatitis?
→ What are the most important bedside tests in the context of pancreatitis?
→ What is a pancreatic pseudocyst?

Clinical features

- Acute, severe **abdominal pain**; usually **constant, epigastric** and **radiating into the back**, and relieved by sitting forwards
- **Vomiting** is early and profuse
- **Patient usually shocked** with rapid pulse, cyanosis
- **Abnormal temperature**: either subnormal or pyrexial
- Examination of the abdomen reveals **generalized tenderness** and usually **guarding** with or without rebound
- **30 per cent of cases** have **mild jaundice** as a result of oedema of the pancreatic head obstructing the common bile duct
- After a severe attack, patient may develop a bluish discoloration in the loins from extravasation of blood-stained pancreatic juice into the retroperitoneum (**Grey Turner's sign**)

↑ **Example viva question**

What is pancreatitis?

Acute pancreatitis: **acute inflammation** of the **pancreas** is a common cause of **acute abdominal pain** with considerable associated morbidity and mortality. It can be divided into mild, moderate and severe, depending on presentation.

A mnemonic to remember the causes of pancreatitis is **GET SMASHED**:

G: **gallstones** (probably the **most common cause**, impacted at the ampulla of Vater and causing backwash of activated pancreatic enzymatic juice into the parenchyma of the pancreas, leading to pancreatic autolysis and haemorrhage)

E: **ethanol** (alcohol is a very common cause of pancreatitis and people with alcohol problems often develop chronic pancreatitis after a number of bouts acutely)

T: **trauma**

S: **steroids**

M: **mumps** (paramyxoviruses)

A: **autoimmune** (panarteritis nodosa or PAN, systemic lupus erythematosus or SLE)

S: **scorpion** sting/snake bite!!

H: **hypercalcaemia**, hyperlipidaemia/hypertriglyceridaemia and hypothermia

E: **ERCP (endoscopic retrograde cholangiopancreatography)**

D: **drugs** (e.g. sulphonamides, frusemide, azathioprine, non-steroidal anti-inflammatory drugs or NSAIDs)

Less common causes: carcinoma of the head of pancreas, pancreas divisum, long common bile duct, fat necrosis, pregnancy, pancreatic ischaemia as a result of bypass surgery.

- Bluish discoloration and bruising may occur in the periumbilical region (**Cullen's sign**).

Investigations

Tests **confirm the diagnosis** and utilize the criteria below to **determine the severity**. In addition to arterial blood gases and venous sampling for amylase, liver function tests (LFTs), full blood count (FBC) and urea and electrolytes (U+Es):

- **ECG: flattened T waves** or arrhythmias may cause confusion with cardiac ischaemia.

- **Abdominal radiograph**: not usually helpful in acute pancreatitis but can show **pancreatic calcification** in cases of acute-on-**chronic pancreatitis**. In some cases a '**sentinel loop**' of proximal jejunum may be seen to be dilated.
- **Erect chest radiograph** to exclude a perforation, which can present in a similar manner.
- **Ultrasonography**: may show gallstones and/or dilated common bile duct and pancreatic duct. Often gives poor views of the pancreas. Good for looking for collections in the acute setting – can also be used to look for pleural effusions.
- **Abdominal computed tomography (CT)** is the **investigation of choice** for acute pancreatitis but is not usually **performed before 48 hours** of onset of the episode. Diagnostically, **fat streaking** is seen around the pancreas or fluid may be seen in the lesser sac, and this may be confirmatory in cases where the serum amylase is normal. Further, **later imaging** may reveal **necrosis** in the pancreas or the **formation of a pancreatic pseudocyst**.
- **Serum calcium**: may well be lowered as a result of fat saponification, and may lead to **tetany** and **cardiac arrhythmias** in severe cases.

ASSESSMENT OF PANCREATITIS SEVERITY

It is **essential to perform arterial blood gas sampling** in all patients with pancreatitis to assess their **acid–base status** (see 'Acid–base balance', Chapter 84, page 349) and to keep a regular check on their arterial P_{O_2}. **Serum amylase** is used as a diagnostic criterion but, in **10 per cent of cases**, it is **normal**, particularly in **acute-on-chronic pancreatitis**, where there is a loss of acinar cell mass, or in severe pancreatitis with pancreatic necrosis.

Scoring systems: two very well-known and used methods are the **Ranson** and the **Glasgow** criteria.

Glasgow criteria for severe pancreatitis

The following criteria are assessed over the first 48 hours. Three or more indicate severe pancreatitis with a high mortality:

- **Age > 55** years
- Hyperglycaemia (**glucose > 10 mmol/L** in the absence of a history of diabetes)
- **Leukocytosis** ($> 15 \times 10^9/L$)
- **Urea > 16 mmol/L** after adequate rehydration
- $P_{O_2} < 8$ kPa on arterial blood gases
- **Calcium < 2.0 mmol/L**
- **Albumin < 32 g/L**
- **Lactate dehydrogenase (LDH) > 600 IU/L**
- Raised **aspartate transaminase (AST) > 100 IU/L**.

Ranson's criteria for pancreatitis

Ranson's criteria on admission

- Age > **55 years**
- White blood cell count (WCC) > **16 000/μL**
- Glucose > **11 mmol/L** (> 200 mg/dL)
- Serum **LDH > 400 IU/L**
- Serum **AST > 250 IU/L**.

Ranson's criteria after 48 hours of admission:

- **Fall in haematocrit** by more than **10 per cent**
- **Fluid sequestration** of > **6 L**
- **Hypocalcaemia** (serum calcium < 1.0 mmol/L (< 8.0 mg/dL))
- Hypoxaemia (PO_2 < 80 mmHg)
- **Increase in urea** to > 1.98 mmol/L (> 5 mg/dL) after intravenous fluid hydration
- **Hypoalbuminaemia** (albumin < 32 g/L (< 3.2 g/dL) in the first 48 hours of admission
- **Base deficit of > 4**.

The prognostic implications of Ranson's criteria are as follows:

Score 0–2: 2 per cent mortality rate
Score 3–4: 15 per cent mortality rate
Score 5–6: 40 per cent mortality rate
Score 7–8: 100 per cent mortality rate.

PATHOPHYSIOLOGY OF MARKERS OF SEVERITY

- **Hypoxia**: a result of acute respiratory distress syndrome (**ARDS**) and **pleural effusions**.
- **Hypocalcaemia**: calcium is **chelated** after the **saponfication** of **omental fat** by pancreatic lipases.
- **Acidosis: anaerobic respiration** of tissues as a result of poor perfusion leads to a lactic acidosis.
- **High urea**: reflects **dehydration**.
- **High WCC**: acute inflammatory response and probable **pancreatic necrosis ±** supervening **bacterial infection**.

TREATMENT

This is largely **conservative** and **non-surgical** but **aggressive**, consisting of:

- **Fluid resuscitation** and replacement with either **colloid or blood** transfusion to **treat profound shock** that can result from acute pancreatitis. Electrolyte replacement is often required, with particular attention to **potassium** and **calcium** if necessary. All patients should be **catheterized** and a **urometer should be used** to produce a strict record of **hourly urine output**. Fluid sequestration can be very severe in acute pancreatitis, requiring **many litres of fluid replacement** to keep up. It is not uncommon for **initial resuscitation volumes** of an individual with acute pancreatitis to be of the order of **10–15 L** over **several hours**.

- **Analgesia**: pain relief with **pethidine commonly**. Morphine is said to produce sphincter of Oddi spasm but there is little evidence to support this theory. Patient-controlled analgesia (PCA) can be useful in this context.
- **Antibiotics**: if profound **pyrexia, positive blood cultures** or associated with **gallstones**. Antibiotic of choice is **imipenem** (very broad spectrum with good Gram-negative cover). Some centres use a second-generation cephalosporin and metronidazole. Many clinicians will put all patients with acute pancreatitis on antibiotics.
- **Pancreas is rested** by making the patient **nil by mouth** with a low threshold for **nasogastic aspiration** to prevent vomiting. The bowel is also rested because acute pancreatitis often results in a generalized ileus.
- **Early liaison with the intensive therapy unit (ITU)** to ensure that smooth handover can occur if ventilatory support or inotropic support is required.
- **H_2-receptor prophylaxis** many be used in the stomach with ranitidine or a proton pump inhibitor (PPI).
- **ERCP ± sphincterotomy** performed **early improves outcome** in the case of proven impacted gallstones at the ampulla. (Note that ERCP can itself worsen or cause pancreatitis.)
- **Surgery** for the **drainage** of an **abscess** or **pseudocyst**. **Exploratory laparotomy** in the context of acute pancreatitis **massively increases mortality and should be avoided**.
- **Late necrosectomy** for débridement of a necrotic pancreas is sometimes required in very severe cases.
- **Nutrition**: **total parenteral nutrition** (see 'Nutrition', Chapter 115, page 477) is instituted in severe cases, although there is a move towards **early enteral feeding wherever possible**. Drugs to reduce pancreatic secretion or enzyme activation are of no proven benefit.
- After an attack of pancreatitis secondary to gallstones, **cholecystectomy is advised** as an elective interval procedure.

COMPLICATIONS

These can be systemic or regional.

Systemic

- Death

- **ARDS** and acute lung injury (see 'Acute respiratory distress syndrome', Chapter 105, page 419)
- **Renal failure** and/or **multiple organ dysfunction syndrome (MODS)** (see 'Sepsis and SIRS', Chapter 121, page 505).

Regional

- **Abscess formation**: seen best on abdominal CT with contrast; associated with persistently raised WCC and swinging pyrexia
- **Pseudocyst**: persistently raised amylase and pain, usually in the second week, presenting as an epigastric mass
- **Gastrointestinal bleeding**: acute gastric erosions or peptic ulceration
- **Splenic artery pseudoaneurysm** formation
- **Venous thrombosis**: splenic vein, superior mesenteric vein, portal vein
- **Diabetes mellitus** as a result of β-islet cell destruction.

105 Acute respiratory distress syndrome

Example viva question

What is the definition of ARDS?

ARDS is a **clinical syndrome** of **acute respiratory failure** with **non-cardiogenic pulmonary oedema** leading to decreased lung compliance and hypoxaemia **refractory to oxygen therapy**. It is characterized by:

- **Diffuse pulmonary infiltrates** seen on chest radiograph
- A **normal** pulmonary artery **wedge pressure** (PAWP < 18 mmHg) – important for excluding pulmonary oedema secondary to elevated left atrial pressure
- PaO_2/FiO_2 ratio of < 26.6 kPa

DEFINITION OF LUNG COMPLIANCE

This is the **change in volume of the lung per unit change in pressure**; thus a lung with low compliance will need greater pressure to inflate it than a highly compliant lung.

CLINICAL FEATURES

- Dyspnoea
- Tachypnoea and increased work of breathing
- Hypoxia
- Bilateral diffuse infiltrates on chest radiograph
- No clinical evidence of a raised left atrial pressure.

CAUSES

- Sepsis
- Multiple trauma
- Aspiration
- Fat embolism
- Chest injury
- Burns (both skin and airway)
- Pancreatitis
- Massive transfusion
- Disseminated intravascular coagulation (DIC)
- Cardiopulmonary bypass.

PATHOLOGY

ARDS can be considered to be the **respiratory component** to the multiorgan effects of the **systemic inflammatory response syndrome or SIRS** (see 'Sepsis and SIRS', Chapter 121, page 505). An **acute inflammatory response** is seen with an **immediate exudative phase,** involving **activated neutrophils** and **activated macrophages** secreting a number of **cytokine** mediators of acute inflammation, including interleukin 6 (Il-6), tumour necrosis factor α (TNFα), proteases, prostaglandins and oxygen radicals. In turn, the **complement system is activated** along with local activation of the **clotting cascades.** This increases capillary permeability by local endothelial injury, manifesting as a decrease of **type II pneumocytes** and reduced pulmonary surfactant production. This **reduces lung compliance** further by increasing the force required to open the alveoli.

A **proliferative phase** is seen some days later with a hyperplasia of both type II pneumocytes and the local fibroblast population, leading to a **progressive interstitial fibrosis**. This may **persist** even **after** the patient has **recovered**.

These pathological changes result in:

- **Decreased lung compliance** increasing work of breathing
- Increased local atelectasis leading to **reduced functional residual capacity**
- **Increased shunt** and ventilation–perfusion ($\dot{V}$/Q) mismatch
- **Increased pulmonary vascular resistance**, as a result of **pulmonary oedema compressing the vessels**, and **local vasoconstriction**, as a reaction to **localized hypoxia**, in an effort to **improve the $\dot{V}$/Q mismatch**
- **Pulmonary hypertension** can lead to right heart dysfunction.

PRINCIPLES OF MANAGEMENT

- **Transfer to ITU**
- **Management of the initial** causative factor (if known)
- Nutritional support (see 'Nutrition', Chapter 115, page 477)
- **Mechanical ventilation** to aid in **oxygenation**, decrease the work of breathing for the patient and **improve the clearance of CO$_2$. High levels** of positive end-expiratory pressure (**PEEP**) can be used to **splint open the stiff alveoli** to prevent collapse during the respiratory cycle and **improve alveolar recruitment**. Note that high **PEEP increases the risk** of alveolar **barotrauma**
- **Reversed inspiratory:expiratory (I:E) ratios** to **increase inspiratory phase** at the expense of the expiratory phase (may allow a moderate degree of hypercapnia)
- **Prone ventilation: redistributes secretions, minimizes basal atelectasis** with regular turning and **improves $\dot{V}$/Q mismatch**, thereby improving oxygenation
- **Strict fluid management – low threshold for monitoring PAWP** (using **Swan–Ganz catheterization**) and ensure that patient does not develop cardiogenic pulmonary oedema as a result of fluid overload
- Others: inhaled **prostacyclin**, **nitrous oxide** and **steroids** may be of help but are **unproven**.

PROGNOSIS

Outcome usually **poor**:

- **50–60 per cent mortality rate** overall
- 90 per cent mortality rate if associated with sepsis.

Morbidity can be a considerable problem with **progressive interstitial fibrosis** and **pulmonary hypertension** being relatively common sequelae of ARDS.

↑ **Example viva question**

What is the role of decreased surfactant and inhaled nitric oxide in ARDS?

Surfactant: there are, to date, no randomized controlled trials showing a mortality benefit from the administration of exogenous surfactant in the adult population. There are, however, a number of case series of its **successful use in the neonatal population**.

Nitric oxide: in theory, **inhaled nitric oxide** acts as a **potent local pulmonary vasodilator**, improving perfusion to better-ventilated areas of lung. There is, however, **no class 1 evidence** to show any mortality benefit from its use.

106 Brain-stem death and transplantation

Possible viva questions related to this topic

→ What is brain-stem death?
→ Why is brain-stem function important for life?
→ Why it is an important concept?
→ How is brain-stem death diagnosed?
→ What medical criteria need to be satisfied in order for a diagnosis of brain-stem death to be valid?
→ Who can diagnose brain-stem death?
→ When should these cases be referred to the coroner?
→ What is the pathway to organ explantation and harvesting?
→ What is a persistent vegetative state? Does it constitute brain-stem death?

Related topics		
Topic	Chapter	Page
Renal transplantation	40	140

With the advent of transplantation medicine, brain-stem death has become an important economic and resource-based concept, although the diagnosis also gives important prognostic information to the relatives and treating doctors.

Example viva question

What is brain stem death?

The Department of Health working party on brain-stem death in 1998 defined it in these terms:

'... irreversible loss of the capacity for consciousness, combined with irreversible loss of the capacity to breathe. The irreversible cessation of brain stem function (brain stem death) whether induced by intra-cranial events or the result of extra-cranial phenomena, such as hypoxia, will produce this clinical state and therefore brain stem death equates with the death of the individual.'

WHY IS BRAIN-STEM FUNCTION IMPORTANT?

The brain stem includes nuclei controlling the body's major **homoeostatic mechanisms** including:

- **Respiratory centres**
- **Cardiovascular centres** (autonomics – particularly **vagus nerve** nuclei)
- **Arousal centres** (reticular activating system)
- + Cranial nerve nuclei IV–XII.

Loss of these nuclei is **incompatible with life.**

CRITERIA FOR BRAIN-STEM DEATH

All brain-stem reflexes are absent:

- **The pupils are fixed** and **do not respond to light** (mediated by cranial nerves II and III).
- There is **no corneal reflex** (sensory Va, motor VII cranial nerves).
- The **vestibulo-ocular reflexes** are **absent**. (No eye movements are seen during or following the slow injection of at least 50 mL of ice cold water over 1 minute into each external auditory meatus in turn.) **Clear access to the tympanic membrane must be established** by direct inspection and the head should be flexed at 30°.
- **No motor responses** within the cranial nerve distribution (**cranial nerves VII and Vc**) can be elicited by **adequate stimulation** of any **somatic area**. There is **no limb response to supraorbital pressure.**
- There is **no gag reflex (sensory IX, motor X cranial nerves)** or reflex response to bronchial stimulation by suction catheter placed down the trachea.
- **No respiratory movements** occur when the patient is **disconnected from the mechanical ventilator**. During this test it is necessary for the arterial CO_2 to exceed the threshold for respiratory stimulation, i.e. the $PaCO_2$ **should reach 6.65 kPa**. This should be ensured by measurement of the blood gases. If 6.65 kPa is not reached as the patient becomes anoxic the test must be stopped: brain-stem criteria are not met.

Note on the apnoea test

The patient may be moderately hypothermic, flaccid and with a depressed metabolic rate such that the $PaCO_2$ rises slowly during apnoea. **Hypoxia** during disconnection should be **prevented** by delivering oxygen at 6 L/min through a **catheter in the trachea**. The patient should **first be ventilated with 100 per cent oxygen** for **10 min, then** with **5 per cent CO_2 in O_2 for 5 min**. The ventilator should then be disconnected for 10 mins. During this period, O_2 should be delivered through a catheter at the carina.

Those patients with **pre-existing chronic respiratory disease**, who may be responsive only to supranormal levels of CO_2 and who depend upon hypoxic drive, are special cases who should be managed in consultation with an expert in respiratory disease.

A number of medical criteria must be satisfied before brain-stem death testing is deemed to be lawful and valid:

- **No sedation (barbiturates** and **benzodiazepines** can accumulate and **need to be stopped for some time** before brain-stem testing can begin)
- **No muscle relaxants** (this must be confirmed by the use of a standard **neuromuscular stimulator** on one of the limbs)
- Patient must be **normothermic** (hypothermia must be excluded)
- Patient must have **normal electrolyte levels** and be **normoglycaemic**
- **Decerebrate or decorticate posturing** is **incompatible** with brain-stem death although **true spinal-mediated reflexes** may be **compatible** with the diagnosis.

The **diagnosis** of brain-stem death should be made by at **least two medical practitioners** who have been **registered for more than 5 years**, are competent in this field and are **not members of the transplant team**; at least one of the doctors should be a consultant. **Two sets of tests should always be performed**; these may be carried out by the two practitioners **separately** or **together**.

The timing between these two sets of tests will vary according to the pathology in question and the individual situation but brain-stem death can be diagnosed only after two full sets of criteria have been met.

ORGAN TRANSPLANTATION

If the patient is deemed to be a potential organ donor then the **transplant coordinator** for the unit should be **contacted as soon as possible** after the diagnosis of brain-stem death. If they are contacted **before the diagnosis** is made, the **patient's relatives should be informed** of this. The **transplant coordinator** will ensure that **appropriate informed assent** is gained from the relatives and that all **virology, serology** and **tissue typing** is performed appropriately after this (see 'Renal transplantation', Chapter 40, page 140, for an example of this process).

DONOR CARDS

Although a **signed donor card** of the patient's intentions is, by law, **binding** and **overrides any concerns voiced by the relatives**, in practice organs are rarely harvested against the relative's wishes.

PATHWAY TO TRANSPLANTATION

- Brain-stem death diagnosed
- ± Coroner informed
- Transplant coordinator involved
- Relatives consulted
- Blood tests, virology and serology, and other screening tests
- Donor must be screened for malignancy including glioblastoma
- ± Surgical and anaesthetic interventions to assess viability of organs (e.g. Swan–Ganz catheterization is often performed if heart–lung or heart explantation is expected)
- Organ harvesting by dedicated transplant team (heart–lung last).

INFORMING THE CORONER

In any case where the cause of brain-stem death is not clearly the result of natural causes the coroner, coroner's officer or, in Scotland, the procurator fiscal must be consulted. The medical staff involved in the care of the patient ought to be the ones who contact the coroner if this is necessary, although the transplant coordinator is the person usually responsible for identifying who is in lawful possession of the body and for obtaining the necessary authorization for organ removal.

PERSISTENT VEGETATIVE STATE

This should on no account be confused with brain-stem death. This is a state where there is no evidence of higher brain function but brain-stem reflexes are intact. There is much controversy about the definition and prognosis of persistent vegetative state (PVS) and there are reports of PVS being at least partially reversible in the literature. Some functional brain studies have shown some of these patients to have higher brain activity as a result of somatic stimuli despite no outward clinical evidence of this.

107 Burns

Possible viva questions related to this topic

→ How would you determine the area of a burn?
→ How would you determine the thickness of a burn?
→ Which burns patients need intravenous fluid resuscitation?
→ What is Parkland's formula? How is it used?
→ Which burns patients need transfer to a regional burns centre?
→ How would you manage a patient with a 70 per cent burn?
→ What are the principles of escharotomy?
→ What are the complications of burns?
→ What sort of burns require skin grafting?

Related topics

Topic	Chapter	Page
Wound healing, scarring and reconstruction	83	342
Acute respiratory distress syndrome	105	419
Compartment syndrome	108	433
Skin grafting and flap reconstruction	78	320
Sepsis and SIRS	121	505

BURN THICKNESS

Burns can be **full thickness** or **partial thickness**. The thickness of a burn is determined by the level of the **dermis** affected. **Superficial partial-thickness** burns involve the epidermis and a thin layer of the dermis. **Deep dermal burns** are limited to, but not involving the entire thickness of the dermis, and **full-thickness burns** involve the entire thickness of the dermis and can also involve underlying structures.

Burn thickness	Characteristics
Superficial partial thickness	Blistering – note that erythema without blistering (e.g. mild sunburn) is NOT counted as a burn Colour – pink skin Capillary return – blanches and refills rapidly Pain – painful No fixed (non-blanching) staining of skin Soft skin
Deep dermal	Colour – pink skin Capillary return – blanches and refills Pain – painful Texture – soft skin Some fixed (non-blanching) staining in tissues
Full thickness	Colour – white or brown skin Capillary return – none. Skin does not change colour on pressure Pain – painless

AREA OF A BURN

Accurate assessment of the area of a burn (measured as percentage of total body surface area) is critical to acute burn management. There are three ways to determine the area:

1. Wallace's rule of 9s: the body is divided into seven zones, each of which is either 9 per cent or a multiple thereof. The head and each upper limb count as 9 per cent, the front of the torso, the back of the torso and each lower limb count as 18 per cent. The genital area is the final 1 per cent, bringing the total to 100 per cent.
2. Patient's hand: a quick and easy method of calculating relatively small burns is to use the patient's hand area. The area of the closed palm is approximately 1 per cent of the total body surface area.
3. Lund and Browder charts: these charts give the most accurate estimations of burn area. They also have the advantages of being able to correct for different age groups (children have age-dependent head and limb proportions), and they provide documentation of the burn for the patient's notes.

BURNS MANAGEMENT

First aid at the scene

- Ensure your and the patient's safety – remove any causative factors (e.g. chemical burns, electrical burns)

- Remove any overlying or affected clothes, which can trap heat close to the skin
- Cool the burn in cold, running water up to 2 hours post-burn (avoid iced water which can cause vasospasm and further compromise of perfusion).

Immediate management

Airway
Always check for signs of **airway burns or inhalational injury,** which can cause rapid and dramatic airway oedema. Have a **low threshold** for an early anaesthetic opinion and **intubation.** Mucosal oedema can occur up to 8 hours after the burn, so **re-assess** regularly. Risk factors include:

- History of fire in enclosed space
- Soot around nostrils, in nose or mouth
- Singeing of nasal hairs
- Carbonaceous sputum
- Hoarseness
- Stridor or wheeze
- Drooling
- COHb > 10 per cent.

Breathing
Ensure that adequate respiration can be achieved. Tracheal or pulmonary burns can impair effective gas exchange (see 'Acute respiratory distress syndrome', Chapter 105, page 419). Full-thickness **chest burns** can impede chest wall expansion – consider **escharotomy.**

Circulation
Fluid loss and shock are common in major burns. **Early intravenous fluid resuscitation** is essential in management of any significant burn.

Then the next stages are:

- **Remove** any precipitating cause: dilute a caustic or acid burn with water
- **Clean and cover** the burn: aqueous chlorhexidine wound toilet and a Clingfilm dressing
- Send blood for Hb, U+Es, albumin, COHb, blood gases, cross-match
- Beware of **hypothermia.**

Subsequent management and prognosis

- Goal is to **minimize scarring** and **contractures** causing loss of function:
  - scarring occurs if burnt skin has not **re-epithelialized by 2 weeks**
  - usually **partial-thickness** burns will **heal by 2 weeks** unless healing is delayed by infection or concurrent morbidity

- **Full-thickness** burns and non-healing partial thickness burns require **burn excision** down to healthy tissue
- Skin grafting may be required to cover areas of skin loss.

Late management

- Re-orientation of contractures to increase range of joint movement:
  - Z-plasties
  - local flaps
- Excision of contractures and reconstruction:
  - split-thickness skin grafting
  - tissue expansion
  - synthetic dermal grafting (Integra)
  - flap reconstruction.

INTRAVENOUS FLUID RESUSCITATION

Any burn **> 15 per cent in adults** or **> 10 per cent in children** requires intravenous fluid **resuscitation**. The most common algorithm for resuscitation is **Parkland's formula**.

↑ **Example viva question**

What is Parkland's formula? How is it used?

Parkland's formula

Volume of crystalloid required (mL) = 4 × % burn × Patient's weight (kg)

This gives the volume of crystalloid needed for resuscitation within the first 24 hours. **Half** is given in the first **8 hours** and **half** in the subsequent **16 hours**. **If time has elapsed** since the burn, initial fluid infusion rate should be increased to meet the **resuscitation deficit** rapidly. Close monitoring of **fluid balance is essential** in these patients (see 'Fluid balance', Chapter 111, page 452).

The **Muir and Barclay formula** was described for **albumin** as the resuscitation fluid. It tends to give **less fluid per unit time** than **Parkland's formula** favoured by the British Burns Association, and is now little used.

National Burns Care Review guidelines recommend that the following patients be transferred to a **burns centre** or **burns unit**:

- Adults with burns > 15 per cent or 10 per cent with dermal loss
- Children with burns > 5 per cent (note that not 10 per cent as required for fluid resuscitation)
- Burns at extremes of age

- Airway burns or patients at risk of airway obstruction
- Facial burns
- Perineal burns
- Hand or feet burns
- Burns requiring escharotomy
- Other **complex** burns (burns in patients with significant associated injuries or pre-existing medical conditions, chemical, radiation, high pressure or high tension electrical burns and burns of flexures, especially the neck)
- When non-accidental burn injuries are suspected
- EXCEPT when specialist management of the burn is redundant (moving a patient who will die from the burn away from friends and family causes unnecessary additional distress).

SPECIFIC CONSIDERATIONS

- **Acid or alkali** burns: copious water **irrigation** until the burn area reaches pH 7. Test repeatedly with appropriate litmus or universal indicator paper
- **Hydrofluoric acid** burns: apply **calcium gluconate** gel
- **Electric burns**: identify **entry** and **exit wounds** and consider that the entire tract between these points will be burnt. Severe internal organ burns can occur with even minor skin electrical burns

---

⬆ **Key learning point**

Escharotomy is the excision of burnt skin to relieve constriction.

It must be considered in **circumferential burns** or **chest wall burns** where constriction of overlying skin can cause **compartment syndrome** (see 'Compartment syndrome', Chapter 108, page 433) or **respiratory compromise** (see 'Respiratory failure and respiratory function tests', Chapter 119, page 495).

Escharotomy is performed as an emergency and involves **incisions down to healthy tissue**:

- **In limbs**: **medial** and **lateral** incisions that may need to be extended into individual digits
- **On chest wall**: bilateral midclavicular incisions and two transverse incisions to make the '**noughts and crosses**' release

It may be required as an emergency procedure in the accident and emergency department (A&E) resuscitation unit and may not reach theatre.

Consider combining **escharotomy with fasciotomy** if compartment syndrome is suspected.

- Burns in **children**: consider **non-accidental injury**
- **Circumferential** burns: these can contract causing **compartment syndrome**. **Escharotomy** may be required.

COMPLICATIONS OF BURNS

Early

- Death
- Renal failure
- Sepsis and DIC
- Infection
- Compartment syndrome
- ARDS.

Late

- Limb loss
- Scarring and contractures
- Cosmesis
- Chronic regional pain syndromes
- Functional disabilities.

108 Compartment syndrome

Possible viva questions related to this topic

→ What is compartment syndrome?
→ What do you understand by the term 'abdominal compartment syndrome'?
→ How do you measure the pressure in the abdominal compartment?
→ Where can compartment syndrome occur?
→ What are the clinical features of a compartment syndrome in the lower limb?
→ What are the systemic consequences of a compartment syndrome?
→ Discuss the management of compartment syndrome.
→ What are the complications of compartment syndrome?
→ What are the causes of compartment syndrome?

Related topics

Topic	Chapter	Page
Shock	122	510
CVP lines and invasive monitoring	110	443
Acid–base balance	84	349
Burns	107	427

Example viva question

What is compartment syndrome?

A **progressive condition** in which the **elevated tissue pressure** within a **myofascial compartment exceeds** the **capillary pressure** and compromises blood flow to structures within that compartment.

It most commonly occurs in the fascial compartments of the limbs, although an abdominal compartment syndrome is recognized where the intra-abdominal pressure exceeds the capillary pressure within the abdominal viscera, most notably the renal capillary bed.

COMPARTMENT SYNDROME WITHIN A LIMB

This can result from factors that either increase the volume of the compartment contents or decrease the volume of the compartment itself.

Increase in volume of compartment contents

- **Large haematoma** as the result of vascular injury or coagulopathy
- **Haemorrhage** and **oedema** after a **fracture** and soft tissue injury
- **Swelling of muscle** tissue post-**ischaemic** insult
- Limb compression.

Decrease in volume of compartment

- Overly **constricting** dressing or **cast**
- **Full-thickness burns**
- Closure of fascial defects after surgery.

The **four compartments of the lower leg** are most commonly affected, although compartment syndrome can occur in the:

- shoulder
- arm
- forearm
- hand
- buttocks
- thigh
- foot.

Therefore, after orthopaedic surgery or vascular surgery to these areas, careful clinical observation must be utilized to assess for a rise in compartment pressure.

Clinical signs of raised intracompartment pressure

Early signs
- Paraesthesia
- Pain on passive movement of distal joints
- Generalized pain in the limb
- Loss of distal sensation.

Late signs
- Obvious compartmental swelling
- Loss of muscle power
- Decreased pulse pressure or loss of pulse in distal limb (**very late sign**).

Muscle creatine phosphokinase (CPK) can be measured – massively **elevated in muscle necrosis**.

It can be seen from the signs above that, in answer to this question, **confusion with the 'pain, pale, paraesthetic, pulseless, perishingly cold'** description of the acutely ischaemic limb **is unwise!** Indeed **increasing pain** associated with **exacerbation of** pain on **passive flexion and extension** of distal joints is a **sensitive test** for early compartment syndrome.

If there is any doubt, **pressure monitors** can be placed in each compartment directly to monitor the pressure, although the **diagnosis** is a **clinical** one with monitoring only a confirmatory step.

A compartment pressure of **40 mmHg below** the **mean arterial pressure** is enough to cause compartment syndrome.

Management

Keep the patient **nil by mouth** if the diagnosis is suspected and measure the compartmental pressures if necessary.

Urgent **decompressive fasciotomies** to decompress the compartments (ensure that all compartments are decompressed).

Urgent **escharotomies** in circumferential burns (see 'Burns', Chapter 107, page 427).

Formally split any orthopaedic **plaster casts**.

Wounds are left open and covered with saline-soaked gauze.

A **re-look** and exploration in **24–48 hours** are usually necessary to **excise** any **necrotic tissue** and débride the wounds. In extreme cases more than one re-look may be necessary.

Closure of fasciotomies may well require skin grafting and early liaison with a plastic surgeon should be the norm.

Complications

These can be divided into systemic and local.

Systemic (mostly as a result of *muscle death*)
- **Rhabdomyolysis** leading to myoglobinaemia and subsequent renal failure
  - treated by prompt hydration and the maintenance of an alkaline urine using sodium bicarbonate, provided that urine output is adequate (preventing dissociation of myoglobin into more toxic metabolites)
- **Shock** as a result of massive peripheral vasodilatation (see 'Shock', Chapter 122, page 510)
- Hyperkalaemia
- Hyperphosphataemia
- Hyperuricaemia

- **Metabolic acidosis** as a result of **anaerobic respiration** (see 'Acid–base balance', Chapter 84, page 349)
- Death.

Local

- Chronic regional pain syndromes
- Contractures
- Muscle weakness
- Limb necrosis leading to requirement for amputation.

Note that **early diagnosis** and **prompt treatment** are the key to the prevention of complications. A **difference** between compartmental pressure and mean arterial pressure of just **30–40 mmHg** for **15 min** is enough to create **functional changes** in **muscles** and **nerves**; **4–8 hours** with this pressure difference can lead to **ischaemic necrosis**.

ABDOMINAL COMPARTMENT SYNDROME

↑ **Example viva question**

What do you understand by the term 'abdominal compartment syndrome?'

Abdominal compartment syndrome is defined as the adverse physiological effects of increased intra-abdominal pressure (IAP). Prolonged, unrelieved, increased IAP > 20 mmHg can produce pulmonary compromise, renal impairment, cardiac failure, shock and death.

Abdominal compartment syndrome (ACS) can be categorized into **primary**, **secondary** and **chronic**.

ACS occurs when the **IAP** is **too high**, similar to compartment syndrome in an extremity. The three types of ACS have different and sometimes overlapping causes.

Primary (i.e. acute with abdominal pathology)

- **Penetrating trauma**
- **Gastrointestinal haemorrhage**
- **Pancreatitis**
- External compressing forces, such as debris from a motor vehicle collision or after explosion of a large structure
- **Pelvic fracture**
- **Rupture** of abdominal **aortic aneurysm**
- **Perforated peptic ulcer**
- **Closure of abdominal fascia in gastroschisis and exomphalos neonatally**.

Secondary

Secondary ACS may occur in patients **without an intra-abdominal injury**, when **fluid accumulates** in volumes sufficient to cause a rise in IAP.

- **Sepsis**
- Large areas of **full-thickness burns**
- Penetrating or **blunt trauma** without identifiable injury
- **Postoperative**
- Packing and **primary fascial closure** after **emergency laparotomy**
- **Large-volume resuscitation**.

Chronic

- Peritoneal dialysis
- Morbid obesity
- Cirrhosis
- Meigs' syndrome (ovarian fibroma associated with ascites/pleural effusion).

Pathophysiology of abdominal compartment syndrome

Direct effects of compression on intra-abdominal and other viscera:

- **Gut: compression** of vasculature and portal system leads to **thrombosis** and **mucosal oedema**, ultimately resulting in translocation of bacteria across the mucosal wall and **systemic sepsis**; this causes more **fluid secretion** in the intra-abdominal compartment and a **further rise in pressure**
- **Kidneys:** renal perfusion is impaired and **urine output drops**
- **Liver: portal vein collapses** along with the inferior vena cava (IVC), causing congestion
- **Respiratory:** increased IAP makes it harder to breathe and **ventilation becomes more difficult**
- **Cardiac:** rise in abdominal pressure causes **CVP (central venous pressure)** and PAOP (pulmonary artery occlusion pressure) (see 'CVP lines and invasive monitoring', Chapter 110, page 443) **to rise despite** a **hypovolaemic state**, leading possibly to **inadequate fluid resuscitation**.

History

- Pancreatitis and/or alcohol abuse
- Emergency laparotomy
- NSAID use
- Melaena
- Syncope.

Signs and symptoms

- Abdominal pain – not always present and not always useful (particularly in sedated and ventilated obtunded patients in the ITU!)

- Decreased urine output – a frequent and early sign of abdominal compartment syndrome
- Melaena
- Progressively difficult ventilation
- Increased abdominal girth (not always easy to see).

Measurement of IAP is by the use of a **Foley catheter** introduced into the **bladder**; 50 mL saline is injected into it and then it is connected to a manometer to measure **intracystic pressure**, which is thought to be a reflection of IAP.

Abdominal CT can be useful to look for radiological signs of raised pressure such as **collapsed IVC**, **bilateral inguinal hernias**, and **enhanced and thickened gut wall**.

Management

- The best management of abdominal compartment syndrome is **prevention** and early treatment of any intra-abdominal hypertension
- Consider **avoiding primary closure** in emergency laparotomies, which are at high risk from abdominal compartment syndrome (extensive dead bowel, liver lacerations and packing, necrosectomy for pancreatitis)
- **Percutaneous drainage** of fluid collections
- **Laparoscopic decompression** may be used in abdominal blunt trauma
- **Laparostomy** remains the mainstay of treatment in the UK.

Complications

These can be split into complications from the compartment syndrome and complications from immediate decompression.

Direct complications from compartment syndrome
- Respiratory failure (increasing airway pressures and decreasing tidal volumes in ventilated patients)
- Renal failure (see above)
- Bowel ischaemia and infarction
- Increased ICP
- Decreased cardiac output and refractory shock.

Complications from immediate decompression
- **Massive and precipitous fall in blood pressure**:
  - caused partly by reperfusion syndrome with a fall in systemic vascular resistance and partly by inadequate fluid resuscitation as a result of a falsely elevated CVP (see above)
  - extensive **fluid resuscitation preceding decompression** reduces the incidence of refractory hypotension.

109 Criteria for admission to the ITU and HDU

Possible viva questions related to this topic

→ What are the criteria for admission to the ITU?
→ What are the main differences between the ITU and the high dependency unit (HDU)?
→ How do you go about making an ITU referral?
→ What investigations will be expected on making an ITU referral?
→ Do you know of any ITU scoring systems? What is the principle behind them?
→ What is level 1, 2 and 3 care?

↑ Example viva question

What are the criteria for admission to the ITU?

A common question. The main criteria are set out below but the principles here are that the ITU is the main place in the hospital for **invasive ventilatory support** and the support of two or more failing organ systems (including respiratory system).

In many hospitals, non-invasive ventilation such as continuous positive airway pressure (CPAP) (see 'Intubation and ventilation', Chapter 114, page 470) can be performed in an HDU setting.

CRITERIA FOR ADMISSION TO THE ITU

- Patients requiring or likely to require **advanced respiratory support** (usually in the form of endotracheal intubation and ventilation)
- Patients requiring support for **two or more organ systems**:
  - respiratory: ventilation/CPAP
  - renal: haemofiltration/haemodialysis
  - cardiac: ECG monitoring and **inotropic** support
  - hepatic: blood transfusion
  - neurological: intracranial pressure monitoring
- Patients with **chronic impairment** of one or more systems sufficient to restrict daily activities (**co-morbidities ASA III and above**) and who require support for an **acute, reversible failure of another organ system**
- Patients who also require **one-to-one nursing care**.

CRITERIA FOR ADMISSION TO THE HDU

- Patients requiring support for a **single failing organ system** excluding those requiring advanced respiratory support
- Patients who would benefit from **more regular and detailed observation** than can be safely provided on a general ward
- **Postoperative** patients who need **close observation and monitoring** for longer than a few hours.

DEFINITIONS OF SYSTEM FAILURES

Cardiovascular failure (see 'Shock', Chapter 122, page 510)
- Heart rate > 140 beats/min
- Systolic blood pressure < 100 mmHg
- ± Cardiac arrest.

Respiratory failure (see 'Intubation and ventilation', Chapter 114, page 470)
- Airway compromise
- Respiratory rate > 36 breaths/min
- SpO_2 < 90 per cent on > 40 per cent O_2 (via non-rebreather O_2 mask on the ward)
- ± Respiratory arrest.

Renal failure (see 'Oliguria and renal replacement', Chapter 116, page 482)
Urine output < 120 mL in 4 h with associated hyperkalaemia/acidosis.

Central nervous system (CNS) dysfunction
- Glasgow Coma Score (GCS) < 9 or a fall of 2 points
- Seizures, new or sustained > 10 min (status epilepticus).

MAKING AN ITU REFERRAL

Differs between hospitals but either the **senior house officer (SHO) or specialist registrar** usually makes referral directly to **clinician on call for ITU** specifically, registrar on call for anaesthetics or **consultant on call for ITU**. History, pertinent examination findings and laboratory tests/radiology/arterial blood gases will usually be required.

SIGNS AND INVESTIGATIONS

Respiratory failure

This cannot be adequately diagnosed without the use of **arterial blood gas** (ABG) and this is a simple bedside test that should be performed in the case of **all sick patients**, regardless of whether they appear to have respiratory compromise (see 'Respiratory failure and respiratory function tests', Chapter 119, page 495).

Respiratory failure can be split into **type I** which is a failure of **oxygenation** and **type II** which is a failure of **ventilation**:

- **Type I**: $PaO_2 < 8\,kPa$ (PCO_2 will be normal or low)
- **Type II**: $PaCO_2 > 6.5\,kPa$ and $PaO_2 < 8\,kPa$.

Note that normal PaO_2 on air should be around 13 kPa, assuming normal lungs.

Subtract 10 from FiO_2 (per cent) to obtain predicted PaO_2 for that FiO_2.

Severe respiratory failure is defined as one-third of the predicted value.

Thus, it is **essential to know what FiO_2 the patient is on** when the ABG is taken. Therefore, **flow rate and type of mask** must be recorded to determine the FiO_2 (see 'Intubation and ventilation', Chapter 114, page 470, and 'Acid–base balance', Chapter 84, page 349).

Circulatory failure

See 'Shock', Chapter 122, page 510 and 'Inotropes', Chapter 113, page 466.

To exclude compensated shock, all of the following should be fulfilled:

- Capillary refill < 10 s
- Patient not confused or thirsty
- Heart rate < 100 beats/min
- Mean arterial pressure (MAP) $> 80\,mmHg$ (see 'CVP lines and invasive monitoring', Chapter 110, page 443)
- Urine output $> 0.5\,mL/kg$ per h
- Base excess < 2 (see 'Acid–base balance', Chapter 84, page 349)
- Normal CVP/PAWP: obviously not available on the ward but jugular venous pressure (JVP) may be used as a non-invasive surrogate for ward assessment.

Oliguria

See 'Oliguria and renal replacement therapy, Chapter 116, page 482.

- Urine output $< 0.5\,mL/kg$ per h
- Beware blocked catheters, diuretics and nephrotoxics on drug chart!

CNS

Basic assessment on the ward:

- Can the patient defend the airway and is there a cough reflex present?
- Is GCS < 7? Immediate intubation for airway protection
- Adequate ventilation? (Check $P\text{CO}_2$)
- Clearing secretions?
- Is GCS deteriorating? (Fall by 2 points or more is significant)
- Presence of sepsis – confusion?

SCORING SYSTEMS IN ITU AND HDU

Various systems have been developed over the years in an attempt to quantify the severity of a patient's illness, the most widely used of which is the APACHE II (Acute Physiology And Chronic Health Evaluation) system.

This is calculated by computer from data on a dozen physiological parameters (BP, [Hb], etc.) + GCS. It is weighted for age, diagnosis and co-morbidities.

↑ **Example viva question**

What is level 1, 2 and 3 care?

1 Acute postoperative care (excluding respiratory support)
2 HDU
3 ITU

---

110 CVP lines and invasive monitoring

Possible viva questions related to this topic

→ How can blood pressure be monitored?
→ How do you assess the cardiovascular status of a patient?
→ What are the indications for central venous access?
→ What are the complications of central venous access?
→ Draw the CVP waveform and label the various components.
→ Is absolute CVP a useful measurement?
→ In what circumstances might CVP not represent overall filling?
→ How do you put in and take out a central line?
→ What are the indications for insertion of a pulmonary artery flotation catheter (PAFC)?
→ Draw the trace of a PAFC as it passes though the heart and wedges.
→ What parameters can be measured and what parameters can be calculated from a PAFC (Swan–Ganz)?
→ What methods are there for measuring cardiac output in the intensive care setting?
→ What do you understand by Fick's principle?
→ How can an arterial waveform tell you about the patient's fluid balance?

Related topics

Topic	Chapter	Page
Shock	122	510
Acute respiratory distress syndrome	105	419
Sepsis and SIRS	121	505
Blood pressure control	87	358
Starling's law of the heart and cardiovascular equations	102	403
Fluid balance	111	452
Acid–base balance	84	349
Nutrition	115	477
Oliguria and renal replacement	116	482

↑ **Example viva question**

How can blood pressure be monitored?

Categorized into **non-invasive** and **invasive** measures:

Non-invasive
- *Traditional sphygmomanometer*
  - intermittent, cumbersome and time-consuming
  - **non-invasive** method is manual (using stethoscope)
- *Dynamap* system (still uses arm cuff but based on **oscillometry**)
  - automatic, quicker, less time-consuming
  - probably slightly less accurate than manual measurement
  - intermittent but can be set to retake BP every minute
- **Radial artery tonometry**
  - based on superficial pressure sensors and therefore highly positional
  - new technology but may eventually replace an arterial line for short-term monitoring (e.g. in local anaesthetic procedures such as carotid endarterectomy)
  - continuous monitoring, produces BP waveform as with an arterial line
- **Finometer**
  - largely for research, based on measurement of 'finger blood pressure'

Invasive
- **Arterial line**
  - commonly a 20 G catheter inserted into the radial artery.
  - invasive – risks of clotting of line, infection
  - most accurate, continuous waveform
  - allows accurate, **beat-to-beat assessment** of MAP and **BP**
  - allows assessment of arterial waveform to see if it is 'swinging', indicating underfilling (see 'Fluid balance', Chapter 111, page 452)
  - allows regular aspiration of arterial blood for ABGs

ASSESSING THE CARDIOVASCULAR STATUS

Remember that in **most cases**, cardiovascular status is assessed **clinically**:

- Pulse:
  - **rate**
  - **rhythm**
  - **character** (palpable radial suggests systolic $\geq 80\,mmHg$)
- **Skin temperature** (cold peripheries indicating poor **peripheral perfusion**)

- **Skin colour** (look for peripheral cyanosis, signs of early skin necrosis)
- **Urine output** (see 'Fluid balance', Chapter 111, page 452)
- Respiratory rate
- Mental status (evidence of brain perfusion, i.e. alert and coherent, confused, obtunded, in coma).

FURTHER BEDSIDE TESTS AND OBSERVATIONS

- Pulse oximetry (see 'Pulse oximetry', Chapter 118, page 491)
- BP (as above)
- ECG
- **ABGs**: with particular attention to **acid–base balance** looking for any evidence of a **metabolic acidosis** (see 'Acid–base balance, Chapter 84, page 349).

CENTRAL VENOUS ACCESS

Indications

- Monitoring of **CVP** (see 'Fluid balance', Chapter 111, page 452)
- Passage of a pulmonary artery flotation catheter **(Swan–Ganz)**
- Infusion of **inotropes** and venosclerotic drugs centrally (usually via triple- or quadruple-lumen CVP lines)
- Administration of total parenteral nutrition **(TPN)** (see 'Nutrition', Chapter 115, page 477)
- **Haemofiltration** (large, double-lumen Vascath) (see 'Oliguria and renal replacement, Chapter 116, page 482)
- Insertion of **pacing wire**.

↑ Example viva question

How do you put in and take out a central line?

Insertion
- **Three** standard approaches:
  - ○ internal jugular
  - ○ subclavian approach
  - ○ femoral (not usually the preferred route for most access – higher incidence of deep venous thrombosis [DVT])
- **Patient positioning**:
  - ○ **head down** and turned to **opposite side** – particularly important in underfilled patients to improve chances of cannulating the vein and **decrease** the chances of an **air embolism**
  - ○ aseptic technique

- ○ local infiltration with local anaesthetic
- ○ prepare and drape the skin
- **Seldinger** technique the most common:
  - ○ or **internal jugular**: **high** or **low** approach.
    - – **high**: puncture the skin at the midpoint of the posterior border of sternocleidomastoid with needle held at 30° to the skin, heading a little laterally. Displace the internal carotid artery medially with a finger. Continue, aspirating regularly until the vein is entered
    - – **low**: puncture the skin between the two heads of sternocleidomastoid – careful, do not go too deep!
  - ○ for **subclavian**: puncture skin at a point between the lateral one-third and medial two-thirds of the clavicle, heading for the sternoclavicular joint ipsilaterally. 'Walk' the needle along the underside of the clavicle, aspirating regularly until the vein is entered
  - ○ after the vein has been entered, pass the guidewire in through the needle, checking that it advances freely – watch the ECG if you have one and do not put the guidewire in too far!
  - ○ remove the needle and railroad dilators followed by the CVP line over the guidewire (you will need to make a tiny incision in the skin to pass the line dilator). Ensure that you don't lose the guidewire when pushing in the CVP line – keep some part of the wire in sight at all times
  - ○ after the line has been advanced to the required length (usually 15–20 cm), remove guidewire, ensure that line aspirates and flushes freely through all lumina, and then suture in place
  - ○ **chest radiograph** to ensure that no **pneumothorax** has been caused and that line is in the correct position (just above the right atrium)

Removing a central line

- Ensure that patient is **flat/head down** to **prevent air embolus**. Check that **clotting** and **platelets** are **normal**. Remove line and immediately place a dressing over the area. **Send the tip** for microbiology and culture
- Indwelling, **tunnelled lines** may need to **removed** in theatre as a larger incision down to a retaining plastic cuff may be required

Complications of central venous access

- **Line-related sepsis**
- **Problems** associated with **insertion**:
  - ○ pneumothorax
  - ○ haemopneumothorax
  - ○ air embolus

- **Damage** to surrounding structures:
  - ○ **arterial damage**: puncture of carotid artery or cannulation of subclavian artery, leading to false aneurysm formation, arteriovenous fistula or haematoma
  - ○ **cannulation** of the **thoracic duct**
- **Central venous thrombosis**
- **Catheter embolization**
- **Malposition** of catheter (e.g. into neck veins from subclavian approach or into contralateral vein)
- **Cardiac** complications:
  - ○ **arrhythmias**
  - ○ perforation of the right atrium.

THE CVP WAVEFORM

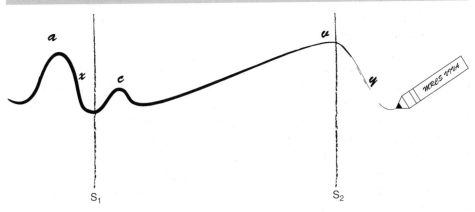

Figure 110.1

The **a wave** is caused by **atrial contraction**.

The **x descent** follows **atrial relaxation**.

The **c wave** is formed by the intrusion of the **tricuspid valve** leaflets into the atrium at the start of ventricular systole.

The **v wave** is a measure of the **venous return** to the atrium. It marks the point of ventricular systole but it is NOT caused by it.

The **y descent** occurs when the tricuspid valve opens and the **atrium empties**.

The waveform can be affected by various conditions:

- **Atrial fibrillation** (AF): **absent a waves** (lack of coordinated atrial contraction)

- **Tricuspid regurgitation**: **large v wave** caused by a jet of blood coming into the atrium during ventricular systole as a result of an incompetent valve
- **Tricuspid stenosis**: **large a wave** caused by arteriovenous outflow obstruction. **Slow y descent** results from slow atrial emptying
- **Complete heart block**: **'cannon' a waves** caused by uncoordination of atria and ventricles, leading to occasional contractions where the atrium contracts against a closed tricuspid valve.

↑ **Example viva question**

Is absolute CVP a useful measurement? In what circumstances might CVP not represent overall filling?

Absolute CVP depends on ensuring that the patient is properly positioned each time that it is measured (at 45° or at least the same angle for all measurements with the transducer set at the same height.) **It is not as useful** a clinical tool as the **response of the CVP to a fluid challenge** (see 'Fluid balance', Chapter 111, page 452).

In circumstances where the **right heart** is **not functioning normally** (particularly in valvular heart disease) or the overall myocardial compliance (e.g. **right-sided heart failure** or **pulmonary hypertension**) is affected, the CVP may not give a true reflection of the patient's filling. In these cases, the parameter has to be considered in the light of **other physiological parameters** and a **PAFC may be considered**.

THE PAFC (SWAN–GANZ)

This is a **flow-directed catheter** that is floated through the heart on an inflatable balloon until it wedges in a branch of the pulmonary artery. When the balloon is inflated, there is a **continuous column of blood** between the **tip of the catheter** and the **left atrium**, so that the **wedge pressure** reflects **left atrial pressure**.

Indications

The indications for a PAFC are **controversial** and some clinicians believe that they should not be used at all! There is ongoing research in this area and these devices are **likely** eventually **to be** completely **replaced** by less invasive systems (see later).

- Measurement of the **SVR** (systemic vascular resistance) in **septic shock**, severe sepsis or SIRS to guide inotrope management (see 'Inotropes', Chapter 113, page 466)
- Measurement of wedge pressure to guide **fluid management** in difficult cases (severe sepsis and/or acute right heart failure)

- **Post-cardiac surgery** in cases of **poor left ventricular function**
- Multiorgan failure
- **ARDS** with or without concomitant pulmonary oedema
- Measurement of **cardiac index** and **cardiac output** in an ITU setting.

Insertion technique

Common approaches are **internal jugular** and **subclavian** as with all central venous access. Once in the right atrium, the **balloon is inflated** to float through the tricuspid valve and into the right ventricle. The line is advanced through the right ventricle, through the pulmonary valve and into the pulmonary artery. As it is advanced, the **balloon wedges** in one of the branches of the pulmonary artery and the trace become essentially flat (see below.)

As this line is indwelling, the **balloon is kept deflated** until a measurement of wedge pressure is required.

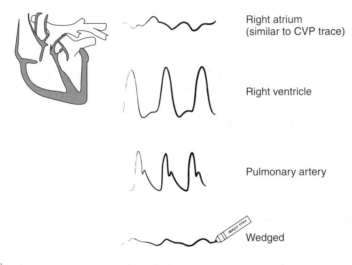

Right atrium
(similar to CVP trace)

Right ventricle

Pulmonary artery

Wedged

Figure 110.2

Complications of PAFC insertion

- All central line insertion complications (see above)
- **Cardiac arrhythmias**:
  - commonly atrial and ventricular ectopics
  - can cause ventricular tachycardia, ventricular fibrillation and heart block in irritable myocardium
  - if encountered, balloon must be deflated before catheter is pulled back to prevent valvular or myocardial damage
- **Pulmonary artery rupture**: usually presents as haemoptysis
- **Pulmonary artery infarction**: if balloon has been left up too long

• **Pulmonary embolus** from catheter tip
• **Knotting** of catheter.

Directly measured physiological parameters

• MAP
• Heart rate
• **Cardiac output** (measured by either thermodilution or indicator dilution techniques – see below)
• Mean pulmonary artery pressure (MPAP)
• **PAOP** or PAWP
• Heart rate.

Derived physiological parameters

• **Cardiac index** (cardiac output/body surface area)
• Stroke volume
• SVR:

$$SVR = (MAP - CVP)/CO \times 80$$

  ○ **normal range 900–1400 dyn/s per cm^{-5}**
• Pulmonary vascular resistance (PVR):

$$PVR = (MPAP - PAOP)/CO \times 80$$

  ○ normal range is 150–250 dyn/s per cm^{-5}
• Indexed SVR and PVR (divided by body surface area)
• Oxygen delivery.

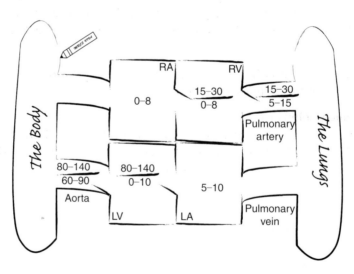

Figure 110.3   Schematic of pressures found within the heart and cardio-pulmonary circulation.

Example viva question

What methods are there for measuring cardiac output in the intensive care setting? What do you understand by Fick's principle?

Swan–Ganz (PAFC)

- Continuous cardiac output measurement is now available with the **thermodilution technique** and is based on **Fick's principle**. A **bolus of cold saline** is injected and a **thermistor at the catheter tip** measures the **drop in temperature** of the blood. More modern systems use a small heater coil some distance down the catheter and a thermistor at the tip

- **Fick's principle**:
  Classically described for **oxygen consumption**, it has been generalized to:

  Organ blood flow/time = Amount of marker taken up/Concentration
                            difference between supply and drainage

  Thus, cardiac output is proportional to change in temperature of the blood divided by time.

PiCCO

- Uses a **thermodilution technique** from cold fluid infused through a CVP line and analysed via a **modified arterial line** containing a thermistor
- **Commonly used** in modern ITUs – allows continuous CO monitoring

LiDCO

- Uses principle of **lithium dilution** similar to Fick's principle. Small doses of lithium, as an indicator, are picked up by a lithium electrode in a modified arterial line. CO is calculated from pulse contour analysis

Echo Doppler

- Measures **blood flow** in the aorta using an **oesophageal probe**. CO can be derived from the Doppler waveform

Echocardiography

- Not a continuous technique and operator dependent but allows direct visualization of the myocardium and an assessment of ejection fraction

111 Fluid balance

Possible viva questions related to this topic

→ What are the daily maintenance requirements of common cations and anions in a healthy 70 kg man?

→ How is body fluid homoeostasis achieved and regulated?

→ Discuss water balance in terms of intake and output in a healthy individual.

→ What is the physiological consequence of dehydration?

→ What clinical measures do we have to assess fluid balance?

→ Discuss distribution of total body water with respect to intracellular and extracellular compartments.

→ Discuss the ion composition of extracellular and intracellular fluid.

→ What's in a bag of physiological (0.9%) saline?

→ What is Hartmann's solution and what advantages does it have over saline?

→ What is the difference between a colloid and a crystalloid? When might you choose one over the other? Is there any evidence to support your decision?

→ What is the osmolality of plasma? How would you calculate it roughly?

→ How can loss of extracellular fluid (ECF) volume be calculated?

→ How can loss of plasma volume be calculated?

→ What are the principles behind the prescription of fluid regimens for maintenance and in the setting of an acutely unwell surgical patient?

→ What are the possible complications of giving a colloid?

→ Explain the effects of fluid resuscitation in terms of Starling's curve and explain how the CVP response to a fluid challenge is explained by the curve.

↑ **Example viva question**

What is in a bag of Hartmann's solution, 0.9% (normal) saline and 5 per cent dextrose?

Name of fluid	Commonly referred to as	Na$^+$	Cl$^-$	HCO$_3^-$ (all mmol/L)	K$^+$
NaCl (0.9 per cent)	**Normal (physiological) saline**	150	150	–	–
Ringer's lactate	**Hartmann's**	131	111	29 (as lactate)	5
Glucose (5 per cent)	**5 per cent dextrose**	–	–	–	–

BODY WATER

There is approximately **45 litres** of total body **water** in a healthy **70 kg man**. This is **split into extracellular and intracellular** compartments:

- **Intracellular: 30 litres** in total
- **Extracellular: 15 litres** in total:
  - lymph = 1.5 litres
  - transcellular = 1.5 litres
  - extracellular fluid proper = 10 litres
  - **intravascular fluid (plasma) = 5 litres**.

The **transcellular** compartment is separated by a layer of epithelium (e.g. CSF, gut lumen). In some pathological processes, this space is increased and referred to as the third space.

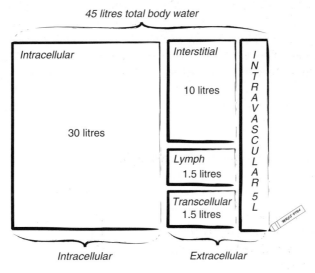

Figure 111.1

Ion composition of ECF and intracellular fluid (ICF)		
Ion	ECF (mmol/L)	ICF (mmol/L)
Na^+	135–145	4–10
K^+	3.5–5.0	150
Ca^{2+}	1.0–1.25	0.001
Mg^{2+}	1.0	40
HCO_3^-	25	10
Cl^-	95–105	15
PO_4^{3-}	1.1	100

The **distribution** of the **ECF** between the plasma and the interstitial space is **regulated** by the **capillaries** and **lymphatics** (see 'Starling forces in the capillaries/oedema', Chapter 101, page 401).

WATER AND ELECTROLYTE BALANCE

As well as gastrointestinal intake of water, the human body **makes approximately 350 mL water/day** as a result of the oxidization of carbohydrates. This is known as **metabolic water** and, added to approximately **1500 mL from drink** and **750 mL from food**, makes up the **average daily intake of 2600 mL.**

Approximately **1000 mL of water are lost each day** through the **skin** and the **lungs**; **1500 mL** are lost in the **urine** and approximately **100 mL** in the **faeces**, thus balancing the input and output.

More correctly, **individual water requirements** in a healthy individual are calculated according to the patient's **weight** and **age**. Thus, **adults** require about **30–40 mL/kg per day**, whereas **children require relatively more:**

- 0–10 kg: 4 mL/kg per h
- 10–20 kg: 40 mL/h + 2 mL/kg per h for each kg > 10 kg
- > 20 kg: 60 mL/h + 1 mL/kg per h for each kg > 20 kg.

The **average requirements** of **sodium** and **potassium** are **1 mmol/kg per day** of each. It is particularly important to keep up with the potassium requirement because the kidney is much more efficient at conserving sodium than potassium. Indeed, **there is an obligatory loss of potassium** in both **urine and faeces**, and patients with diarrhoea or polyuria can quickly become hypokalaemic. It should be noted that there is a considerable intracellular potassium load and that there can be a steep fall in total body potassium before it is noted as a fall in plasma potassium.

THE PHYSIOLOGY OF DEHYDRATION

See 'Functions of the kidney II', Chapter 93, page 377)

- **One-fifth of the cardiac output** is filtered by the kidney
- In dehydration, there is **increased production of ADH** by the neurohypophysis (a direct effect by osmoreceptors in the hypothalamus)
- Leads to **synthesis of more water channels** in the **distal collecting duct** of the kidney, leading in turn to **increased H_2O reabsorption** and a concentrated urine (see 'Functions of the kidney II', Chapter 93, page 377)
- Renin is produced by the juxtaglomerular apparatus in response to a decrease in the afferent arteriolar pressure and decreased Na^+ delivery.
- **Activation of the renin–angiotensin–angiotensin II axis** leads to **aldosterone** promoting Na^+ **retention** and K^+ **excretion**; angiotensin II is a potent vasoconstrictor
- **Two systems** above achieve **blood pressure homoeostasis.**

ASSESSING FLUID BALANCE CLINICALLY

Bedside observations

- **Pulse**
- **BP** (including pulse width)
- **Urine output** (and assessment of bedside fluid chart)
- **JVP**
- Weight (particularly of relevance in renal patients)
- Peripheral capillary return
- Mental status
- Skin turgor
- Sunken eyes in dehydration
- Dry mouth in dehydration.

Invasive measurements

See 'CVP lines and invasive monitoring', Chapter 110, page 443).

- **CVP** and response to a fluid challenge: **if inadequately filled**, a patient's **CVP will initially increase** with a fluid bolus but rapidly **fall again** as the fluid equilibrates between the **intra- and extracellular** compartments. If **adequately filled**, the **CVP will rise to a new level** and be maintained at this level over time. This can be explained in terms of Starling's law of the heart (see 'Starling's law of the heart and cardiovascular equations', Chapter 102, page 403)

- **PAWP**: in some instances, this can be used as a surrogate for left atrial filling pressure, particularly in instances where the function of the right side of the heart is in doubt or where the peripheral vascular resistance is very low in an acutely septic patient.

ASSESSMENT OF LOSS IN VOLUME OF PLASMA AND ECF

The key to this assessment is the **plasma albumin concentration** and the **blood haematocrit**.

In the context of a **loss in plasma volume**, the **plasma albumin** concentration remains constant but, as no erythrocytes have been lost, the **blood haematocrit** will **increase**. The percentage loss of plasma volume can be calculated as below, where $H1$ = initial value of haematocrit and $H2$ = value to which haematocrit rises.

$$\text{Percentage fall in plasma volume} = 100 \times \{1 - [H1/(100 - H1)] \times [(100 - H2)]/H2\}$$

In the context of a **loss in ECF volume**, the **total albumin remains the same**, although the **albumin concentration goes up**. The percentage loss of ECF volume can be calculated as below, where $A1$ = initial albumin concentration and $A2$ = concentration of albumin following dehydration.

$$\text{Percentage fall in ECF volume} = (1 - [A1/A]) \times 100$$

FLUID REPLACEMENT STRATEGIES

There are **three factors** to consider when prescribing fluid regimens:

1. Basic **basal requirements** of water and ions (as discussed above)
2. Continuing **abnormal losses** in addition to basal requirements
3. Correction of any **pre-existing fluid or electrolyte deficit,** and maintenance of an adequate left atrial filling volume to **maintain blood pressure,** and therefore tissue perfusion and peripheral oxygen delivery.

Basic requirements

An **average 70 kg man** requires **70 mmol/day** of **sodium** and **potassium** and three possible regimens are shown below:

1. 1 L 0.9% (normal) saline and 2000 mL 5 per cent dextrose (70 mmol Na^+)
2. 2000 mL 5 per cent dextrose and 500 mL Hartmann's (65.5 mmol Na^+, 2.5 mmol K^+)
3. 2500 mL dextrose saline (75 mmol Na^+).

It should be noted that K^+ **will need to be added to the above regimens** and commonly now fluids are available with 20 mmol K^+ added to each bag. In the past, ampoules of 20 mmol KCl in 10 mL were available to add to fluid bags, but unfortunately these have been **used in error** as saline flushes, causing **fatal arrhythmias**. Thus, concentrated KCl is now **not routinely available on wards**, although it is of course still available as a controlled drug in an ITU/HDU setting.

It should never be given at a rate faster than 40 mmol/h.

Abnormal losses

A great deal of **water is lost** in an unwell patient, through the **skin** as a result of **pyrexia** and through the **lungs** as a result of **tachypnoea** or **ventilation with non-humidified air**. Two of the most common surgical conditions leading to massive fluid and electrolyte deficits are **pancreatitis** (see 'Acute pancreatitis', Chapter 104, page 413) and **acute bowel obstruction**.

The **fluid secreted into the bowel** and aspirated from the nasogastric tube is **rich in Na^+ and K^+** and therefore 0.9% (normal) saline with added K^+ should be used to replace it. **Inappropriate management** with dextrose saline or 5 per cent dextrose can lead to a rapid and profound **hyponatraemia**.

It is essential that an **accurate input–output chart** be kept in this type of patient and that a **daily positive or negative balance** be calculated and recorded, taking into account any insensible losses.

All too often, fluid management is careless and this can lead to both postoperative and preoperative disasters.

Pre-existing fluid or electrolyte deficit

To assess this, the techniques described above are crucial to assess the fluid status of the patient and their immediate electrolyte requirements (see 'CVP lines and invasive monitoring', Chapter 110, page 443).

Postoperatively, for the first 36 hours there is **sodium and water retention** although **obligatory loss of potassium continues**. Remember to **check postoperative drains, nasogastric tube aspirates,** etc. and ensure that this loss is **added to the input–output chart** and factored in when prescribing fluids.

TYPES OF COLLOIDS

- Blood
- HAS available in 4.5 per cent and 20 per cent
- Dextrans: 40 or 70 depending on molecular mass
- Gelatins: relatively short plasma half-life, e.g. Gelofusin, Haemaccel
- Starches, e.g. hetastarch or pentastarch – risk of coagulopathy.

COMPLICATIONS OF COLLOIDS

- Transmission of infection – particularly with blood and blood products
- Coagulopathy: Dextran 70, gelatins and starches can interfere with the clotting cascade and platelet adhesion
- Anaphylaxis
- Worsening oedema (if capillary integrity is lost, larger molecules can leak into the interstitial space taking water with it).

↑ **Key learning points**

Colloids and crystalloids

Colloids: composed of **large molecules** with a molecular mass of $> 30\,000$ daltons (30 kDa). Can be **natural or synthetic**. Confined to the plasma for **longer**.

Crystalloids: easily able to **pass between compartments**. Exert much **less osmotic pressure than colloids**. Following the metabolism of dextrose, 5 per cent dextrose is distributed evenly as total body water.

A **loss of plasma volume** in the past has resulted in the use of **human albumin solution** (HAS) to replace the large protein content of plasma, providing much of the osmotic pressure of the plasma. Not only is this **expensive and limited**, but it has also been shown in many studies **not actually to improve outcome**! Thus, colloids have been developed with osmotic activity, their **larger molecules** attempting to **hold water and sodium** in the **intravascular space** longer than crystalloids such as 0.9% (normal) saline.

Although controversial, most surgeons would use **colloids to maintain blood pressure** and plasma volume in an acute situation, in an attempt to keep volume in the intravascular compartment for longer. There is, however, **little evidence** to suggest that colloid administration over crystalloid improves overall outcome.

Five per cent dextrose is a **poor choice for resuscitation** in any setting because the fluid is distributed as **total body water** between **all compartments** after the metabolism of dextrose. Colloids are (in theory) confined for longer to the intravascular space.

112 Head injury and intracranial pressure

Possible viva questions related to this topic

You're a general surgical registrar called to see a 28-year-old man who has been in a road traffic accident (RTA) with a head injury.

→ How would you assess him?

→ His GCS falls to < 6 (E1 V1 M3). What would you do?

→ Right pupil becomes fixed and dilated. Why and what would you do?

→ Why does the pupil dilate in raised intracranial pressure (ICP)?

→ What now? How would you attempt to measure his ICP?

→ What is CPP (cerebral perfusion pressure)? Why is it useful? What is the theory behind it?

→ What manoeuvres can be performed to control ICP and how do they work?

→ What reversible factors could be responsible for a transient rise in ICP?

→ What do you understand by the Monro–Kellie doctrine?

→ Should you ever perform a lumbar puncture in head injury?

RAISED ICP

Physiology

In order to understand the physiology of head injury, one must know the principles of the **Monro–Kellie** doctrine: the **brain** is in a **closed box**, the skull. It contains **three things** inside, namely **blood, brain and CSF**. The pressure in the head is related to the balance among these three. If the **brain volume increases**, e.g. in cerebral oedema, in order for the pressure to remain normal, **one of the other two (blood and CSF) must be decreased** in volume.

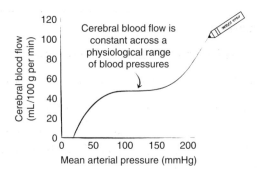

Figure 112.1

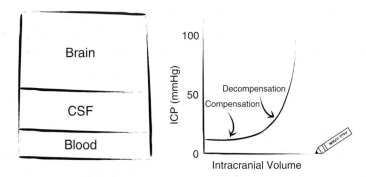

Figure 112.2

Causes of raised ICP

Surgical
Infection
• **Empyema**.

Head injury
• **Extradural haematoma**: classic lucid interval; not necessarily associated with cortical damage if evacuated in a timely manner; classically, an arterial injury stripping pericranium away from the skull (**mass effect increases ICP**)
• **Subdural haematoma**: the result of tearing of **dural bridging veins**; indicates underlying cortical damage (**mass effect increases ICP**)
• **Subarachnoid haemorrhage**: usually the result of direct contusional injury to the brain and not the result of rupture of an underlying vascular malformation (aneurysm/arteriovenous malformation) (**blockage** of **arachnoid granulations** impairing CSF reabsorption, along with **cerebral oedema**, as a result of hypoxia **increases ICP**)

↑ **Example viva question**

What is CPP? Why is it useful? What is the theory behind it?

$$CPP = \text{mean arterial pressure (MAP)} - ICP$$

where MAP = one-third of pulse pressure + diastolic blood pressure

Thus, either **decreasing ICP** or **increasing MAP** should **increase CPP**. This relationship holds true only for brain in which cerebral autoregulation is lost, as in traumatic brain injury.

Write down these formulae in a viva when asked about factors that affect ICP, e.g. in **hyperventilation** there is a **decreased P_{CO_2}**:

As an **increase in P_{CO_2}** will cause **vasodilatation**, a **decrease** will cause **vasoconstriction**, thus **decreasing** the **cerebral blood volume** and therefore **reducing ICP** according to the Monro–Kellie doctrine (see above).

Similar questions could be devised for all factors that can affect ICP, e.g. hydrocephalus involves an increase in the volume of CSF as a result of obstruction, over-production or decreased absorption.

Caveats to the CPP model: although CPP is a useful concept, blood pressure is not necessarily equivalent to blood flow or, even more fundamentally, oxygen transfer and a tissue's ability to utilize that oxygen. Thus, brain may be ischaemic despite an adequate CPP of > 70 mmHg.

- **Contusions**: the result of rapid deceleration of the brain against the inside of the cranium (classically **coup contre-coup**). Bifrontal contusions common and likely to evolve and **swell**, leading to a delayed drop in GCS. The initial CT scan almost always underestimates the eventual size of contusions, leading to the requirement for a low threshold for repeat imaging (**contusions** exert **mass effect** as a result of **blood** and **oedema** to increase ICP)
- **Diffuse axonal injury**: this carries with it a poor prognosis and is a shearing of the white matter against the grey matter, leading to significant fibre disruption (increases ICP as a result of **generalized cerebral oedema** secondary to parenchymal disruption).

Medical
- Electrolyte imbalance (cerebral oedema)
- Ischaemia (cerebrovascular accident or CVA)
- Infection: meningitis, cerebritis.

Symptoms of raised ICP

- Decreased conscious level (see below)
- Headache
- Nausea and vomiting.

A fall in GCS

- **Pressure symptoms**: evolving **haematoma**, evolving **contusions** (remember classic lucid interval suggestive of extradural haematoma)
- **Ischaemic cause**: loss of **autoregulation** and decreased blood pressure may lead to cerebral ischaemia
- **Post-ictal**: **seizures** are common after blunt head injury and can lead to a temporary drop in GCS
- **Remember metabolic causes**: sudden **hypoglycaemia** in a patient with diabetes can lead to a profound drop in GCS.

Signs of raised ICP

- A **suddenly dilated pupil, unreactive to light** is suggestive of a **third nerve palsy**. Paralysis of lateral rectus (**sixth nerve**) leading to a defect in lateral gaze is also a sign of **raised ICP**. This is a manifestation of a **traction injury** on the sixth nerve because it has a long intracranial course.
- **Fall in GCS** usually a result of pressure on the brain stem (see other causes above).
- **Papilloedema**.

↑ **Example viva question**

Why does the pupil dilate in raised ICP?

This occurs in raised ICP because the nerve is **pushed** against the free edge of the tentorium and is a sign of **impending tentorial herniation (coning)**.

The fibres that are damaged are the **parasympathetics** that travel with the **third nerve** from the **Edinger–Westphal nucleus** in the **midbrain** to supply **sphincter pupillae**, leading to **unopposed sympathetic dilatation** of the pupil.

Without a CT, in a suspected extradural haematoma, a **burr hole** would be drilled on the **same side as the pupil**. However, in some cases the opposite side can be dilated (false localizing sign).

CT signs

- **Extradural**: this respects the skull sutures because an extradural haematoma will strip the pericranial dura away from the skull, classically creating a relatively localized **convex haematoma**; often causes a **midline shift**

- **Subdural**: this does not respect skull sutures as with extradurals and will lie in a relatively **thin sheet of blood** over the cortex. As this is the result of damage to bridging veins, underlying cerebral damage usually leads to significant **oedema** and **midline shift**
- **Subarachnoid**: blood is seen in the **subarachnoid space**, often in the **perimesencephalic cisterns** and extending into the **ventricles**. Blood in the ventricles **increases** the risk of **hydrocephalus** and a 'full' third ventricle along with visible temporal horns are signs of this
- **Midline shift:** seen in many pathologies that result in mass effect; suggestive of raised ICP if acute
- **Grey/white differentiation:** loss of grey/white differentiation on the CT is suggestive of acute ischaemia.

MEASURING ICP

Invasive methods

- **External ventricular drain (EVD)** or ventriculostomy, passed into the anterior horn of the lateral ventricle via usually a frontal burr hole, is still considered the **gold standard**
- **Brain parenchymal ICP transducer** through a cranial access device (usually referred to as 'a bolt')
- **Subdural catheter**: little used now and has been shown to correlate poorly with 'actual' ICP
- **Palpation** of a **craniotomy flap** when the bone is left out (obviously not very accurate but can be a useful sign if there is no ICP monitor *in situ*).

Non-invasive methods

Not well validated but transcranial Doppler (**TCD**) can be used to measure velocities in the middle cerebral artery and derive a 'pulsatility index' that may correlate with ICP.

↑ **Example viva question**

What factors can cause a transient rise in ICP?

To answer this question, draw out the **Monro–Kellie diagram** and explain that an increase in either **cerebral blood volume, CSF** or **brain** matter will increase ICP. Transient factors to do this may include **hypoventilation** (including $P\text{CO}_2$) as a result of a **mucus plug** or migrated **tracheostomy** in the ITU setting, traumatic **hydocephalus** or **seizures**. (There are of course many others.)

MEDICAL MANAGEMENT OF RAISED ICP

Always remember ABC first!

Note that these are the factors that are most important when **considering transfer of the patient to a neurosurgical centre**.

- **Mannitol** bolus (20 per cent) or **hypertonic saline after discussion** with neurosurgeon
- **Intubation** if not protecting airway (remember ABC) and **sedation**
- Possibly load with **phenytoin**/use of benzodiazepines to **control seizures**
- **Head up** 30° (taking care to immobilize C-spine)
- **Mild hypothermia**
- An anaesthetist may aid with **mild hyperventilation** to keep the $P\text{CO}_2$ **around 4.5 kPa** (dangerous if allowed to fall too low because this causes local cerebral **vasoconstriction** and can lead to **ischaemia**)
- **Increase CPP** by increasing MAP with inotropes (dopamine, noradrenaline [care as causes vasoconstriction], adrenaline) (see 'Inotropes', Chapter 113, page 466).

SURGICAL MANAGEMENT OF RAISED ICP

- **External ventricular drain (EVD)** to drain off CSF, so decreasing ICP transiently
- **Surgical craniectomy** ± evacuation of mass lesions
- **Bifrontal craniectomy** for intractably raised ICP.

↑ **Example viva question**

Should you ever perform a lumbar puncture in head injury?

For the purposes of the viva, the answer to this question should be no!

A more correct answer is that lumbar puncture should not be performed in the context of head injury **unless an intracranial infection** is suspected. Furthermore, in the **presence of a mass lesion** with raised ICP, **lumbar puncture is absolutely contraindicated** for fear of precipitating **coning**.

In rare cases, lumbar puncture is performed in head injury but **only after a CT** to ensure **no mass lesion** and **open basal cisterns**.

ROLE OF IMAGING IN HEAD INJURY

Any drop in GCS initially warrants a **CT of the head** and any **further deterioration** should result in **repeat imaging**. CT appearances of traumatic brain injury evolve over time and must be monitored. Small subdurals and extradurals can easily expand and contusions can evolve. Thus clinical vigilance and a very **low threshold for repeat imaging** is required.

Currently there are no indications in traumatic brain injury for emergency magnetic resonance imaging (MRI) because this is both costly and time-consuming, adding little acute information in most cases. Contusions of the brain stem and posterior fossa are better imaged with MRI but this information is prognostic on a more long-term basis.

↑ **Key learning point**

All questions related to 'how should you manage' and a clinical scenario involving an acute patient should immediately result in 'A, B, C' and in this case 'D' for disability. In advanced trauma life support (ATLS), the AVPU score is taught but many surgeons will use the GCS (eyes/voice/movement).

---

113 Inotropes

DEFINITION

An **inotrope** is a drug that **increases myocardial contractility** and therefore shifts Starling's curve up (see 'Starling's law of the heart and cardiovascular equations', Chapter 102, page 403).

VASOACTIVE COMPOUNDS

These are drugs used artificially to support a failing or dysfunctional cardiovascular system. Via their actions on various receptors, they affect either heart rate or force of contraction, or alter systemic vascular resistance. Effects are predominantly mediated by either α-, β_1- or β_2-receptors.

They are divided into the following groups:

• Inotropes: increase the force of contraction of the heart
• Pure chronotropes: increase heart rate
• Vasodilators
• Vasoconstrictors.

RECEPTORS, POSITION AND ACTION

- α-receptors: expressed in the vasculature; agonists cause **vasoconstriction**
- β_1-receptors: expressed in the heart, agonists are **positively chronotropic** (increase heart rate) and **positively inotropic** (increase force of contraction)
- β_2: expressed predominantly in the vasculature; agonists cause **vasodilatation**.

Adrenaline

Actions on: α, β_1, β_2 – 'dirty drug'.

Used at **cardiac arrest** and turns patient into '**heart–brain preparation**' attempting to **spare the brain and myocardium** from ischaemia by causing **massive** peripheral **vasoconstriction** (α effects) and strong **positive chronotropia** (β_1 effects).

Noradrenaline

Not an inotrope strictly because **no increase** in **force of contraction**.

Actions on: α.

- Causes **peripheral vasoconstriction**, so **increasing SVR**. An inotrope given in the context of septic shock (see 'Shock', Chapter 122, page 510, and 'Sepsis and SIRS', Chapter 121, page 505)
- Must be administered centrally
- At low doses, invasive arterial monitoring and urine output may be all that is required. However, in the context of severe sepsis with high inotrope/multiple inotrope requirements, some measure of SVR must be available to titrate the dose. This can be derived from traditional Swan–Ganz (pulmonary artery or PA) catheter measurements or, more commonly now, less invasive measures such as LidCo (lithium dilution) (see 'CVP lines and invasive monitoring', Chapter 110, page 443).

Note that SVR is never directly measured but is derived from PA measurements in the case of the PA catheter.

Dopamine

Actions on: **D-receptors in the gut and kidney.**

In small doses: renal arteries dilate, so increasing urinary output. Splanchnic blood flow increases.

In medium doses: predominantly β_1 effects resulting in a tachycardia and increased force of contraction.

In large doses: predominantly α effects, causing peripheral vasoconstriction and an increase in SVR.

> **↑ Key learning point**
>
> Note that increasing **evidence does not support** the use of 'low or renal dose' dopamine in the context of a **poor urinary output** and failing cardiovascular system as a renal-sparing inotrope, but it is still used in some units around the country. You should be aware of the **controversy** surrounding its low dose usage.

Many ITUs no longer use dopamine as their first-line inotrope and instead use more selective dopamine derivatives, such as dobutamine or dopexamine.

Isoprenaline

Actions on: β_1 and β_2.

This affects the β-receptors in the heart, bronchi, skeletal muscle and gut vasculature. It reduces the SVR by vasodilatation in the vascular beds of the skeletal muscles, kidney and mesentery. It is positively chronotropic and inotropic so increasing cardiac output.

Its strong β_1 effects produce a tachycardia, however, and this limits its clinical effectiveness.

Dobutamine

Actions on: predominantly β_1 (with some β_2 action)

A synthetic analogue of isoprenaline with its main advantage being that it causes less of a tachycardia, so increasing its usefulness. The drug is used for cardiogenic shock on cardiac care units because β_2 action offloads the heart and β_1 action increases force of contraction.

Nitrates (vasodilators – not inotropes)

Actions: venodilatation.

In circumstances where the heart needs to be 'offloaded', such as pulmonary oedema or left ventricular failure, nitrates can be used. Their action is to reduce SVR and venodilate, thereby reducing both afterload and preload.

Note that, if arterial vasodilatation is required, **hydralazine** may be used (this of course reduces afterload alone).

MONITORING AND CHOICE OF INOTROPE

The **choice of inotrope** will depend on the patient's condition, and the **specific physio-logical parameters**. **Invasive monitoring** is usually required with at least a **urinary catheter**, an indwelling **arterial line** and some form of **central venous access**.

A measure of **SVR, PA** pressure and pulmonary capillary wedge pressure (**PCWP**) or right atrial pressure (**RAP**) is often required. These can be measured (and derived, in the case of SVR) from invasive **PA catheters**, less invasive **PICCO** or **LidCo** systems, or even **oesophageal Doppler** measurements (see 'CVP lines and invasive monitoring', Chapter 110, page 443).

Possible viva questions related to this topic

→ What are the indications for intubation?
→ What apparatus can be used for endotracheal intubation? Describe the technique for orotracheal intubation.
→ What is meant by 'rapid sequence induction'?
→ How does cricoid pressure assist in rapid sequence induction?
→ What is the definition of anatomical and physiological dead space?
→ Draw a standard spirometry trace and label the key values.
→ How can oxygen be delivered to the patient?
→ What is a Venturi connector?
→ How does a reservoir bag increase the FiO_2 given to a patient?
→ What modes of mechanical ventilation are available and what are their uses?
→ What do you understand by the term 'CPAP'?
→ What is PEEP?
→ What are the complications of mechanical ventilation?

Related topics		
Topic	Chapter	Page
Sedation	120	500
Acute respiratory distress syndrome	105	419
CVP lines and invasive monitoring	110	443
Control of respiration	91	373
Criteria for admission to the ITU and HDU	109	439
Pneumothorax	117	488
Respiratory failure and respiratory function tests	119	495
Tracheostomy	42	148
Starling's law of the heart and cardiovascular equations	102	403

TYPES OF DEFINITIVE AIRWAY

- Endotracheal airways:
  - orotracheal intubation – most commonly used
  - nasotracheal intubation
- Laryngeal mask

↑ **Example viva question**

What are the indications for intubation?

Endotracheal (ET) intubation is performed for the express purpose of securing the airway. The use of an ET tube should prevent silent aspiration with the cuff inflated.

Indications
- Apnoea and/or respiratory failure
- Protecting the airway from impending obstruction (e.g. burns/facial oedema/facial trauma, low GCS)
- Protection from aspiration pneumonitis (e.g. in abdominal surgery)
- Head injury with risk of raised ICP and a need for tight control of $PaCO_2$
- Inability to maintain an airway by less invasive methods
- Hypoxia refractory to oxygen therapy
- Vocal fold paralysis
- ET intubation is indicated in elective abdominal surgery

- Surgical airways:
  - cricothyroidotomy
  - tracheostomy (surgical or percutaneous) (see 'Tracheostomy', Chapter 42, page 148).

METHODS OF OXYGEN DELIVERY

Oxygen delivery to the lungs depends on:
- Patent airway
- Concentration of inspired oxygen (FiO_2)
- Adequate ventilation.

Patent airway

Although a definitive airway is often used in surgical practice, an obstructed airway can be managed with escalating levels of invasive care:
- **Chin lift** and **jaw thrust** (as per ATLS): maintain patency of the upper airway when the tongue has fallen back
- **Guedel airway**: not suitable for fully alert patients but useful for temporary bag-and-mask ventilation of the unconscious patient before intubation. Situated above the vocal folds so cannot prevent aspiration and can initiate the gag reflex
- **Nasopharyngeal airway**: more suitable for drowsy patients and less likely to initiate the gag reflex than the Guedel airway. Contraindicated in facial trauma and suspected base of skull fractures.

↑ **Example viva question**

Describe the technique for orotracheal intubation.

Orotracheal intubation
- **Check** all equipment **before starting**: laryngoscope, suction, ET tube (size 7–8 for females and size 8–9 for males), Ambu bag and mask, oxygen supply, muscle relaxant, intravenous sedation, intravenous access and ensure that you have an assistant
- **Preoxygenate** the patient **with 100 per cent O$_2$** for several minutes – if breathing on their own, hold the mask close to the face and allow them to preoxygenate without sedation or muscle relaxation. In an acute setting, give sedation and/or muscle relaxant before attempting to preoxygenate
- Allow a **maximum of 30 seconds** per insertion attempt
- Use **laryngoscope directly** to **visualize** the **vocal folds** and pass the ET tube between them. In difficult intubations where an unobstructed view of the folds cannot be achieved, the use of a **bougie may be helpful**, railroading the tube on the bougie, having passed it between the folds
- **Inflate cuff** and **check position of tube** by **auscultation** of the **lungs** and epigastrium. End-tidal CO$_2$ monitors are also useful in verifying tube position
- **Secure tube** by tying in place with tapes (average length to teeth in females is 21–23 cm, 23–25 cm in males)

Rapid sequence induction
This process involves the intubation of a patient with **suspected gastric contents**:

- Recent meal
- Delayed gastric emptying: **trauma**, sepsis, **gastroparesis**
- Incompetent lower oesophageal sphincter: **pregnancy**, hiatus hernia
- After administration of the muscle relaxant, **cricoid pressure** is initiated by the assistant. This **collapses the oesophageal lumen** behind and **prevents aspiration**. The cricoid pressure is released only when the tube position has been confirmed and the ET cuff inflated

Concentration of inspired oxygen

A simple **Hudson mask** delivers an **unreliable** FiO$_2$ to the patient and its use should be **avoided** in the acute setting if at all possible.

Venturi connectors are useful and reliable methods of delivering a relatively **constant** FiO$_2$ to a patient and rely on the Venturi effect.

The **Venturi effect** is a special case of **Bernoulli's** principle, in the case of fluid flow or airflow through a tube or pipe with a constriction in it. The fluid must **speed up in the** restriction, **reducing its pressure** and **producing a partial vacuum** via Bernoulli's effect. This vacuum encourages air to mix with the oxygen flow at a set rate, thereby setting the FiO_2. It is essential, when using Venturi connectors, to ensure that the rate from the wall is the same as that printed on the connector.

The **most oxygen** that can be delivered on the ward is through a **reservoir bag**. As the **flow of oxygen from the wall cannot match the minute volume of the patient**, air mixes with each breath around the sides of the Hudson mask and through the holes in it. A mask with a reservoir bag must be close fitting and, with each breath, the **extra air** that cannot be supplied by the wall is **supplied by the 100 per cent oxygen** in the **reservoir bag**, thus **increasing** the FiO_2. Despite this, a reservoir bag can still produce only around a **60–70 per cent FiO_2** as a result of imperfections in the fitting of the mask.

In the case of most modern mechanical ventilators, the FiO_2 can be set through the ventilator.

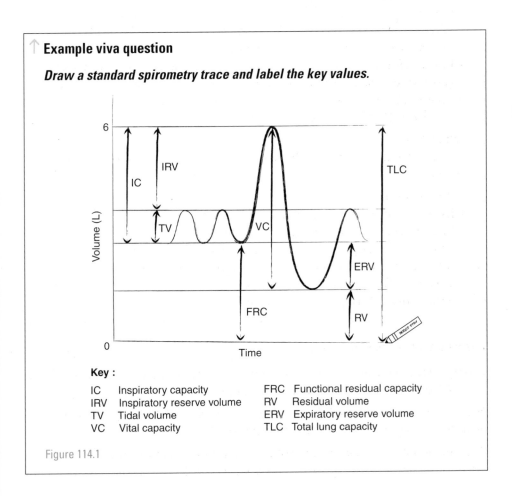

Example viva question

Draw a standard spirometry trace and label the key values.

Key :

IC	Inspiratory capacity	FRC	Functional residual capacity
IRV	Inspiratory reserve volume	RV	Residual volume
TV	Tidal volume	ERV	Expiratory reserve volume
VC	Vital capacity	TLC	Total lung capacity

Figure 114.1

ASSISTED VENTILATION

Assisted ventilation can be split into **non-invasive** and **invasive** ventilation.

Non-invasive ventilation

- **CPAP (continuous positive airway pressure)**: delivered by an airtight mask over the nose and mouth, which provides a continuous positive pressure in the airways, thus **splinting open alveoli** and **improving recruitment**, **reducing the work of breathing**
- **Pressure support**: can be delivered by a CPAP mask. Closely monitors the airflow in the circuit and **provides a positive pressure increase when** it senses that the **patient wishes to take a breath. Used** together **with CPAP** it can drastically **reduce the work of breathing** and may be termed 'BIPAP' (bilevel positive airway pressure).

Invasive ventilation

Invasive ventilation provides the most **reliable way** of providing a **constant** FiO_2 to the patient, along with **reducing the anatomical dead space** and in some cases increasing the **efficiency of ventilation**.

- **CPAP** may be administered invasively.
- **BIPAP** and/or **pressure support** may be administered invasively.
- **IPPV** (intermittent positive-pressure ventilation) is an **obligatory** ventilatory mode requiring **apnoea**. It is the most used form of ventilation in acute trauma or surgery where patients are anaesthetized and paralysed at the same time.
- **SIMV** (simultaneous intermittent mechanical ventilation) allows synchronization with any respiratory effort that the patient may make, but guarantees a number of breaths per minute.

↑ **Example viva question**

What is PEEP?

PEEP stands for **positive end-expiratory pressure** and is used to ensure a positive pressure at the end of expiration, **splinting open the alveoli** and preventing the usual alveolar collapse. This **decreases the work of breathing** by obviating the initial force on inspiration required to open the alveoli and **overcome the surface tension of alveolar water**.

High levels of PEEP **increase the risk of barotrauma**.

A further subdivision of invasive ventilation is **pressure-controlled** and **volume-controlled** ventilation.

Volume controlled

A **less sophisticated** method of ventilation, this allows the user to **set a tidal volume** that must be delivered **regardless of the airway pressures** involved, and thus **increase the risk or barotrauma** to the lungs (see 'Complications' below). Pressure limits can be used to help prevent this. Volume-controlled ventilation does **provide a constant minute volume.**

Pressure controlled

A **more sophisticated** method of ventilation, it allows the user to set a **peak inspiratory pressure (PIP)**. Inhalation occurs until this PIP is reached, after which passive exhalation is allowed. The delivered volume with each respiration is dependent on the pulmonary and thoracic compliance. A major advantage of pressure-controlled ventilation is a **decelerating inspiratory flow pattern**, in which **inspiratory flow tapers off** as the **lung inflates**. This usually results in a more homogeneous gas distribution throughout the lungs and a **decrease in the incidence of barotrauma.**

However, **tidal volumes are not constant** in this method of ventilation, although mixed modes with volume-assured, pressure-controlled ventilation are now available on some ventilators.

Complications of mechanical ventilation

Pulmonary effects
- **Barotrauma** results in **pulmonary interstitial emphysema**, pneumomediastinum, pneumoperitoneum, pneumothorax and/or tension pneumothorax. High peak inflation pressures ($> 40\,cmH_2O$) are associated with an increased incidence of barotrauma.
- **Alveolar cellular dysfunction** occurs with high airway pressures. The resultant **surfactant depletion** leads to **atelectasis**, which requires further **increases in airway pressure** to **maintain lung volumes**.
- **High airway pressures** result in **alveolar over-distension (volutrauma)**, increased **microvascular permeability** and **parenchymal injury**.
- High-inspired concentrations of oxygen ($FiO_2 > 50$ per cent) result in **free-radical formation** and **secondary cellular damage**. These same high concentrations of oxygen can lead to alveolar nitrogen washout and **secondary absorption atelectasis**.

Cardiovascular effects
- **Increased intrathoracic pressures** result in a **decrease in cardiac output** as a result of **decreased venous return** to the heart (see 'Starling's law of the heart and cardiovascular equations', Chapter 102, page 403), right ventricular dysfunction and altered left ventricular distensibility.

- Exaggerated respiratory variation on the arterial pressure waveform ('**swinging of the arterial line waveform**') is a clue that positive pressure ventilation is significantly affecting venous return and cardiac output. In the absence of an arterial line, a good pulse oximetry waveform can be equally instructive. A reduction in the variation after volume loading confirms this effect (see 'Fluid balance', Chapter 111, page 452).

Renal, hepatic and gastrointestinal effects

- Positive pressure ventilation is responsible for an overall **decline in renal function** with **decreased urine volume** and **sodium excretion**.
- **Hepatic function** is adversely affected by **decrease** in **cardiac output**, increased hepatic vascular resistance and elevated bile duct pressure.
- The gastric mucosa does not have autoregulatory capability. Thus, **mucosal ischaemia** and secondary bleeding may result from a decrease in cardiac output and increased gastric venous pressure.

↑ **Example viva question**

What is the definition of anatomical and physiological dead space?

The dead space is the **total volume** of the parts of the lung and airways that **does not participate in gaseous exchange**:

- Anatomical: mouth, nasopharynx, larynx, trachea and bronchi
- Physiological: diseased lung unable to perform gaseous exchange (either collapsed alveoli or poorly perfused alveoli, i.e. $\dot{V}/\dot{Q}$ mismatch)

---

115 Nutrition

Possible viva questions related to this topic

→ Why is nutrition important in the context of surgical disease?
→ How can nutrition be administered?
→ What are the clinical signs of malnutrition?
→ How can nutritional status be assessed?
→ What are the advantages of enteral feeding over total parenteral nutrition (TPN)?
→ What are the complications of TPN?
→ What are the nutritional requirements of a 70 kg man before and after elective surgery? What would happen to them if he developed a post-operative pyrexia/sepsis?
→ How do severe burns affect nutritional requirements?
→ What trace elements are required and which are associated with wound healing?

NUTRITION IN SURGERY

In an **elective context**, the nutrition of a patient both **pre-** and **postoperatively** is crucial. An undernourished patient will suffer from **poor wound healing**, a **dampened immune system** and eventually **organ dysfunction**.

In an emergency context, the nutrition of an **acutely unwell patient** is even **more critical** because ill, septic patients in a **catabolic state** have a much **increased** nutritional requirement (see 'Systemic response to surgery', Chapter 123, page 574).

ASSESSMENT OF NUTRITIONAL STATUS

- History
- Examination
- Anthropometric and dynamometric measurements

- Biochemical assessment (e.g. albumin, liver function, U+Es)
- Immune function.

↑ **Key learning point**

When asked how to assess the nutritional status of a patient, **don't jump to the common answer 'plasma albumin',** which has, in fact, been shown to **very poorly correlate** with nutritional status. However, consistent drops in plasma albumin in the context of acutely unwell patients have been shown to correlate quite well with poor outcomes. (Note that this is not purely attributable to nutrition.)

SIGNS OF MALNUTRITION

Early signs (loss of 15 per cent body weight)

Na^+ and water retention leading to peripheral oedema.

Severe signs (loss of > 15 per cent body weight)

- Loss of muscle mass and fat
- Anaemia
- Diarrhoea.

Pre-terminal signs

- Decreased albumin synthesis and antibody production
- Poor wound healing (particularly zinc, magnesium and selenium trace elements important)
- Acidosis
- Hyperkalaemia
- Decreased cough reflex – leading to possible pneumonia.

ENTERAL NUTRITION

This utilizes the GI tract and so a prerequisite for this type of nutrition is an intact and functional gut. Methods of enteral feeding are:

- Oral
- Nasogastric tube (NGT) or nasojejunal tube (NJT)
- Percutaneous endoscopic gastrostomy (PEG)
- Percutaneous endoscopic jejunostomy (PEJ)
- Surgical jejunostomy.

Indications for enteral feeding

- Severe catabolic states (e.g. burns)
- Malnutrition pre-surgery
- Postoperative oesophagogastric surgery
- The unconscious patient
- Anorexic elderly patient with inadequate intake
- Mild-to-moderate GI disease (pancreatitis, short-gut syndrome, Crohn's disease).

Monitoring

- Clinical
- Fluid balance
- Daily weights
- Electrolytes and twice-weekly trace elements.

Advantages over TPN

- Safer
- Cheaper
- Fewer complications
- Prevents atrophy of gut mucosa (occurs within 48 h of fasting)
- Continues to encourage adequate immunological barrier across gut mucosa (IgA levels and intact endothelium).

Complications of enteral feeding

- Blockage/misplaced tube
- Aspiration (either silent or overt) and subsequent pneumonia
- Irritation of gut lining and ulceration/bleeding

↑ **Example viva question**

What are the nutritional requirements of a 70 kg man before and after surgery? How does this change if he develops a pyrexia or sepsis?

Normal nutritional requirements are approximately 30 kcal/kg, which works out to roughly 2000 kcal in the 70 kg man.

Postoperatively this increases to 35 kcal/kg, and increases by a further 10 per cent per degree increase in temperature.

In the septic state, requirements go up further still to 40–45 kcal/kg and in hypercatabolic states, such as severe burns, can rise to as high as 60 kcal/kg!

- Nausea and vomiting
- Diarrhoea
- Deranged LFTs
- 'Re-feeding syndrome' in patients who have not been fed for significant period of time.

PPN AND TPN (PARTIAL OR TOTAL PARENTERAL NUTRITION)

This is delivery of **nutrition** via the **intravenous** route. Its advantages are that it **does not require an intact gastrointestinal system**.

Indications

- Absolute or relative intestinal failure
- Hypercatabolic states
- Postoperative (in some selected cases – particularly with prolonged gastroparesis and failure of absorption).

↑ **Example viva question**

What does TPN contain?

TPN is made up for the **individual patient** and is changed according to their individual requirements (e.g. more potassium, less lipids, etc.).

However, essentially TPN is a mixture of **hypertonic sugars** with **fat emulsions**, **nitrogen, electrolytes, vitamins** and **trace elements**:

- > 50 per cent carbohydrates
- 30–40 per cent fat emulsions
- 1–2 g/kg by body weight per day of fat
- nitrogen: synthetic crystalline amino acid preparation in *laevo* form
- water: 30–35 mL/kg per day
- electrolytes: Na^+, K^+, Cl^-, Ca^{2+}, Mg^{2+}, PO_4^{3-}
- vitamins: A, D, E, K (fat soluble), B, C

MONITORING TPN

- Weight
- U+Es, glucose, FBC, LFTs
- Fluid balance
- Temperature and signs of sepsis
- Trace elements.

ROUTES OF ADMINISTRATION

This is usually via an **indwelling central venous access device**, be that a Hickman line or simple non-tunnelled CVP line. TPN can be given by long/peripheral lines, usually sited in the antecubital fossa.

COMPLICATIONS

- Line sepsis
- Metabolic derangement
- Na^+ retention, acidosis
- TPN jaundice
- Expense
- Venous access problems.

116 Oliguria and renal replacement

Possible viva questions related to this topic

→ What are the common causes of postoperative oliguria?
→ What are the principles of management of oliguria?
→ What are the indications for renal replacement therapy?
→ What are the various varieties of renal replacement therapy?
→ What is the minimum acceptable urine output for a patient?
→ How would you classify acute renal failure?
→ What factors determine the urine output?
→ What is creatinine clearance? How can it be measured?

ACUTE RENAL FAILURE AND CHRONIC RENAL FAILURE

Acute renal failure (ARF) is a relatively common postoperative surgical condition and it in most cases a **surgical disease** as a result of **shock from any cause** (see 'Shock', Chapter 122, page 510) whereas **chronic renal failure (CRF)** is a **medical disease**.

Factors that determine urine output

- Renal **perfusion pressure** (proportional to glomerular filtration rate or GFR)
- Renal **tubular function**
- **Patent urinary tract**
- Neurohormonal mechanisms affecting **electrolyte** and **water retention** (see 'Function of the kidney II', Chapter 93, page 377).

Example viva question

How would you classify acute renal failure?

Acute renal failure is a syndrome of **rapidly deteriorating renal function**. There is **no consensus** as to its exact definition and over **30 different definitions** have been published.

One possible definition is: 'Acute renal failure (ARF) is a syndrome characterised by a rapid decline in glomerular filtration rate (hours to days), retention of nitrogenous waste products, and perturbation of extracellular fluid volume and electrolyte and acid–base homeostasis.'

Acute renal failure can be classified as:

- **Pre-renal** (haemodynamic instability, **low cardiac output** and **hypotension** leading to **low renal perfusion**)
- **Renal** (**parenchymal damage** and **glomerulonephritis**)
- **Post-renal** (**obstructive** – stones, strictures, tumours in the wall of the ureter, e.g. transitional cell carcinoma, iatrogenic [ligation of the ureters intraoperative])

Example viva question

What is creatinine clearance? How can it be measured?

Definition: The inverse of the time constant that describes the removal rate of creatinine from the body divided by its volume of distribution (or total body water).

It is used as a **surrogate for GFR** but correctly is **NOT the volume of plasma cleared of creatinine per unit time.** Thus:

$$CrCl = (uCr \times uV)/(sCr \times 1440)$$

where: uCr = urine creatinine concentration, uV = volume of urine in 24 h, sCr = serum creatinine concentration.

This method, known as '24-hour urine' because **required only** in circumstances of **altered protein intake** or **decreased body mass**. In other cases, the **Cockcroft and Gault formula** is usually sufficient:

- **Altered protein intake** – malnutrition, vegetarian diet, creatinine supplementation
- **Altered body mass** – amputation, malnutrition or muscle wasting

DETERMINATION OF GFR AND CREATININE CLEARANCE

Clinically, the **Cockcroft and Gault formula** can be used to estimate the creatinine clearance for a given patient and thus their GFR:

$$\text{Male: GFR} = [(140 - \text{Age}) \times (\text{Weight})]/(\text{sCr} \times 72)$$

$$\text{Female: GFR} = [(140 - \text{Age}) \times (\text{Weight}) \times 0.85]/(\text{sCr} \times 72).$$

Common causes of postoperative oliguria ($< 30\,\text{mL/h}$ or $< 0.5\,\text{mL/kg}$ per h in adults and $< 1.0\,\text{mL/kg}$ per h in children)

- **Stress response** (see 'Systemic response to surgery', Chapter 123, page 514). Sodium and water retained as a result of ADH, aldosterone and cortisol secretion as a stress response
- **Poor renal perfusion** (pre-renal):
  - **hypotension** as a result of **underfilling** (dehydration or inadequate fluid replacement in patients nil by mouth) or continued **blood loss**
  - **low cardiac output** state
  - **vasodilatation** secondary to SIRS or septic shock (see 'Sepsis and SIRS', Chapter 121, page 505)
  - **intra-abdominal compartment syndrome** (see 'Compartment syndrome', Chapter 108, page 433)
- Established acute tubular necrosis (**ATN**) (**renal**) from a bout of perioperative hypotension
- **Renal tract obstruction** (**post-renal**) iatrogenic, **blocked urinary catheter**, stones, extrinsic compression.

PRINCIPLES OF MANAGEMENT OF POSTOPERATIVE OLIGURIA

ARF as a result of ATN postoperatively is potentially fully reversible if caught in time. It is therefore most important to exclude ATN as a cause of oliguria postoperatively.

- **Obstruction** must be excluded:
  - **urinary catheter flush ± replacement. Bladder scan** can be useful to measure the volume of urine in an obstructed bladder
  - there are only two causes of **anuria**: one is a **blocked catheter** and the other **advanced ATN**.
- **Hypovolaemia** should be **excluded** (see 'Fluid balance', Chapter 111, page 452).
- If necessary, a **CVP line** should be sited and **response to a fluid challenge** should be assessed.
- Measure the patient's **urine osmolality**. If the urine is **isosmolar** to plasma (280–320 mosmol/L) this is suggestive of **renal failure**. Fluid should then be **restricted to 20 mL/h** plus the previous hour's output and a careful eye must be

placed on the serum **potassium**, treating above **6 mmol/L** with an **insulin** and **dextrose** infusion ± calcium resonium/calcium gluconate. ECG should be performed to see if hyperkalaemia has associated **ECG changes** (peaked T waves, etc.).

- Low threshold for liaising with ITU early.
- Check **ABGs** to monitor any development of a **metabolic acidosis** (see 'Acid–base balance', Chapter 84, page 349).
- Measure **serum creatinine** at least **daily**.
- Ensure that **accurate fluid balance chart** is kept and that urine osmolality and electrolyte content are measured daily.
- Ensure that there are **no nephrotoxic agents** on the drug chart (e.g. **aminoglycosides** and **NSAIDs** in particular).
- There is no evidence to suggest that so-called 'renal dose' dopamine improves outcome or prevents renal failure.
- Consider **inotropic support** (see 'Inotropes', Chapter 113, page 466) and/or a **frusemide infusion** (in HDU/ITU setting usually).
- Arrange **ultrasonography of kidneys** to exclude an obstructive cause.

RENAL REPLACEMENT THERAPIES

In an acute setting, renal replacement is indicated if:

- It is impossible to control the serum potassium with conventional measures such as an insulin and dextrose infusion (**hyperkalaemia > 6 mmol/L**)
- The **patient is overloaded** and in **pulmonary oedema** with the intention of taking fluid off and creating a negative fluid balance
- There is a symptomatic uraemia (**serum urea > 30 mmol/L**)
- There are signs of **encephalopathy**
- There is a profound **metabolic acidosis** (pH < 7.2)
- Hepatorenal syndrome is developing
- Serum creatinine is rising very steeply (although this is perhaps the most controversial indication).

Methods of renal replacement

These can be continuous or intermittent and are broadly split into three categories.

Haemofiltration
- Continuous convection of molecules across a semipermeable membrane results in removal of not only solutes but also fluid. This **fluid is replaced** with an isotonic buffered solution. The technique is very useful in an ITU setting for **restoring fluid balance** relatively quickly, and requires only one vascular access port in its simplest venovenous configuration (usually in the femoral vein but

can be via a central line or surgical arteriovenous fistula in the case of chronic patients)
- **Good for fluid removal** but not as efficient as haemodialysis in clearing smaller molecules
- **Continuous system.**

Haemodialysis
- Blood interfaces with a dialysate across a semipermeable membrane, permitting passage of molecules smaller than 5 kDa down a diffusion gradient
- **Less good for fluid removal** (see above)
- **Continuous or intermittent.**

Peritoneal dialysis
- **No longer used** in an acute setting
- Commonly used in patients with CRF
- Peritoneum and omentum becomes semipermeable membrane, dialysate is infused into the abdominal cavity via a Tenckhoff indwelling catheter and is drained off after several hours
- Slow and less efficient than either of above systems
- Does not require vascular access
- Spontaneous bacterial peritonitis a serious complication. Dialysate is infused with broad-spectrum antibiotics to treat this condition.

Modalities of continuous renal replacement

These are categorized according to the vascular pattern utilized and the type of replacement, either dialysis or filtration:

- **Continuous venovenous haemofiltration (CVVH):** flow is produced by roller pumps. Patient needs good vascular access but one Vascath in the femoral vein is common in ITU renal replacement strategies.
- **Continuous arteriovenous haemofiltration:** flow relies on patient's arterial blood pressure and is thus driven by the arteriovenous pressure difference. Less commonly used in most ITUs.
- **Continuous arteriovenous or venovenous haemodialysis.**
- **Haemodiafiltration:** provides the best urea clearance by the combination of the two techniques but can remove large volumes of fluid and needs careful management to prevent the patient from becoming haemodynamically unstable.

Complications of renal replacement

These can be split into the following.

Infections
- Line sepsis
- Bacterial peritonitis in peritoneal dialysis.

Technical problems with the circuit
- Clotted circuit
- Loss of connection leading to air embolus
- Haemorrhage.

Systemic complications
- SIRS
- ARDS.

Complications as a result of fluid and electrolyte shifts
- Hypotension
- **Disequilibrium syndrome: cerebral oedema** following massive shifts in serum osmolality after filtration of large numbers of urea molecules. Presents as headache, nausea and vomiting, and occasionally **seizures**.

117 Pneumothorax

Related topics		
Topic	**Chapter**	**Page**
CVP lines and invasive ventilation	110	443
Starling's law of the heart and cardiovascular equations	102	403
Systemic response to surgery	123	514

DEFINITION

Abnormal air in the intrapleural space.

CLASSIFICATION OF PNEUMOTHORAX

- Closed (spontaneous)
- Open
- Tension.

Closed pneumothorax (spontaneous)

- **Pressure within alveoli > intrapleural pressure** and if weakened alveolus ruptures, and air passes from the lung into the intrapleural space until the pressure in the two spaces equilibrates.
- The **air will reabsorb** if the source of the pneumothorax is **sealed**.

Clinical features
- SOB (shortness of breath)
- Chest pain (often pleuritic in nature)

- Tachycardia
- Reduced chest wall expansion on the affected side
- Hyperresonance on percussion of the affected side.

Causes
- Primary (no known cause – spontaneous)
- Rupture of bullae
- Marfan's/Ehlers–Danlos syndrome and other connective tissue diseases
- Asthma
- Iatrogenic (e.g. CVP line, barotrauma with excessive ventilation)
- Blunt trauma.

Management
Twenty per cent of closed pneumothoraces **do not require** invasive management and may be managed expectantly. **Increasing the FiO_2** of the patient will increase the speed of **reabsorption** as nitrogen is replaced with oxygen in the intrapleural space and this is reabsorbed faster.

Those patients who do require surgical management will require an **intercostal chest drain** with an underwater seal. In a small number of cases, **aspiration** of the pneumothorax may be sufficient.

Open pneumothorax

- Caused by **penetrating trauma** to the chest wall
- Enables air from the outside to communicate with air in the intrapleural space
- If hole in the chest wall is greater than the cross-sectional area of the trachea/larynx, the mediastinum will shift to the contralateral side because air will preferentially enter the hole.

Management
First the wound must be **sealed** either by **surgical closure** or temporarily by an **occlusive dressing**, so converting the open pneumothorax to a closed pneumothorax. A chest drain is then inserted. The danger in this is that, before the chest drain can be inserted, the open pneumothorax may be converted to a tension pneumothorax.

Tension pneumothorax

- Occurs when the **hole in the pleura is unsealed** and a **valve is formed** which **allows air into** the pleural space on **inspiration** but **does not allow it to escape** on expiration
- Pressure in the intrapleural space therefore rises and the mediastinum is pushed into the contralateral space in the chest cavity.

Management
This requires **immediate needle decompression** (without waiting for confirmatory radiology) followed by a chest drain.

> ↑ **Example viva question**
>
> *Why is a tension pneumothorax universally fatal if untreated?*
>
> As the intrapleural pressure rises and the mediastinum is further shifted over to the opposite side of the chest cavity, so the high pressure reduces venous return (Vret) and therefore cardiac output (CO). Eventually, Vret falls to 0, so reducing CO to 0 and causing cardiac arrest. **A heart that cannot fill cannot empty!**

INSERTION OF A CHEST DRAIN

- Unless an emergency, **pre-procedure a chest radiograph** should be performed
- Patient has arm fully abducted behind neck
- 'Triangle of safety' is identified (lateral border of pectoralis major, anterior border of latissimus dorsi and a line superior to the horizontal level of the nipple)
- Skin is prepared and draped and local anaesthetic is infiltrated
- 3 cm incision in rib space (classically fifth intercostal space in the midaxillary line)
- Spencer–Wells forceps used to dissect tissue down to rib
- Chest wall and pleura breached above rib to **avoid neurovascular bundle**
- Drain is placed through track guided with forceps (**never use a trocar!**)
- Stitched in place with 1/0 silk and mattress suture or purse string **inserted but not tied** in anticipation of removal
- Occlusive dressing placed around drain site
- Drain connected to underwater seal ± suction in some instances
- **Chest radiograph** to confirm drain position.

REMOVAL OF A CHEST DRAIN

- Remove in **forced expiration**
- **Tie mattress suture/z-suture/purse-string suture**
- **Occlusive dressing** over wound
- **Chest radiograph post-procedure** to check for **pneumothorax**.

118 Pulse oximetry

Possible viva questions related to this topic

→ What is a pulse oximeter and what is it used for?
→ What are the principles of pulse oximetry?
→ What does pulse oximetry measure?
→ How does the SaO_2 relate to PO_2 on ABGs?
→ What other parameters need to be known to interpret a pulse oximeter reading?
→ What are the pitfalls and sources of error in pulse oximetry?
→ In what circumstances might the percentage saturation be erroneously high?
→ What is methaemoglobin and how does its presence in the blood affect a pulse oximeter?

Example viva question

How does pulse oximetry work?

Pulse oximetry is widely used in the postoperative surgical HDU patient. It **calculates the percentage oxygen saturation** of the arterial blood (SaO_2).

Oxygenated and **deoxygenated haemoglobin** optimally **reflect different wavelengths** of incident **light**. Thus, the pulse oximeter uses two different light-emitting diodes at two wavelengths:

• 660 nm (red light) – measures total amount of haemoglobin
• 940 nm (infrared or IR light) – measures oxygenated haemoglobin

Thus, a **percentage of saturated haemoglobin** can be calculated from a **ratio of the two**.

Probes are attached to either **fingers** or **ear lobes** and measure not only SaO_2 but also **pulse rate**, and estimate **pulse volume** in some cases.

PULSE OXIMETRY AND ABGs

> ↑ **Key learning point**
>
> *FiO₂ is key!*
>
> Note that either SaO_2 or PaO_2 is absolutely **meaningless without** know-ledge of the **concentration of inspired oxygen** or oxygen flow (i.e. FiO_2).
>
> A saturation of **95 per cent on air** may be considered **reasonable** but the same saturations on **high-flow oxygen** with a non-rebreather reservoir bag could indicate **very poor** gas transfer. Likewise, a PaO_2 of **12.0 kPa** on room air would be considered **normal** but the same PaO_2 on **100 per cent humidi-fied** O_2 through an ET tube reflects **severe respiratory failure**.
>
> Therefore, **pulse oximetry does not assess ventilation** and other tests such as **end-tidal CO_2** and **capnography** should be used for this purpose.
>
> *What is the A–a gradient?*
>
> Put simply, the **A–a gradient** is a **measure** of how well **oxygen is transferred from** the **alveolus to the blood** and is defined as:
>
> $$\text{A–a gradient} = PAO_2 - PaO_2$$
>
> where PAO = partial pressure of oxygen in the alveolus and PaO_2 = partial pressure of oxygen in arterial blood.
>
> PaO_2 is obtained from ABGs and PAO_2 is estimated from the alveolar gas equation:
>
> $$PAO_2 = [(760 - 47) \times FiO_2 - PaCO_2]/0.8$$
>
> where FiO_2 is expressed as a fraction.
>
> A normal **A–a gradient** on air is estimated by:
>
> $$(\text{Age} + 10)/4.$$
>
> A **higher gradient** indicates **shunting** and/or a **ventilation–perfusion mismatch**.

The **delivery of oxygen** to the tissues depends on **three factors** (see 'Oxygen transport', Chapter 99, page 394):

1. Cardiac output
2. Haemoglobin concentration
3. Oxygen saturation (SaO_2).

A drop in SaO_2 can be picked up more quickly with pulse oximetry than clinical observation for peripheral cyanosis (where SaO_2 needs to drop to 60–70 per cent before cyanosis is observed).

The PaO_2 has a **non-linear relationship** to SaO_2 (see 'Oxygen dissociation curve', in 'Oxygen transport', Chapter 99, page 394), although the two are often confused. Remember that SaO_2 can be normal despite a low PaO_2 in acute pulmonary embolus, reinforcing the need for ABGs in such a case.

PITFALLS AND SOURCES OF ERROR

- **Cold peripheries** and poor tissue perfusion can lead to an inability of the pulse oximeter to get a reading
- **Abnormal pulses** such as **atrial fibrillation** and **tricuspid regurgitation** can affect the reading because the signal is averaged over a number of heart beats
- **Changes to Hb** or **pigments** in the blood:
  - **CO poisoning** in fire victims and **smokers** (this binds haemoglobin and changes its light reflectance properties to that of oxyhaemoglobin; thus, SaO_2 is reported as erroneously high despite a low O_2 saturation displaced by the CO)
  - **bilirubin** in high concentrations can have a similar effect but it causes the pulse oximeter to **underestimate the true SaO_2**
  - **methaemoglobinaemia** (see below)
- **Delay**: SaO_2 is calculated over a number of heart beats and so there is approximately a **20-second lag** between physiological values and SaO_2
- **Nail varnish:** prevents penetration of light and must be removed preoperatively
- **Electrical interference**: diathermy
- **High ambient light** can interfere with the incident light from the pulse oximeter
- **Movement**/shivering can affect the signal
- Remember that **pulse oximetry is not a measure of ventilation!**

METHAEMOGLOBINAEMIA

Methaemoglobin (Met-Hb) has **iron in a ferric state (Fe^{3+})** within the haem moiety instead of the ferrous state (Fe^{2+}) as in normal haemoglobin. The result of this is that the Met-Hb molecule has a **reduced oxygen-carrying capacity**. This may be a congenital problem with a deficiency of Met-Hb-reducing enzymes (NADH methaemoglobin reductase) or an acquired problem as a result of **nitrate pollution** in the water supply or use of the local anaesthetic agent **prilocaine.**

Treatment is by administration of a **reducing agent** such as methylene blue.

119 Respiratory failure and respiratory function tests

Possible viva questions related to this topic

→ What is the definition of respiratory failure?
→ How can it be classified?
→ Why is P_{CO_2} normal or low in type I failure but high in type II failure?
→ What is the difference between type I and type II respiratory failure?
→ What are the principles of treatment of respiratory failure?
→ How is respiratory function measured?
→ Define the functional residual capacity (FRC). Name some factors that increase and decrease it.
→ What parameters are affected in obstructive versus restrictive disease?
→ What is a flow–volume loop?
→ What do flow–volume loops look like in respiratory disease? Draw some examples.

CLINICAL SIGNS OF RESPIRATORY DISTRESS

A diagnosis of respiratory distress should be made on the following:

- Use of accessory muscles of respiration
- Tachypnoea
- Tachycardia
- Sweating
- Pulsus paradoxus
- Inability to speak full sentences
- Signs of CO_2 retention.

↑ **Key learning point**

Respiratory failure is when pulmonary gas exchange is sufficiently impaired to cause hypoxaemia with or without hypercapnia.

That is, $PaO_2 < 8\,kPa$ (60 mmHg) or $PaCO_2 > 7\,kPa$ (55 mmHg)

Normal ranges for an individual breathing air at sea level:

$$PaO_2 = 10.6-13.3\,kPa,\ PaCO_2 = 4.7-6.0\,kPa$$

Respiratory failure can be classified into two types.

Type I

A **failure of oxygenation** where PaO_2 **is low** on ABG sampling but $PaCO_2$ remains **normal** or is slightly low. Examples:

- Pneumonia ($\dot{V}$/Q mismatch)
- Pulmonary embolism ($\dot{V}$/Q mismatch)
- Cyanotic heart disease (right-to-left shunt)
- Pulmonary oedema ($\dot{V}$/Q mismatch)
- Bronchiectasis and asthma ($\dot{V}$/Q mismatch)
- ARDS ($\dot{V}$/Q mismatch)
- Fibrosing alveolitis ($\dot{V}$/Q mismatch).

Type II

A **failure of ventilation** where PaO_2 is low and $PaCO_2$ is abnormally high. Examples:

- COPD (chronic obstructive pulmonary disease)
- Chronic emphysema
- Chest wall deformities including flail chest trauma
- Respiratory muscle weakness (e.g. Guillain–Barré syndrome)
- Neuromuscular junction: myasthenia gravis
- Respiratory depression: opioids, barbiturates, head injury.

PATHOPHYSIOLOGY OF RESPIRATORY FAILURE

Type I

Pathology is the result of either a **right-to-left shunt** or a $\dot{V}$/Q **mismatch**:

- Initial elevation of $PaCO_2$ increases H^+ in the CSF (see 'Cerebrospinal fluid and the blood–brain barrier', Chapter 90, page 369) and **stimulates the central chemoreceptors** to increase the respiratory rate

- Results in CO_2 blown off maintaining $PaCO_2$
- As the O_2 dissociation curve is sigmoidal, **increasing the ventilation** does **little to the already low PaO_2.**

Type II

Pathology is the result of **alveolar hypoventilation**, leading to a **progressive increase in PCO_2.**

- **No compensation of $PaCO_2$** as a result of **respiratory apparatus failure** or a **resetting** of the central chemoreceptors in the case of COPD, thereby tolerating a higher $PaCO_2$.

MANAGEMENT OF RESPIRATORY FAILURE

Remember A, B, C!

- **Airway and breathing**: ensure that the **airway is patent** and **secure** using ET intubation if necessary
- **Low threshold** for **assisted** or **mechanical ventilation**
- Ensure **adequate ventilation**: progress from non-invasive ventilation such as NIPPV (non-invasive positive-pressure ventilation) by mask to invasive mechanical ventilation as required (see 'Intubation and ventilation', Chapter 114, page 470)
- Ensure **adequate oxygenation**: increase FiO_2 and use **humidified oxygen**
- **Antibiotics** for underlying infective processes
- Management of other underlying causes (e.g. **bronchodilators in asthma, chest physiotherapy** in bronchiectasis and cystic fibrosis)
- **Regular airway management,** e.g. **suction of secretions** and lavage if necessary
- FiO_2 tailored to the results of regular ABG sampling
- Changing of mechanical ventilator parameters (such as PEEP, I:E ratio and minute volume – see 'Acute respiratory distress syndrome', Chapter 105, page 419 and 'Intubation and ventilation', Chapter 114, page 470).

INVESTIGATIONS FOR ASSESSING RESPIRATORY FUNCTION

Non-invasive

- **Peak flow: bedside measure** of respiratory muscle function and airway resistance
- **Pulse oximetry**: estimates **arterial oxygen saturation** and is based on using two wavelengths of light and the different reflective properties of oxyhaemoglobin and deoxyhaemoglobin; depends on FiO_2

- **Capnography**: end-tidal CO_2 is measured as a **marker of ventilatory function** – a facility available on all modern anaesthetic ventilators
- **Spirometry**: a measure of **lung volumes** and **forced expiration** (FEV_1 – forced expiratory volume in 1 s)
- **Gas transfer function**: a measure of the **diffusing capacity** across the alveolus
- **$\dot{V}/\dot{Q}$ scanning** and **CT pulmonary angiography** if pulmonary emboli are suspected
- **Echocardiography**: assessment of **PA pressure** and **right heart function** in pulmonary hypertension
- Other imaging modalities: plain radiology, CT and MRI.

Invasive

- **ABGs**: **gold standard** measurement of **arterial oxygenation** and **Pa_{CO_2}**. Also crucial for assessment of **acid–base balance** (see 'Acid–base balance', Chapter 84, page 349)
- **Bronchoscopy**: for assessment of **lesions** and/or **secretions**; can be flexible or rigid
- **Lung biopsy**: CT guided or open via thoracoscopic procedure or open thoracotomy.

FUNCTIONAL RESIDUAL CAPACITY

This is the **volume of gas remaining in the lungs** after a **quiet expiration** (not forced.)

Factors increasing FRC

- Obstructive disease (e.g. asthma, bronchiectasis, COPD)
- Increasing PEEP – increases intrathoracic pressure.

Factors decreasing FRC

- Increasing age and body mass index (BMI)
- Limitation of lung inflation (e.g. pneumothorax, pleural effusion, empyema, thoracic incision, interstitial lung disease, increased intra-abdominal pressure).

FLOW–VOLUME LOOPS IN OBSTRUCTIVE AND RESTRICTIVE PULMONARY DISEASE

Plotting the relationship between airflow and lung volume over the respiratory cycle gives an indication of the type of pulmonary disease. **Obstructive diseases**, such as asthma, bronchiectasis and COPD, show an **increase in the total lung capacity** and **residual volume** as a result of **air trapping** and hyperinflation.

Restrictive disease shows a **reduction of all volumes** because of an **alteration in lung parenchyma** (e.g. idiopathic pulmonary fibrosis, fibrosing alveolitis), or a **disease of the pleura, chest wall** (e.g. kyphoscoliosis) or **neuromuscular apparatus** as seen in Fig. 119.1.

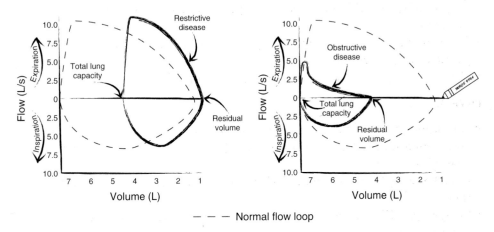

Figure 119.1

120 Sedation

Possible viva questions related to this topic

→ What is a sedative? How do a sedative, an anxiolytic and an anaesthetic differ?
→ What are the indications for sedatives in the acute setting?
→ What classes of sedatives are there and what is their action?
→ What sedatives are used in the ITU setting?
→ What sedative regimen would you use for minor procedures such as a small fracture manipulation not requiring an anaesthetic?
→ What types of sedative reversal are there?
→ What are the complications of sedative use?
→ Should analgesia be withheld before initial examination of the acute abdomen?

INDICATIONS FOR SEDATION

Indications for sedation in surgery are **many and varied** although any invasive procedure can be made easier by some light sedation:

• Light sedation for **minor procedures** (e.g. manipulation of dislocations and fractures, colonoscopy)
• Anxiolytic and light sedative can be used as a **premedication** before major surgery
• Can be useful for a **confused patient** on the ward, although great care must be taken to **investigate the cause** of the confusion (e.g. hypoxia, sepsis) and watch for respiratory depression
• Sedation is **mandatory** (if patient is not in arrest) on **ET intubation** (see 'Intubation and ventilation', Chapter 114, page 470)

↑ **Example viva question**

What is a sedative? How do a sedative, an anxiolytic and an anaesthetic differ?

- Anxiolysis is relief of apprehension and uneasiness without alteration of awareness
- Amnesia is loss of memory of an event or period and can be anterograde or retrograde
- Sedation is depression of a patient's awareness of the environment and reduction of his or her responsiveness to external stimulation:
  - conscious sedation is light sedation in which the patient maintains his or her airway reflexes and ability to cooperate
  - deep sedation is a more profound depression of the response to stimulation in which airway reflexes are not maintained
- Analgesia is relief of pain without sedation or alteration of the state of awareness (although analgesics may have a sedative effect)
- Anaesthesia is a state of unconsciousness

- After administration of neuromuscular blockers to paralyse the patient either for intubation or in ventilatory modes that require paralysis, adequate sedation is essential to prevent the patient from being aware of the paralysis. Further, in ventilatory modes that do not accommodate the patient's breathing effort (e.g. intermittent positive-pressure ventilation or IPPV), if inadequately paralysed and sedated, ventilation may be affected by 'fighting against' the ventilator
- An injured, stressed and uncooperative patient may benefit from sedation, although care must be taken in the context of a head injury; sedation in this context can help to decrease the acute physiological stress response (see 'Systemic response to surgery', Chapter 123, page 514)
- Sedation for MRI in children (must be done by paediatric anaesthetist).

CLASS OF SEDATIVE

Benzodiazepines (diazepam, lorazepam, midazolam)

The benzodiazepines act by stimulating GABA (γ-aminobutyric acid) receptors in the CNS. Stimulation of the receptor results in chloride influx, hyperpolarization and decreased neuronal excitation. Actions include:

- Anxiolysis and sedation
- Amnesia (most profound with midazolam)
- Anticonvulsant

- No analgesic properties
- Respiratory and cardiovascular depression (much greater risk if administered with centrally acting analgesic).

The major differences among the available agents concern the route of administration, time of onset, duration of action, mechanism of metabolism and accumulation of metabolites. In non-intubated patients, they are titrated, starting at the lower end of the range of recommended doses, followed by the administration of incremental doses until the desired effect is achieved. These sedatives are also **first-line agents** for **acute seizure management**.

Midazolam
- **Most commonly used** benzodiazepine for **minor procedures**
- Water soluble
- Short half-life
- **Profound amnesic effect** in many patients
- Rapid onset
- Metabolized by hepatic microsomal system, so suitable for use in renal failure
- In **overdose** can cause **respiratory** and **cardiac depression**
- **All patients having midazolam sedation** should have **intravenous access** and **pulse oximetry** (see 'Pulse oximetry, Chapter 118, page 491); **ECG monitoring** and **resuscitation facilities** should be available (including flumazenil). Patients should **not drive** or operate heavy machinery for **48 hours** afterwards.

Lorazepam
- **Water soluble**
- Intermediate half-life
- Intermediate onset
- **Suitable for infusion** as little accumulation
- Cleared by hepatic conjugation.

Diazepam
- **Not water soluble** – usually prepared in glycerol
- Intermediate to long half-life
- Can be given intravenously, orally or rectally
- Good **anticonvulsant acutely**
- Hepatic metabolites are active and have long half-lives, so **not suitable for infusion**.

Other sedatives: non-barbiturate and barbiturate

Non-barbiturates
Propofol
- Non-barbiturate sedative

- Substituted isopropyl phenol compound prepared in a 10 per cent lipid emulsion **(white emulsion)**
- **Anaesthetic induction agent**: some short operations can be performed solely on propofol without the use of a volatile agent
- Rapid onset and short half-life
- Clearance not affected by renal or hepatic dysfunction
- **Respiratory** and **cardiovascular depressant**
- Good agent for **sedation** in patients receiving **mechanical ventilation**
- **Prolonged infusion** in **paediatrics** is associated with **lactic acidosis.**

Etomidate
- Non-barbiturate imidazole
- Commonly used on **rapid induction intubation** alongside a muscle relaxant such as suxamethonium
- Rapid onset of action and a short but dose-dependent duration of action
- **Cardiovascular effects minimal**
- Can be used as a short-term sedative for procedures
- Depresses adrenal cortex in the long term – **not suitable for infusion.**

Barbiturates
Barbiturates act on **GABA-a receptors** in the brain and are also **respiratory** and **cardiac depressants** as with most sedative and induction agents. They are **highly addictive drugs**.

Thiopental
- Commonly used **induction agent**
- Given in alkaline solution so **irritant** to the tissues if it extravasates
- Rapid onset and relatively short half-life
- If given in an infusion in the ITU (particularly in the treatment of intractably raised ICP), it **accumulates** in the body's **fat stores** so, **when stopped, several days** must be given **before** any formal **testing** of brain or **brain-stem function**
- **Negative inotrope.**

Phenobarbital
- Older drug
- Used in the past as an induction agent
- Still used in some centres for **intractable epilepsy** and status epilepticus.

Opioids

Opioids are agents that induce **systemic analgesia**, some **anxiolysis** and mild **sedation**. They **do not induce amnesia** of any significance. Examples: **morphine, fentanyl.**

- **Main type of analgesic** used in surgery
- Rapid onset and usually intermediate half-life

- Can cause **respiratory depression in overdose**
- Can be given intravenously, intramuscularly, intrathecally, transdermally or orally in some cases
- **Reversal** using **naloxone** (see below)
- Given as titrated **bolus in acute pain**
- Commonly used in **PCA**
- **Long-acting opioids** (fentanyl patches or MST Continus) given in **palliative care** or chronic pain.

↑ **Key learning point**

Sedative reversal

There are **two** major sedative reversal drugs available for clinical use and they are **naloxone** for **opioid reversal** and **flumazenil** for **benzodiazepine reversal**. **For this reason, many ITUs now use morphine and midazolam for sedation.**

Naloxone
Naloxone is a **competitive antagonist** of the opioid class of drugs. The onset of action after intravenous administration is rapid, with effects appearing within 2–3 min. The duration of action is dose related. This antagonist may have shorter duration of action compared with that of the longer-acting opioids, and observation may be required with **repeated dosing** or **an infusion** in some cases.

Flumazenil
Flumazenil is a **competitive antagonist** of the benzodiazepine class of drugs. The onset of action is within 2 min of intravenous administration, with peak effects within 10 min. The duration of action is dose related, but it is typically shorter than that of longer-acting benzodiazepines. **Repeat dosing may be required**.

Exercise caution in patients receiving long-term benzodiazepine therapy, because **seizures can occur**.

↑ **Example viva question**

Should analgesia be withheld before initial examination of the acute abdomen?

Under no circumstances! There is no evidence to suggest that this is helpful and an uncooperative patient in pain is unlikely to allow a thorough examination. There is evidence to suggest that more information may be found from palpation after adequate analgesia than before it.

121 Sepsis and SIRS

Possible viva questions related to this topic

→ What is the systemic inflammatory response syndrome?
→ How does it differ from sepsis?
→ What is the pathological process involved in SIRS?
→ What are its triggers?
→ Name some of the cytokines implicated in the development of SIRS.
→ What is MODS?
→ What are the possible treatments for MODS, SIRS and sepsis?
→ What is activated protein C? Who should receive it?
→ Why is fluid resuscitation alone usually ineffective in cases of severe sepsis?

↑ Example viva question

What is the systemic inflammatory response syndrome?

The **systemic inflammatory response syndrome** (SIRS) is defined by a number of **clinical criteria** and is the **body's reaction to a critical illness** such as overwhelming infection or trauma (**including surgery**):

- Temperature $> 38°C$ or $< 36°C$
- Heart rate > 90 beats/min
- Respiratory rate > 20/min or $Paco_2 < 4.3$ kPa (32 mmHg)
- WCC $> 12\,000$ or < 4000/mL (or > 10 per cent immature forms)

The concept of SIRS was introduced after it was noted that **less than 50 per cent of patients** showing signs of **sepsis** had **positive blood cultures**.

Sepsis is defined as the body's response to **proven infection** which **includes two of the clinical criteria for SIRS.**

Severe sepsis is defined as **sepsis** with **evidence of organ dysfunction.**

Septic shock is defined as **sepsis + hypotension** with systolic < 90 mmHg or drop in BP of > 40 mmHg that is refractory to fluid replacement.

SEPSIS SYNDROME

This is a term that was coined in the original paper introducing the concept of SIRS. It is defined as **SIRS criteria plus** clinical **evidence** of an **infection** site and **with at least one end-organ** demonstrating **inadequate perfusion** or **dysfunction**, expressed as poor or altered cerebral function, hypoxaemia, elevated plasma lactate or oliguria (urine output < 30 mL/h or 0.5 mL/kg per h without corrective therapy).

SIRS

Split into three phases:

1. A **localized injury** in the body results in the activation of the **local acute inflammatory response.** There is chemotaxis of neutrophils and macrophages which themselves release inflammatory mediators (e.g. cytokines and proteases).
2. **Systemic distribution of inflammatory mediators.** Anti-inflammatory mediators such as IL-10 are downregulated.
3. **Massive cytokine release systemically** causes **endothelial dysfunction** and disruption of tight junctions, leading to **leaky capillaries** and subsequent systemic sequelae: **pyrexia, tachycardia,** increased vascular permeability and **peripheral vasodilatation. A catabolic state** ensues with **reduced delivery of oxygen** to the tissues despite **increased demand.**

Triggers for SIRS

- Severe burns
- Multiple trauma (including surgery)
- Sepsis
- Acute pancreatitis
- Cardiopulmonary bypass.

Cytokines implicated in SIRS response

- IL-6 (involved in acute phase response)
- IL-10 (anti-inflammatory downregulated in SIRS)
- IL-8 (neutrophil chemotaxis)
- IL-1 (pyrogen that activates macrophages and T cells)

- TNFα (pyrogen that increases capillary permeability via the induction of nitric oxide synthase + stimulates leukocytes)
- Platelet-activating factor or PAF (increases capillary permeability and activates macrophages and T cells).

↑ **Example viva question**

Why is fluid resuscitation alone usually ineffective in cases of severe sepsis?

Remember that the effects of sepsis are **threefold**:

- Vasodilatation
- Capillary leak after endothelial damage
- Myocardial depression (caused by an unknown toxin or cytokine)

These three factors dictate that **fluid resuscitation alone** will not solve the problem. **Vasoconstrictors** and **inotropic** support are usually required (see 'Inotropes', Chapter 113, page 466).

MULTIPLE ORGAN DYSFUNCTION SYNDROME

↑ **Key learning point**

This is defined as the presence of an **acute, potentially reversible dysfunction of two** or more **organ systems** such that **homoeostasis cannot be maintained** without intervention.

Multiple organ dysfunction syndrome (MODS) can be divided into:

1. **Primary MODS:** directly attributable to the **initial insult**
2. **Secondary MODS** (more common): failure is secondary to the **effects of SIRS.** It is possible that there may be a latent period between the event triggering SIRS and the onset of MODS.

Organ systems that can be involved in MODS

Any organ system can be involved.

Cardiovascular system
Initially a **hyperdynamic state** with **decreased SVR** as a result of massive systemic vasodilatation and increase in capillary permeability. After this, **myocardial depression** may occur.

Respiratory system

ARDS is one of the potential components of MODS (see 'Acute respiratory distress syndrome', Chapter 105, page 419).

Acute renal failure

This can occur as the result of **acute tubular necrosis** (see 'Oliguria and renal replacement', Chapter 116, page 482) and is therefore **potentially reversible**.

Gut

Decreased absorption is associated with downregulation of secretory IgA. **Bacteria translocate** across the **deficient gut wall, perpetuating sepsis**.

Liver

Deranged liver function and hepatocellular jaundice.

Blood

A **coagulopathy** can eventually lead to **DIC**.

Other systems include **bone marrow failure** giving a pancytopenia and **neurological disturbances** including metabolic encephalopathy.

The **mortality** associated with MODS is **directly related** to the **number of organs** affected. Failure of **one organ** (most commonly renal failure or respiratory failure) has a mortality of about **10 per cent** whereas **renal failure and one other** is around **70 per cent**, with **three or more organs at 95 per cent**.

PRINCIPLES OF TREATMENT FOR MODS, SIRS AND SEPSIS

Always remember **A, B, C!**

- **Removal of any precipitating cause** and treatment of any underlying infection. **Antibiotic** treatment is initially **broad spectrum** and **empirical**. This will be changed depending on **culture results** and **microbiological advice**.
- **Airway and breathing**: ventilatory support for ARDS and respiratory failure.
- **Circulation: intravenous fluids, invasive monitoring** (arterial line, CVP ± PAFC) and **inotropic** support to maintain cardiac index, **noradrenaline** to increase SVR, MAP and organ perfusion, thereby maximizing oxygen delivery to the tissues.
- **Renal support:** maintain urine output and renal perfusion. **Dopamine** and **frusemide** have been used to maintain renal perfusion but there **is no evidence** that either of these improves outcome. **Renal replacement** is the **mainstay of renal support** (haemofiltration, haemodialysis, haemodiafiltration).
- **Nutritional support:** in the presence of **gut failure, parenteral feeding** may be necessary (see 'Nutrition', Chapter 115, page 477) to account for the body's massive calorific demands in MODS and SIRS.

↑ Example viva question

What is activated protein C? Who should receive it?

Activated protein C modulates both inflammation and coagulation in severe sepsis, and reduces mortality.

Activated protein C is an **endogenous protein** that promotes fibrinolysis and **inhibits thrombosis and inflammation**. It is an important modulator of the coagulation and inflammation associated with severe sepsis.

It is converted from its inactive precursor, protein C, by thrombin coupled to thrombomodulin. The conversion of protein C to activated protein C may be **impaired during sepsis** as a result of the downregulation of thrombomodulin by inflammatory cytokines. (**Reduced levels of protein C** are found in most **patients with sepsis** and are associated with an **increased mortality.**)

A large randomized controlled trial has **confirmed the efficacy** of activated protein C. In **patients with severe sepsis**, an intravenous infusion for 96 hours is associated with a **significant reduction in mortality**. The use of this drug is indicated if the patient has a **systemic inflammatory response, at least one organ dysfunction** and **known or suspected infection**.

When using an infusion of activated protein C, it is important to monitor for **signs of bleeding**, an important side effect of therapy with this compound. The value of this agent in **patients with multiorgan failure**, or **outside the first 24 hours of injury, is unknown**.

122 Shock

DEFINITION

'A **sudden** and **generalised** lack of **perfusion** and usually oxygenation of all of the **peripheral tissues** and **end organs**, usually caused by **cardiovascular collapse**.'

CLINICAL FEATURES OF SHOCK

- **Hypotension** (systolic < 90 mmHg or drop of > 40 mmHg)
- Decreased capillary refill
- **Tachycardia**
- **Oliguria** (see 'Oliguria and renal replacement', Chapter 116, page 482)
- Confusion and decreased level of consciousness
- **Pyrexia** and warm peripheries in **septic shock** (see 'Sepsis and SIRS', Chapter 121, page 505).

TYPES OF SHOCK

- Cardiogenic
- Hypovolaemic
- Anaphylactic
- Septic
- Spinal (evidence of spinal injury and no other reason for hypotension).

Cardiogenic shock

'Pump failure causing circulatory collapse'

Causes
- Acute myocardial infarction (MI)
- Arrhythmias, e.g. ventricular fibrillation (VT), fast AF
- Tension pneumothorax
- Massive pulmonary embolus (PE)
- Cardiac tamponade.

Treatment
This should be aimed at **resolution of the cause of the pump failure** and is beyond the scope of this topic. However, in broad terms, MIs should be thrombolysed or stented, arrhythmias should be cardioverted, tension pneumothoraces should be decompressed, massive PEs may be thrombolysed or undergo embolectomy, and cardiac tamponade may be resolved by pericardiocentesis or may require cardiothoracic surgery (e.g. pericardial window/repair of myocardial rupture).

Hypovolaemic shock

Haemorrhage
- Ruptured abdominal aortic aneurysm (**AAA**)
- Ruptured ectopic pregnancy
- **Trauma** (pelvic, long bones, splenic rupture, PA/aortic disruption, liver laceration)
- Upper/lower **gastrointestinal (GI) bleeding** (e.g. varices, duodenal ulcer eroded into gastroduodenal artery, brisk bleeding from colonic neoplasm).

Loss of fluid
- **Pancreatitis**
- Intestinal **obstruction**
- High-output **stoma** (e.g. ileostomy)
- **Iatrogenic**, e.g. post-renal dialysis/haemofiltration.

Treatment
In this case treatment is largely aimed at **stopping the plasma loss** and **replacing appropriately** with blood, crystalloids, colloids and clotting products if necessary.

Anaphylactic shock

Common allergies

- Drugs especially antibiotics (e.g. **penicillin** and **radiological contrast agents**)
- Foods (e.g. **peanuts/shellfish**)
- Medical equipment materials especially latex
- Insect bites/stings.

Treatment

Supportive treatment and **cardiac support** with **adrenaline (epinephrine)**. Patients who have an anaphylactic reaction to everyday substances such as foods should be offered an EpiPen to carry around with them.

↑ **Example viva question**

How do SIRS, sepsis and septic shock differ? What is sepsis syndrome?

See 'Sepsis and SIRS', Chapter 121, page 505

SIRS

Any **two or more** of the following:

Temperature > 38°C or < 36°C

- **Heart rate > 90 beats/min**
- **Respiratory rate > 20/min**
- **WCC > 12 000 or < 4000/mL**

Septic shock

Sepsis + **hypotension** with systolic BP < 90 mmHg or drop in BP of > 40 mmHg that is **refractory to fluid replacement**. This relationship should be clear in your mind when going into the exam.

Sepsis syndrome

This is a term that was coined in the original paper introducing the concept of SIRS. It is defined as **SIRS criteria plus** clinical **evidence of** an **infection** site, **with at least one end-organ** demonstrating **inadequate perfusion** or **dysfunction**, expressed as poor or altered cerebral function, hypoxaemia (PaO_2 < 10 kPa), elevated plasma lactate or oliguria (urine output < 30 mL/h or 0.5 mL/kg per h without corrective therapy).

Septic shock

'Hypotension complicating severe sepsis despite adequate fluid resuscitation.'

Commonly termed 'warm shock' as a result of the peripheral vasodilatation caused by mast-cell degranulation from circulating endotoxin.

Treatment

This is with fluids until adequately filled, then vasoconstrictors such as noradrenaline (norepinephrine) (see 'Inotropes', Chapter 113, page 466) should be used. This will need to be given through central venous access (see 'CVP lines and invasive monitoring, Chapter 110, page 443) in an HDU/ITU setting (see 'Criteria for admission to the ITU/HDU, Chapter 109, page 439).

Classification of hypovolaemic shock				
	Class 1	Class 2	Class 3	Class 4
Volume loss (mL)	0–750	750–1500	1500–2000	>2000
Loss (%)	15	30	40	>40
Pulse (beats/min)	<100	>100	>120	>140
BP	Normal	Normal	Decreased	Decreased
Pulse pressure	Normal	Decreased	Decreased	Decreased
Urine output (mL/h)	>30	20–30	5–15	Anuric
Respiratory rate	14–20	20–30	30–40	>40

↑ Example viva question

How much of the total plasma volume can be lost before the BP drops?

Up to 20 per cent of the entire plasma volume can be lost before seeing significant physiological changes. Thus, a young and fit patient with a mild tachycardia could already be in class 2 shock and already have lost over 1 L of blood!

This relationship is even more important in the paediatric population where children can lose even more before suddenly decompensating: thus a tachycardia in a child in the context of a blunt abdominal injury must be treated very seriously.

123 Systemic response to surgery

Possible viva questions related to this topic

→ How does the body react to surgery?
→ What is the metabolic response to surgery?
→ How are lipids mobilized after trauma?
→ How is carbohydrate metabolism affected by trauma?
→ How is protein metabolism affected by trauma?
→ Why is urine output often low in the first 24 hours after surgery?
→ What happens to the metabolic rate after trauma or surgery?
→ How does the metabolic response to surgery affect the strategy for post operative nutrition?
→ What do you understand by the ebb and flow phase after trauma to the body?
→ What physiological systems are involved in the coordination of the stress response?
→ What do glucocorticoids do?
→ Why might a metabolic alkalosis develop immediately after surgery?
→ How might the systemic response to surgery be minimized?

↑ **Example viva question**

How does the body react to surgery?

Surgery is little more than **highly controlled trauma**. Thus, systems that are activated after acute trauma are also activated after surgery:

- **Sympathetic nervous system** activation as a result of **pain** and **hypovolaemia** leads to an **increase** in **cardiovascular output** via an **increase in circulating adrenaline** (tachycardia) and **noradrenaline** (peripheral vasoconstriction). Also aids activation of **glycolysis** in the liver and the **renin–angiotensin–aldosterone axis** (see 'Starling's law of the heart and cardiovascular equations', Chapter 102, page 403, and 'Functions of the kidney III', Chapter 94, page 381)
- **Endocrine response: ACTH production** is stimulated which, in turn, stimulates **glucocorticoid** release – predominantly **cortisol** (see below)
- **Acute phase response:**
  - **cytokines** released by circulating **monocytes** and **lymphocytes**
  - kinins, interleukins, TNF and interferons likewise released; causes **postoperative fever** and further **increases metabolic demand**
  - **ACTH release** further enhanced
  - **clotting cascade** activated
  - serum levels of **acute phase proteins** increase (e.g. C-reactive protein or **CRP, fibrinogen, complement C3**, ceruloplasmin and haptoglobin)
  - liver **downregulates albumin** and transferrin production
- **Vascular endothelium:** highly complex system able to affect **local vasomotor tone** (via nitric oxide or **NO**) and local **coagulation**; can affect systemic response by **modulation** of **platelet** and **leukocyte** binding

Note that the **six stress hormones** in the response to surgery can be remembered by '**T, A, C, G. These are the bases in DNA!**':

T: trauma
A: ADH, aldosterone
C: cortisol, catecholamines
G: growth hormone, glucagon

METABOLISM AFTER SURGERY

Classically divided into '**ebb and flow**' phases according to the **metabolic rate**:

- '**Ebb**': **reduced energy expenditure** after injury for the first **24 hours** and therefore a reduction in the metabolic rate

- 'Flow': the metabolic rate **increases dramatically** and the **catabolic 'flow' phase** can last **many days** with associated **negative nitrogen balance** and **impaired glucose tolerance**.

Immediately after surgery, patients are **nil by mouth** and therefore **starvation** and the **response to trauma** are **both responsible** for this catabolic state. There is increased **heat production** in this phase, along with increased **oxygen consumption** and **weight loss**. The overall duration and increase in metabolic rate in the 'flow' phase depend on the type of stimulus:

- **10 per cent increase in elective surgical operations**
- **50 per cent increase in polytrauma**
- **200 per cent in major burns**.

Once the 'flow' phase has begun, **correction of the underlying stimulus** (e.g. controlling infection, correcting hypovolaemia, controlling pain) will **not** rapidly **reverse** the metabolic condition of the patient.

Finally, if recovery occurs, an anabolic phase occurs where the body replaces its fat and glycogen reserves and synthesizes more protein.

Clearly this has a major implications for **postoperative nutrition** (see 'Nutrition', Chapter 115, page 477), where calculated daily required nutrition must take into account the **extent** and **severity** of the **'flow' metabolic phase** of the patent.

Lipid metabolism

- **Lipids** are the **principal** source of energy after trauma
- **Lipolysis** stimulated by sympathetic nervous system, ACTH, cortisol, decreased serum insulin levels and glucagons
- **Ketones released** and oxidized by all tissues **except blood and brain**
- **Free fatty acids** and **glycerol** undergo **gluconeogenesis** in the liver to provide energy for all tissues.

Carbohydrate metabolism

- **Insulin levels decrease** and glucagon levels increase, **mobilizing glycogen** stores and initiating **glycolysis** to create a **transient hyperglycaemia**. Increased glucocorticoid levels also result in insulin resistance of the tissues, thereby potentiating the effect.
- **Glycolysis** releases energy for **obligate tissue** (CNS, leukocytes and red blood cells – cells that do not require insulin for glucose transport). This is a very important mechanism because in a **serious injury** or after major surgery, **leukocytes can account for 70 per cent** of all **glucose uptake**.

- **Body glycogen stores** can **last for about 24 hours**, after which blood glucose must be maintained by other methods:
  - ○ **gluconeogenesis** of **lipid** breakdown products
  - ○ **gluconeogenesis** of **amino acids** mobilized from protein breakdown.

Protein metabolism

- Suppressed insulin levels encourage the **release of amino acids** from **skeletal muscle**.
- A **three-** to **fourfold increase** in serum **amino acids** is usually required after major trauma. The requirement reaches a peak at a week after injury, although it may continue for many days after this. In the absence of a constant exogenous supply of protein, the **entire nitrogen requirement** is gained from the **skeletal muscle**. The extent of the nitrogen requirement is directly **proportional** to the **extent of injury** (including trauma and sepsis) and the **muscle bulk**.
- Major protein loss results in endothelial dysfunction and atrophy of the intestinal mucosa, removing the barrier to translocation of pathogenic bacteria. Thus, a **loss of over 40 per cent body protein is usually fatal**.

EFFECT ON RESPIRATION

- Pain causes **splinting** and **hypoxia**, leading to **inadequate ventilation**, basal **atelectasis** and basal lung collapse
- Basal collapse **increases risk of infection**
- Hypoxia drives catabolic state and anaerobic respiration leading to a metabolic acidosis (see 'Acid–base balance', Chapter 84, page 349).

MINIMIZATION OF THE SYSTEMIC RESPONSE TO SURGERY

Preoperative factors

- **Minimize fear and stress** (informed consent and clear, concise explanation, premed anxiolytic if necessary) to **reduce sympathetic activity**
- Good, **high protein load** preoperative nutrition; enteral feeding if possible before period of nil by mouth required for gastric emptying
- Correction and **control of preoperative infection**.

Operative factors

- Good **tissue handling**
- Minimally invasive surgery/**minimal trauma**
- Shorten duration of anaesthesia.

↑ **Example viva question**

Why is urine output often low in the first 24 hours after surgery? Why might a metabolic alkalosis develop immediately after trauma?

After trauma, the activation of the **renin–angiotensin–aldosterone axis** and the **increase** in **ADH secretion** leads to a **retention of sodium** and **water** at the expense of potassium (see 'Functions of the kidney III', Chapter 94, page 381 and 'Fluid balance', Chapter 111, page 452).

Although the **total body sodium** may be **elevated**, a **dilutional hyponatraemia** is not uncommon with an excess of serum ADH, leading to **greater water** than sodium **retention**.

Furthermore, in catabolic cells with a degree of energy failure, **sodium pumps are impaired**, so sodium tends to drift into cells and thereby further decrease the plasma sodium concentration. This sodium and water retention leads to a **low urine output** (despite adequate filling) **in the first 24 hours** after surgery. Although the water retention lasts for only 24 hours, the sodium retention may persist for much longer.

In many cases, **postoperatively** the patient may have an ileus, promoting **fluid extravasation** into the **gut lumen** and intravascular depletion, leading to **dehydration** and **further compounding** the **low urine output** state.

The most common acid–base imbalance is a **metabolic alkalosis** because aldosterone promotes **sodium retention** at the expense of **potassium**. As **potassium is excreted**, so are H^+ **ions** in a **co-transporter** mechanism, leading to an **alkalosis**.

In more **severe trauma**, a metabolic **acidosis** can result as a lactic acidosis caused by poor tissue perfusion and anaerobic metabolism.

Postoperative factors

- Correction of **hypovolaemia**:
  - prompt replacement of fluids and electrolytes (see 'Fluid balance', Chapter 111, page 452)
  - transfusion for haemorrhage if necessary
  - colloids for plasma loss
- Correction of **metabolic alkalosis/acidosis**
- Control of **postoperative infection**:
  - **antibiotics** (see 'Antibiotics in surgery', Chapter 67, page 275)

- ○ **enteral feeding** as soon as possible to maintain gut mucosal barrier (see 'Nutrition', Chapter 115, page 477 and 'Sepsis and SIRS', Chapter 121, page 505)
- ○ **débride wounds, drain pus,** etc.
- Adequate and effective **pain control (reduces sympathetic activation** and **splinting/hypoxia** and their effects)
  - ○ **PCA** if appropriate
  - ○ **local and regional blocks** – ideally given **before** surgical insult occurs
  - ○ **epidurals/spinals**
- Correction of **hypoxia**
- Increased **arginine** and **glutamine** intake can be helpful to improve nitrogen balance, encourage weight gain, wound healing and immune function
- **Trace elements** such as **zinc** to improve wound healing and immune function.

Index

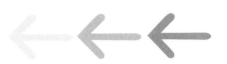